90 0391972 2

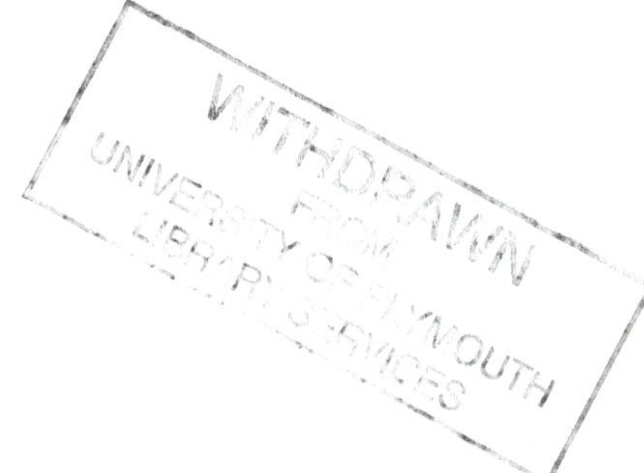
WITHDRAWN
FROM
UNIVERSITY OF PLYMOUTH
LIBRARY SERVICES

D1681030

Immunoassay

A Practical Guide

Immunoassay

A Practical Guide

Edited by

PROFESSOR BRIAN LAW

Zeneca Pharmaceuticals, UK

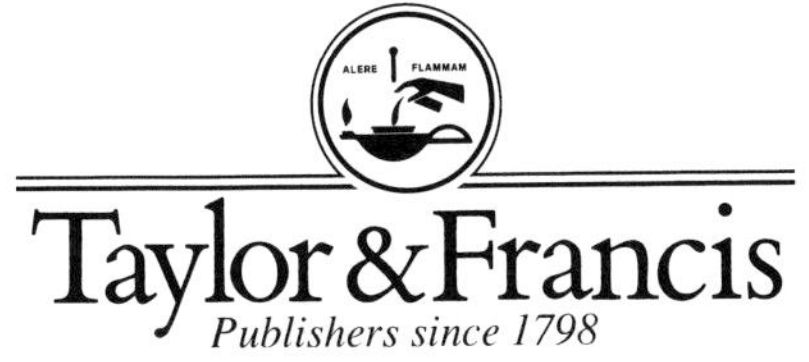

UK Taylor & Francis Ltd, 1 Gunpowder Square, London, EC4A 3DE
USA Taylor & Francis Inc., 1900 Frost Road, Suite 101, Bristol, PA 19007

British Library Cataloguing in Publication Data

A catalogue record for this book is available from the British Library.

ISBN 0-7484-0560-7 (cased)

Library of Congress Cataloguing Publication Data are available

Cover design by Jim Wilkie

Typeset in Times 10/12 pt by Santype International Ltd, Salisbury, Wiltshire

Printed in Great Britain by T. J. Press (Padstow) Ltd

Contents

List of Contributors

BRIAN LAW BSc PhD CChem FRSC
Lead Discovery Department
Zeneca Pharmaceuticals
Alderley Park
Macclesfield
Cheshire
SK10 4TG

CLIVE G. COPLEY BSc PhD MBA
Target Discovery & Infection Section
Zeneca Pharmaceuticals
Alderley Park
Macclesfield
Cheshire
SK10 4TG

ROBERT A. BIDDLECOMBE BSc MSc
Department of International Bioanalysis
Division of Bioanalysis and Drug Metabolism
GlaxoWellcome Research and Development
Beckenham
Kent
BR3 3BS

MICHAEL J. WARWICK BSc PhD
Drug Kinetics Group
Safety of Medicines Department
Zeneca Pharmaceuticals
Alderley Park
Macclesfield
Cheshire
SK10 4TG

MICHAEL D. MALONE BSc PhD
Safety of Medicines Department
Zeneca Pharmaceuticals
Alderley Park
Macclesfield
Cheshire
SK10 4TG

WILLIAM J. JENNER BSc PhD
Department of International Bioanalysis
Division of Bioanalysis and Drug Metabolism
GlaxoWellcome Research and Development
Ware
Hertfordshire
SG12 0DP

Preface

The desire to produce a practical based book on immunoassay came about for a number of reasons. Having been involved in immunoassays for many years my advice was frequently sought regarding the problem of immunoassay development and troubleshooting. A frequent question over the years has been 'are there any good practical books or literature on the subject?' In fact there are only one or two journals which can be said to be devoted to immunoassay or related methods and the number of good books on the subject is similarly limited, both in scope and number. Furthermore virtually none of the books deal with the real nitty-gritty of the subject; i.e. where do I start, what do I do, and how do I do it?

It is interesting to contrast immunoassay with the technique of HPLC which has grown and developed over a similar period. When faced with a similar question regarding HPLC, it is a simple matter to direct the enquirer to one of the innumerable journals, books, programmed texts or even videos on the technique. These cover every aspect of HPLC from column selection to data processing and troubleshooting. Returning to the original question regarding immunoassay therefore, the simple answer was 'no'. Invariably this led one into lengthy discussions on the do's and don'ts of immunoassay development and the intractable problem of assay troubleshooting.

Around the time the ideas for the book were developing, my colleagues and I became involved in producing a training course on immunoassays. This course was run under the auspices of the Drug Metabolism Discussion Group (DMDG). This is an informal organisation, representing the views and interests of all those involved in drug analysis, pharmacokinetics and drug metabolism in the UK and Western European pharmaceutical industry. The first course was successfully run in 1991 and the book more or less developed naturally out of this.

As indicated above, the book is really about the 'how' of immunoassay development and we have assumed that anyone referring to the book has a basic knowledge of the techniques.

This text is very much aimed at research workers who need to get an assay up and running as quickly as possible, or those workers who are reluctant to devote a great deal of time to assay development for fear that the project will be terminated.

What is required therefore is an efficient, reliable and simple guide leading to the rapid development of immunoassay methods – we think this book provides that.

Brian Law

September 1995

Macclesfield, UK

1

Introduction

B. LAW

Zeneca Pharmaceuticals, Macclesfield

It is probably difficult to produce a book on immunoassays without some mention of the history of the technique, more so in the present case since the history and the development of immunoassays has some bearing on the rationale for the writing of this book.

The claim for the development of immunoassays comes from two groups. As a result of studies on the metabolism of ^{131}I-labelled insulin in the late 1950s, Solomon Berson and Rosalyn Yalow working at the Veterans Administration Hospital in New York, developed the technique of radioimmunoassay (RIA) (Yalow and Berson, 1959). The view that antibodies could be raised against a small-molecular-weight material was considered controversial at the time and it was with some difficulty that Berson and Yalow were actually able to publish their initial papers on the subject.

Around the same time Roger Ekins, working at the Middlesex Hospital in London, developed a similar method for the measurement of thyroxine in human plasma (Ekins, 1960). His approach was less wide ranging in its implications as he used a naturally occurring thyroxine binding protein rather than more generally applicable antibodies. It is probably for this reason that Berson and Yalow are credited with the discovery of the technique which was to result in Rosalyn Yalow receiving the Nobel prize for Medicine and Physiology in 1977.

The benefits of the technique were soon recognised by the clinical fraternity, and the use of the technique rapidly grew in the area of clinical biochemistry as it is known today. The fact that the technique was initially confined to the clinical area probably reflects a number of factors. The two discoveries were both made in departments of physics or nuclear medicine within hospitals. One of the discoverers (Berson) was medically qualified and the early publications were confined mainly to clinical journals. The subsequent development of the technique in the 1960s was still very much confined to clinical medicine with assays being developed and reported for a variety of peptide hormones leading to the development of RIAs for steroids in 1969 (Abraham, 1969).

The first immunoassay for a drug compound was reported in 1968 when Oliver and co-workers published an RIA method for digitoxin (Oliver *et al.*, 1968). The expansion of the technique outside the clinical field was relatively slow however. A major spurt in the development of RIA seemed to occur in the 1970s and this coincided with the American involvement in Vietnam (1965 to 1975). It is interesting to speculate on the link between these two events.

The late 1960s and early 1970s saw GIs returning to the USA from Vietnam in increasing numbers. With Vietnam centred in the drug producing region of South-East Asia, the so-called Golden Triangle, recreational drug use had become a way of life for the young soldiers thrown into the horrors of war. As a consequence many of the GIs became addicted or dependent on illicit drugs. Realising they had a major drug problem on their hands, the USA Government set about putting drug screening programmes in place. The techniques available at the time however, being based on solvent extraction of large volumes of biological sample followed by chromatographic analysis, were unsuited to the task of screening massive numbers of samples. It was at this point that the Government invested heavily in the development of immunoassay methods. Finance was provided for companies like Syva and Roche, leading to the development of the RIA for morphine, as a result immunoassay moved from the clinical to the general analytical laboratory beginning its transition into the widely used analytical tool it is today.

Over the past 5 years or so the use of immunoassay has further expanded. It is now being applied to the determination of mycotoxins in grain (Casale *et al.*, 1988), drugs of abuse in hair (Marsh and Evans, 1993; Marsh *et al.*, 1995), gibberellin hormones in plant tissue (Yang *et al.*, 1993), fungicides in potatoes and apples (Brandon *et al.*, 1993), herbicides in drinking and river waters (McConnell *et al.*, 1994; Meulenberg and Stoks, 1995), explosives in ground water and soil (Keuchel *et al.*, 1992), the detection of sulphate-reducing bacteria in oils (Odom and Ebersole, 1994), the determination of the species of origin of milk (Perez *et al.*, 1992), the identification of lung tissue in processed meat products (Smith, 1992) and even the detection of drugs in Egyptian mummies (Balabanova *et al.*, 1992). Thus scientists, previously more concerned with the application of classical analytical procedures are now becoming involved in immunoassay development, and that is where the problems begin.

Although many workers have successfully developed immunoassays, the rapid production of highly optimised procedures requires a very wide range of skills or knowledge, including: an understanding of the biochemical or metabolic fate of the analyte in the matrix or organism of interest; synthetic organic chemistry for the production of functionalised haptens; protein chemistry and purification techniques for the production of immunogens and enzyme conjugates; immunology and veterinary techniques; radiochemistry or enzymology for the production of tracers; and knowledge of general biochemical techniques and statistical principles for the development and optimisation of the assay system. Looking around it is obvious that few laboratories, let alone individuals, possess all these skills in the necessary depth to make immunoassay development a simple and straightforward process.

The purpose of this book therefore is several fold. It should help anyone coming into the technique for the first time to find their way through the mass of contradictory and confusing literature. It should also help instil in those already working in the area a greater sense of confidence. We hope to do this by providing the reader with a clearer understanding of the reasoning behind the techniques they use.

Anyone opening the book and perusing the contents pages will immediately become aware of the extreme bias, particularly with regard to what has been left out. This was deliberate and for this action I make no apologies. However I do feel that some justification is required.

In this present work we have concentrated on radioisotopes and enzymes for two good reasons. The use of these two types of tracer offers a wide range of formats from simple liquid assays to complex sandwich assays with one of the reagents bound to a solid support. Radioisotopic and enzyme tracers have been around for a long time and they have been utilised extensively in commercial kits. For these two reasons there is not only considerable information available, but both assay types are well supported with reagents and instrumentation. High sensitivities are also easily achievable with both these tracers. Radioimmunoassays are also relatively quick to develop and they require the minimum of reagents. The ease with which radioactivity can be detected makes the isolation and characterisation of the tracer somewhat easier than with the alternatives. Enzymeimmunoassays (EIA) in contrast, although more difficult to set up, are capable of full automation.

There are obviously concerns surrounding the use of radioactivity and this has been one of the driving forces behind the evaluation of alternatives. The amount of radioactivity employed in a typical RIA is relatively small, around 20 nCi per assay tube and, given the short half-life of ^{125}I, the problem of disposal of waste can be minimised.

The number of literature reports on RIA (excluding patents) has been declining steadily since 1981, with those for EIA, in all its various forms, increasing over a similar period (Figure 1.1). In 1984 the number of literature reports on EIA (excluding patents) exceeded those on RIA for the first time. RIA appears to have diminished in its significance as judged by the number of recent publications: it only constituted around 16 per cent of the immunoassay literature in 1994. However, this decline probably reflects the maturation of the technique since a similar phenomenon has occurred with EIA since 1990. Despite this, EIA and RIA still made up over 70 per cent of all the immunoassay publications in the early 1990s and both

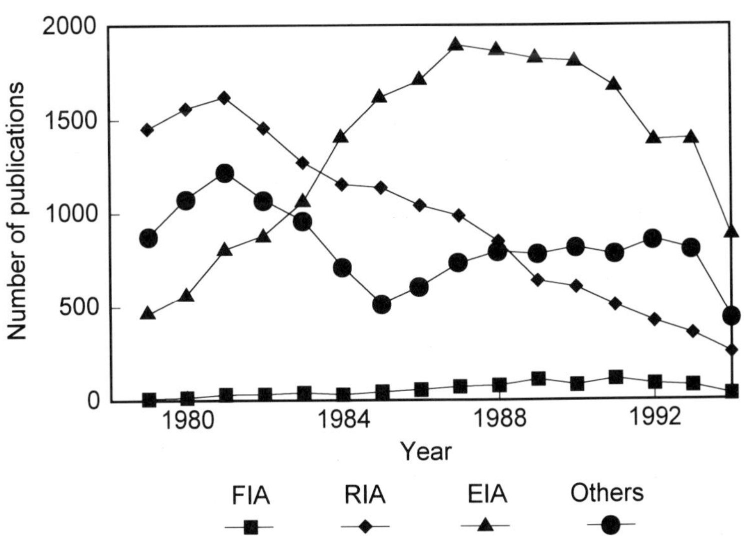

Figure 1.1 The variation in the number of publications related to different types of immunoassay technique between the years 1979 and 1994. The data for 1994 is incomplete.

techniques are still very widely used, particularly in a research environment. It is interesting to note that fluoroimmunoassay (FIA) despite being around for many years has never exceeded 5 per cent of immunoassay publications.

Taken together we believe that the information presented above is ample justification for the continued exploitation of both enzymes *and* radioisotopes as tracers in immunoassays.

The second omission from the book, or to present it more positively, the focus on polyclonal antisera to the total exclusion of monoclonal sera is again deliberate and I feel justifiable. Not all laboratories have access to the necessary facilities and expertise for monoclonal antibody production. The work involved in cloning etc. although automatable, is also very labour intensive. Most importantly, however, monoclonal antibodies probably offer very little advantage over their polyclonal counterparts for the analysis of small molecules. In fact there are even reports of workers having to mix monoclonal sera to obtain the necessary specificity! The major driving force behind monoclonal sera is probably commercial suppliers of kits and reagent antisera, where consistency and quantity are of the utmost importance. However, if sheep are used to raise polyclonal sera, then even with a relatively poor titre of around 1/1000 there would be enough sera from one (non-terminal) bleed to provide 1.5 million tests! This is surely enough to see out most development projects.

The third focus of this book relates to the analysis of small molecules especially of the non-clinical nature. Immunoassay from its inception has enjoyed a wide application in clinical medicine where it has been successfully used for the analysis of peptide and steroid hormones, a wide range of biochemical markers and more recently for the therapeutic monitoring of drugs. Much of the published literature including the books and reviews (e.g. Pratt, 1978; Chan and Perlstein, 1987) have concentrated on these areas which have their own special features. The comparable literature on non-clinical small molecule immunoassay, especially that for drugs, is either dated (e.g. Landon and Moffat, 1976) or of insufficient practical detail (e.g. Smith, 1988) to be of any real practical help to the novice.

It is my desire to see the technique of immunoassay develop in the disciplines of pharmaceuticals, forensic toxicology, agrochemicals, food technology and environmental monitoring etc. To that end I hope this book will further the growth of immunoassay methods and lead to their continued development outside the clinical discipline which hitherto has been their foundation.

The following chapters set out, in logical sequence, the steps that need to be followed for the rapid and effective development of RIAs and EIAs. Where well-established methods are known these are presented as recommended PROCEDURES, with supporting theory and background information where possible. Recommendations are also given with regard to specific equipment and sources of reagents, where these have been used successfully by the authors.

Whilst not actually guaranteeing successful assay development, following the advice presented in the succeeding chapters should at least raise its probability markedly.

References

Abraham, G. E. (1969) *J. Clin. Endocrinol. Metab.*, **29**, 866.

Balabanova, S., Parsche, F. & Prisig, W. (1992) *Naturwissenschaften*, **79**, 358.

Brandon, D. L., Binder, R. G., Wilson, R. E. & Montague, W. C. (1993) *J. Agric. Food Chem.*, **41**, 996.
Casale, W. L., Pestka, J. J. & Hart, L. P. (1988) *J. Agric. Food Chem.*, **36**, 663.
Chan, D. W. & Perlstein, M. T. (1987) *Immunoassay: A Practical Guide.* Academic Press, Florida.
Ekins, R. P. (1960) *Clin. Chim. Acta*, **5**, 453.
Keuchel, C., Weil, L. & Niessner, R. (1992) *Fresenius J. Anal. Chem.*, **343**, 143.
Landon, J. & Moffat, A. C. (1976) *Analyst*, **101**, 225.
Marsh, A. & Evans, M. B. (1993) *J. Pharm. Biomed. Anal.*, **11**, 693.
Marsh, A., Evans, M. B. & Strang, J. (1995) *J. Pharm. Biomed. Anal.*, **13**, 829.
McConnell, R. I., Lamont, J. V. & Fitzgerald, S. P. (1994) *Food Agric. Immunol.*, **6**, 401.
Meulenberg, E. P. & Stoks, P. G. (1995) *Anal. Chim. Acta.*, **311**, 407.
Odom, J. M. & Ebersole, R. C. (1994) *Methods Enzymol.*, **243**, 607.
Oliver, G. C., Parker, B. M., Brasfield, D. L. & Parker, C. W. (1968) *J. Clin. Invest.*, **47**, 1035.
Perez, M. D., Sanchez, L., Aranda, P., Ena, J. M. & Calvo, M. (1992) In: Morgan, M. R. A., Smith, C. J. & Williams, P. A. (eds) *Food Safety and Quality Assurance: Applications of Immunoassay Systems.* Elsevier, London, pp. 41.
Pratt, J. J. (1978) *Clin. Chem.*, **24**, 1869.
Smith, C. J. (1992) In: Morgan, M. R. A., Smith, C. J. & Williams, P. A. (eds) *Food Safety and Quality Assurance: Applications of Immunoassay Systems.* Elsevier, London, pp. 13.
Smith, R. N. (1988) *Forensic Sci. Prog.*, **3**, 1.
Yalow, R. S. & Berson, S. A. (1959) *Nature*, **184**, 1648.
Yang, Y. Y., Yamaguchi, I., Murofushi, N. & Takahashi, N. (1993) *Biosci. Biotechnol. Biochem.*, **57**, 1016.

2

Hazards and safe handling procedures

B. LAW

Zeneca Pharmaceuticals, Macclesfield

Introduction

In developing and working with immunoassays there are three types of hazards that may be encountered, these are: chemical, biological and radiological. All countries have their own legislation dealing with such hazards and furthermore, most laboratories will have their own local rules and interpretation of their respective legislation. It is not the purpose of this chapter therefore to discuss safe handling procedures in detail, but merely to give an indication of the size and scope of the problems and give some general guidance on the precautions to be adopted.

Although each of the above mentioned hazards poses its own special problems, necessitating different precautions and safe handling procedures, there are a number of standard laboratory practices that are applicable to all three and which should be in place in all laboratories.

Facilities and equipment provided in the laboratory should be suitable for the work to be carried out. Rules and regulations, particularly those pertaining to safety, should be accessible to everyone and should be rigorously enforced. All staff should wear laboratory coats and safety spectacles, and there should be no eating, smoking, drinking or applying cosmetics in laboratory areas. Pipetting should *never* be carried out by mouth.

These simple but important rules create a firm foundation for dealing with the more specialised hazards associated with immunoassay work which are outlined below.

Chemical hazards

The chemicals used in immunoassay work present a range of potential hazards. For example, *iso*-butyl chloroformate, which is a widely used conjugation reagent, is a powerful lachrymator; the enzyme substrate 1,2-phenylenediamine, which is used in ELISA procedures, is an irritant and a cancer suspect agent. It is essential therefore that appropriate precautions and handling conditions are employed at all times.

Most laboratories have their own rules for the handling of such substances, but when in doubt operate under the most stringent conditions, e.g. wear disposable gloves and work in a fume cupboard. For further guidance reference can be made to, for example, the Control of Substances Hazardous to Health (COSHH) regulations in the UK and Title 29 of the Code of Federal Regulations (CFR) in the USA.

Biological hazards

All biological samples should be considered as potentially infectious, especially those from primates and man. Fortunately the two species used for antibody raising, i.e. sheep and rabbits, pose minimum threat of serious infection to those developing and working with immunoassays.

The major routes of infection arise through open cuts and sores on the hands, needle stick injuries and the inhalation of aerosols. It is strongly recommended, therefore, when handling any biological samples to ensure that all open sores and wounds, particularly those on the hands, are covered. Always wear gloves and minimise the risk of exposure to aerosols by opening and working with all biological samples in a ventilated area such as a fume hood.

It is generally wise to assume that all samples are potentially infectious and adopt the necessary working practices. However, where samples are definitely known to be infected with serious pathogens such as HIV or hepatitis, then special procedures will be necessary. Under such circumstances the local safety officer should be consulted before any work is undertaken on the samples.

Radiological hazards

Of all the hazards associated with immunoassay work, the most emotive, although not necessarily the most serious, is radioactivity. Unlike chemical hazards it cannot be seen or smelt, and its effects can manifest themselves many years after an exposure incident. The regulations governing the handling of radioactivity are quite rigorous and they are becoming more restrictive as time goes on. In some countries, Japan for example, there are serious limitations on the way radioactivity can be used. The disposal of radioactive waste in the USA has also recently been under review. These international controls on the handling and disposal of radioactivity obviously pose serious limitations on the way radioactivity is utilised in analytical science.

The current legislation in the UK is the Ionising Radiations Regulations 1985 and in the USA the equivalent legislation is Title 10 of the Code of Federal Regulations (CFR). For practical guidance with respect to UK regulation, reference should be made to the Approved Code of Practice, 1985. These, along with the local rules for the laboratory, should be consulted before any work involving radioactivity is undertaken. It is essential also that all staff involved in such work have had suitable training and that this has been documented.

The hazards associated with radioactivity are reduced with decreasing amounts of radioactivity, increased distance from the source and reduced exposure time. Safe handling therefore is concerned with reducing the amounts handled and minimising the exposure both in terms of time and activity.

Hazards associated with the various isotopes require different treatment, so each will be considered separately, however some general points can be made. It is strongly recommended that all work involving radioactivity is carried out in a tray capable of containing any spillage. This tray should be lined with absorbent paper to take up any spilt liquids and minimise the extent of contamination. Such paper lining can be readily disposed of should it become contaminated.

Carbon-14 and tritium

Both ^{14}C and ^{3}H undergo radioactive decay to emit low energy β-particles or electrons. The maximum range of these β-particles in air is only 6 mm for ^{3}H and 240 mm for ^{14}C. In solution the range is much reduced: to less than 1 mm for both isotopes. This means that radioactivity will not escape from containers of reagents and the hazard when working with these isotopes is therefore very much an internal one, i.e. these isotopes will only produce a serious risk if ingested or inhaled. Immunoassay kits contain no more than 10 μCi of radioactivity, which in most cases will be in solution. If normal laboratory procedures are adopted, i.e. no eating or drinking etc., then the actual hazard in handling these isotopes should be minimal.

Iodine-125

The properties of radioiodine and its radiation are quite different to those for the β-emitting isotopes discussed above and the precautions and safe handling procedures are also quite different. First, the radioactive emissions from ^{125}I are γ-rays and although of relatively low energy (around 30 keV) they are still reasonably penetrating and they will pass through glass, plastic and living tissue. Although the interaction between γ-rays and living tissue is minimal, steps should be taken to minimise this potential external radiation hazard. This is normally done through minimising the quantities handled at any one time and by the use of some form of shielding. The small lead pots, which are used to transport commercial samples of radioiodine, are very useful for the storage of stock solutions of radiotracers. Lead in any form is a good shield against the γ-rays from radioiodine: 0.02 mm of lead will reduce the output from a ^{125}I source by half. Once again the amounts used in a typical RIA kit are relatively small, less than 10 μCi, so that with normal working practices such amounts can be safely handled on an open bench.

The greatest potential hazard with ^{125}I occurs when iodination reactions are carried out. Under these circumstances it is necessary to handle relatively large amounts of radioiodine, typically 1 mCi, usually in the form of sodium ^{125}I-iodide. The act of opening a vial of a sodium ^{125}I-iodide solution can release radioiodine vapour which could be inhaled. It is essential therefore when working with significant amounts of ^{125}I to keep containers closed wherever possible and carry out all manipulations in a well-ventilated fume cupboard. A further potential problem exists with sodium ^{125}I-iodide. Potentially harmful radioiodine vapour can be liberated if a solution of sodium ^{125}I-iodide is frozen or iodine containing materials are treated with strong oxidants or acids. Every precaution should be taken to avoid these types of procedure.

Radioiodine in some forms has the ability to penetrate rubber gloves. When carrying out iodination work it is necessary to wear at least two pairs of gloves. During the work the surface of the gloves should be checked at regular intervals for radioactive contamination using a scintillation monitor and if contamination is detected, the outer pair of gloves changed.

As a precursor to the implementation of any new procedure and part of any training programme it is recommended that a dummy run of the iodination procedure is carried out using everything except the radioiodine. This can be particularly useful in identifying 'snags' in the proposed method or the possible inappropriateness of a particular piece of equipment.

When carrying out procedures using large amounts of radioiodine the use of some form of shielding is essential. Traditionally this has been carried out using lead blocks or lead pots as mentioned above. The disadvantage of lead is that it is opaque which can be unfavourable in certain circumstances. Recently however, a number of manufacturers (e.g. Scotlab, Strathclyde, UK and Amersham International, Amersham, UK) have introduced a wide range of transparent containers, shields etc. fabricated from a lead/acrylic copolymer. This material is of optical quality and provides excellent shielding from the γ-radiation produced by ^{125}I.

In the event of a serious spillage when using radioiodine, neutralisation of the radioactive material is first necessary prior to any decontamination. Neutralisation is effectively carried out using a solution consisting of sodium hydroxide (0.1 M), sodium iodide (0.1 M) and sodium thiosulphate (0.1 M). The sodium hydroxide acts to neutralise any acid and the thiosulphate to reduce any 'active' iodine species back to relatively stable iodide. Thus both these agents act to prevent release of volatile iodine vapour. The sodium iodide merely dilutes any radiolabelled iodide thus minimising any subsequent contamination. This solution should be readily available whenever radioiodination work is carried out. Following neutralisation, decontamination should be carried out using a strong alkaline detergent solution.

Monitoring

The monitoring of the work area and personnel is essential when working with radioactivity. In the case of tritium or carbon-14, work surfaces can be swabbed and the swabs counted in a liquid scintillation counter. Alternatively surfaces can be monitored using an appropriate contamination monitor. Where personnel monitoring is required this would usually be carried out by urine analysis. The use of monitoring badges serves little purpose with these low energy β-emitting isotopes.

In the case of ^{125}I the use of badge monitors is recommended when iodination work is carried out. At the beginning and end of every iodination experiment the fume cupboard and other work areas should be checked using a scintillation monitor. The same monitor can be used to check the cuffs and front areas of laboratory coats and aprons, i.e. those areas susceptible to contamination. The thyroid gland, which is the major target organ for ^{125}I, should also be checked at the beginning and end of each experiment using the scintillation monitor.

General monitoring of all work areas should be carried out regularly and comprehensive details of all procedures and results recorded.

Disposal

It has been general practice over the years to recommend disposable equipment for use in radioactive work, and the prompt disposal of all radioactive waste, normally through incineration. At the present time this is still the preferred procedure. However any future changes in the legislation with regard to the disposal of radioactive materials may alter this situation.

Bibliography

HMSO (1985) *Approved Code of Practice, The Protection of Persons Against Ionising Radiation Arising from Any Work Activity*, 40pp., London, HMSO.

HMSO (1988) *The Control of Substances Hazardous to Health (COSHH) Regulations*, London, HMSO.

HMSO (1985) *The Ionising Radiations Regulations*, 83pp., London, HMSO.

DEPARTMENT OF ENERGY (1992) *Federal Register Title 10, Code of Federal Regulations, US Nuclear Regulatory Commission Rules and Regulations* (April 1992), Washington, DC, US Government Printing Office.

DEPARTMENT OF LABOR (1991) *Federal Register, Title 29, Code of Federal Regulations, Occupational Exposure to Hazardous Chemicals in Laboratories* (December 1991), Washington, DC, US Government Printing Office.

DEPARTMENT OF LABOR (1991) *Federal Register, Title 29, Code of Federal Regulations, Occupational Exposure to Bloodborne Pathogens* (December 1991), Washington, DC, US Government Printing Office.

3

Immunogen preparation and purification

W. N. JENNER

GlaxoWellcome Research and Development, Ware

B. LAW

Zeneca Pharmaceuticals, Macclesfield

Introduction

The antiserum is the key reagent in any immunoassay as it governs the selectivity, sensitivity, precision and accuracy of the method. One highly avid and selective antiserum is worth any number of indifferent ones and no matter how good the tracer is and how carefully the assay has been optimised, the deficiencies of a poor antiserum cannot be compensated for in terms of assay performance. It is therefore essential that sufficient care is taken in antiserum production, particularly as months of assay development time can be wasted if the antisera produced are found to be unsuitable, and work on antiserum production has to recommence. This chapter will focus on the first stage of antibody production, namely the preparation of immunogenic conjugates (immunogens). The remaining two steps, namely immunisation and antisera assessment will be discussed in Chapters 4, and 6 and 7 respectively.

High-molecular-weight foreign proteins and polypeptides are naturally immunogenic and when injected into a suitable animal they will elicit an immune response. Low-molecular-weight peptides – in the range 2000 to 10 000 Dalton – are capable of eliciting an immune response on their own but the response is usually weak. This response may be improved considerably by coupling the peptides to larger-molecular-weight carrier proteins which are themselves immunogenic. Peptides with molecular masses of less than 2000 Dalton, steroid hormones, thyroid hormones and most drugs are haptens which must first be covalently attached to a carrier protein (usually foreign to the animal being immunised), before a satisfactory immune response can be elicited. This book is devoted to the immunoassay of small molecules, i.e. compounds with molecular masses of less than 2000 Dalton, hence this chapter will focus on the production of immunogenic hapten–protein conjugates.

For a comprehensive overview of conjugation chemistry the reader is referred to the reviews by Beiser *et al.* (1968), Erlanger (1980) and Brinkley (1992) and also a most comprehensive new book on the subject *Chemistry of Protein Conjugation and Cross-Linking* (Wong, 1993). The catalogue and handbook of *Life Science and Analytical Research Products*, produced by the reagent and equipment company Pierce Warriner (Chester, UK) has long been a valuable source of information on conjugation reagents and procedures. This catalogue has gone from strength to strength and the current edition (1996) lists over 50 cross-linking reagents with full structures and in most cases a number of references to their use.

The various factors which must be considered to produce the right conjugate to give the desired antisera are discussed in turn below.

Point of attachment

The most suitable point of attachment to link the hapten to the carrier is indicated by **Landsteiner's Principle** (Landsteiner, 1945). This states that antibody specificity is directed primarily at the portion of the hapten furthest removed from the functional group that is used to link it to the carrier protein, i.e. that portion of the molecule which will be most accessible to the circulating lymphocytes during the immune response. The parts of the hapten close to the site of attachment can be considered to be sterically hindered by the carrier protein thus preventing their specific recognition.

Clearly, Landsteiner's Principle indicates that the metabolism or chemical degradation of the analyte must be taken into account in considering the point of attachment. To produce an assay specific for a parent analyte, the hapten should be attached to the carrier protein at a site remote from the site of chemical or metabolic change. The targeting of an antiserum to a specific region of an analyte molecule, to avoid interference by related materials, is all very well if the metabolism in the species providing the samples for analysis is known. If this information is not available one could either try and predict the routes of metabolism, which carries an inherent risk, or preferably, prepare antisera to more than one immunogen in which the hapten is attached to carrier proteins through different regions of the (hapten) molecule. In this way, there is a reasonable chance that at least one of the antisera produced will be selective for the parent compound.

The effect which the point of attachment on the hapten has on the specificity of the resulting antisera is illustrated for the drug loxitidine (Figure 3.1). In this case an immunogen prepared by linking an analogue of the drug to a protein carrier via the triazole ring (immunogen 1) led to extensive cross-reactivity with two metabolites (I and II). These metabolites differed in structure to the parent drug in the region of the triazole ring. When a second analogue of the drug was linked to a protein via the piperidine ring (immunogen 2) these metabolites did not cross-react with the resulting antisera and a specific assay ensued. Metabolites III, IV and V did not bind to either antiserum as they lacked the full complement of the parent molecule's structural features required for binding.

It should also be remembered when designing an immunogen, that if metabolism is not too extensive, a non-specific antiserum could still be functionally specific for the parent drug when applied to biological samples. An example of this is shown in the RIA for ranitidine (Jenner *et al.*, 1981). Even though three metabolites had significant cross-reactivity, none of these were present in plasma at sufficiently high

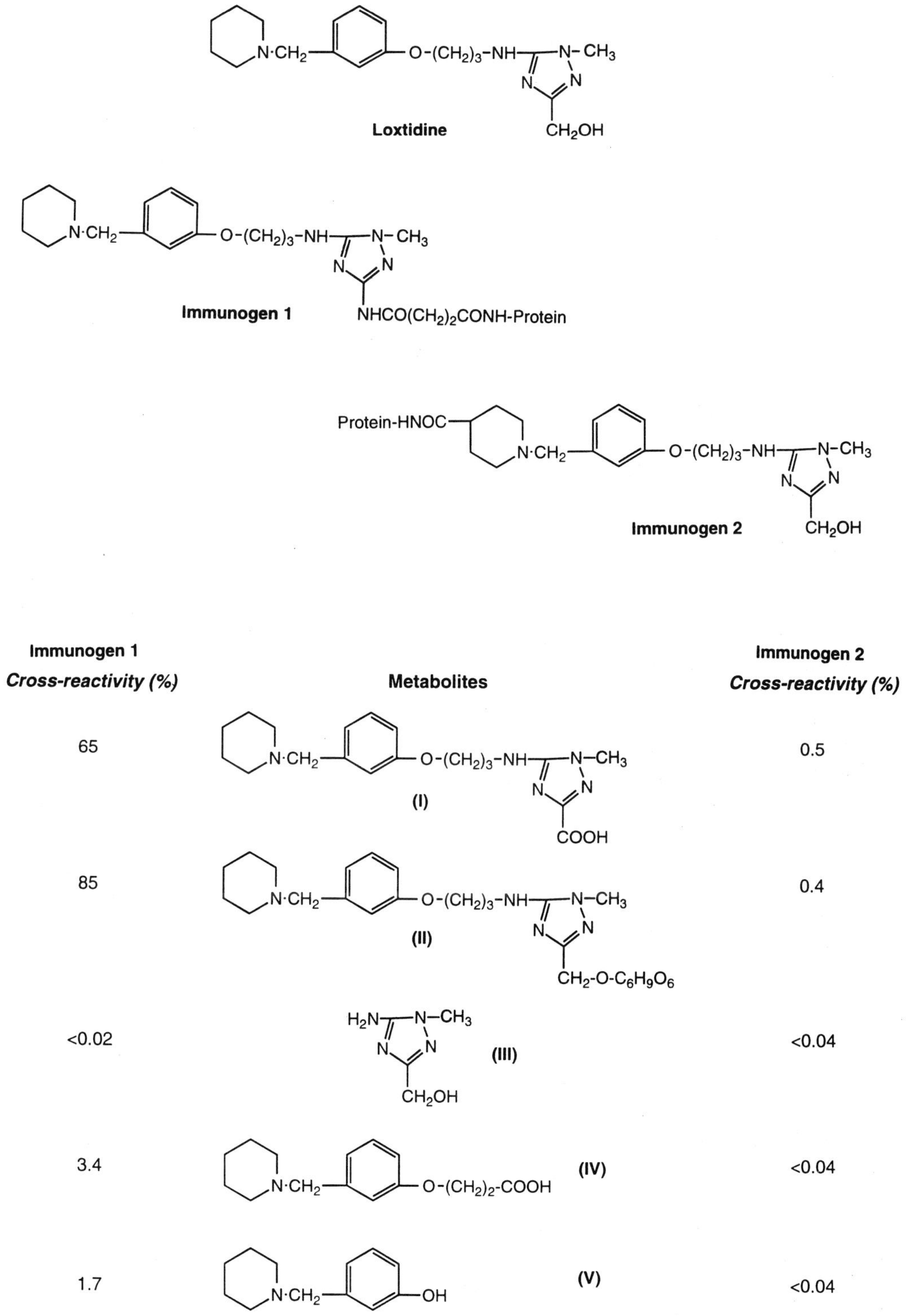

N·CH_2— O-$(CH_2)_3$-NH— N-CH_3 N N CH_2OH

Loxtidine

N·CH_2— O-$(CH_2)_3$-NH— N-CH_3 N N NHCO$(CH_2)_2$CONH-Protein

Immunogen 1

Protein-HNOC— N·CH_2— O-$(CH_2)_3$-NH— N-CH_3 N N CH_2OH

Immunogen 2

Immunogen 1 *Cross-reactivity (%)*	**Metabolites**	**Immunogen 2** *Cross-reactivity (%)*
65	**(I)** N·CH_2— O-$(CH_2)_3$-NH— N-CH_3 N N COOH	0.5
85	**(II)** N·CH_2— O-$(CH_2)_3$-NH— N-CH_3 N N CH_2-O-$C_6H_9O_6$	0.4
<0.02	**(III)** H_2N— N-CH_3 N N CH_2OH	<0.04
3.4	**(IV)** N·CH_2— O-$(CH_2)_2$-COOH	<0.04
1.7	**(V)** N·CH_2— OH	<0.04

Figure 3.1 The effect of position of attachment of the hapten to the carrier protein on the selectivity of the resulting antiserum in the assay for loxtidine.

concentration relative to the parent drug to interfere in the assay. One should never totally reject possible points of attachment, since metabolism in the species of interest may not be too extensive. This is particularly true if there are no alternative coupling sites available on the molecule. Even if cross-reactivity by endogenous compounds or metabolites etc. cannot be avoided, it is often possible to remove these interfering compounds by selective extraction (Wring *et al.*, 1994a) or HPLC fractionation of the sample prior to immunoassay (see Chapter 6).

The determination of metabolite cross-reactivity will be discussed in more detail in Chapter 9 on validation of immunoassays.

Functionalisation of the hapten

The hapten used for covalent attachment to the carrier protein may be the analyte itself or, more commonly, an analogue or a derivative. Whichever is used, a suitable functional group must be present to react specifically with a complementary functional group on the carrier protein. The most commonly used linkage involves the formation of an amide bond between a carboxylic acid moiety and a primary amino group. In practice, it is more usual to react carboxylic acid groups on the hapten with amino groups on the protein as the latter are usually more numerous and enable good levels of incorporation to be achieved.

It is rare for the analyte to carry the necessary functional group for direct attachment to a protein. Usually either a suitable derivative is synthesised or a structural analogue with the required functionality is used. In pharmaceutical or agrochemical development, a suitable compound may already have been synthesised by the project chemists in the search for an active compound. Where a derivative or an analogue has to be synthesised, having someone familiar with the chemistry of the analyte is useful, although in many instances anyone in the immunoassay development team with a chemistry background should be capable of carrying out the necessary chemical modification.

An example of the use of an analogue with the required functionality is shown in Figure 3.2. In this particular case, the molecule of interest sufotidine, could not be coupled to a protein carrier via the triazole ring because there were no suitable functional groups present. However, the structural analogue lamtidine was available with a reactive amino group which could be coupled to a protein, either directly or after further modification. As expected, both sufotidine and lamtidine showed

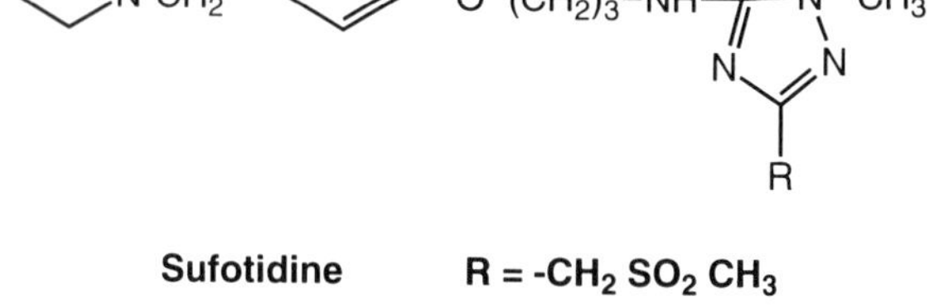

Sufotidine R = $-CH_2SO_2CH_3$

Lamtidine R = $-NH_2$

Figure 3.2 Stuctures of the drug sufotidine and the analogue lamtidine which was used for immunogen production in the development of an assay for sufotidine.

similar levels of immunoreactivity with the antiserum raised against the lamtidine conjugate.

The required chemistry for derivatisation will depend very much on the properties of the particular analyte and a detailed discussion of this is outside the scope of this chapter. A number of the commonly used reactions are shown in Figure 3.3.

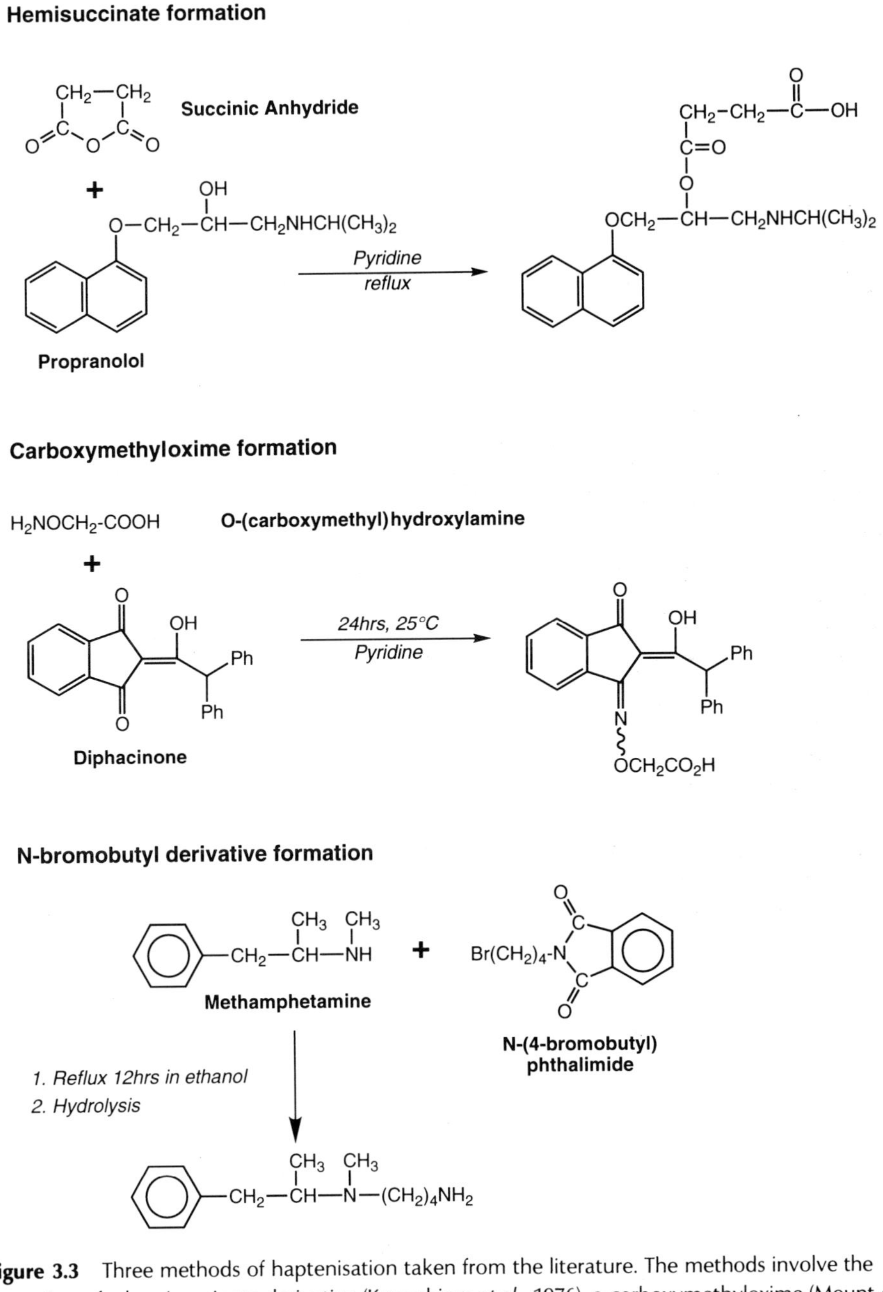

Figure 3.3 Three methods of haptenisation taken from the literature. The methods involve the formation of a hemisuccinate derivative (Kawashima *et al.*, 1976), a carboxymethyloxime (Mount *et al.*, 1988) and an *N*-4-aminobutyl derivative (Cheng *et al.*, 1973).

Succinic anhydride, which has been used since the early days of steroid immunoassay (Erlanger *et al.*, 1957, 1959) reacts with alcoholic or phenolic hydroxy groups to form hemisuccinates (Kawashima *et al.*, 1976; Pontikis *et al.*, 1980) and with primary or secondary amines to form hemisuccinamides (Michiels *et al.*, 1977; Brunswick *et al.*, 1978). Both these reactions result in the introduction of a free carboxylic acid group. *O*-(Carboxymethyl)hydroxylamine reacts cleanly with aldehydes or ketones to give carboxymethyloximes, again with a free carboxylic acid function (Mount *et al.*, 1988). This reagent has been used widely in the formation of steroid conjugates where the ketone group is relatively common, although its use in other areas has been limited. *N*-(4-Bromobutyl)phthalimide is a useful reagent for the conversion of secondary amines to primary amines or for the addition of a bridge into a primary amine whilst maintaining the same functional group (Cheng *et al.*, 1973; Mould *et al.*, 1981).

Other less well-used reactions include the formation of thioethers which have been used to introduce carboxylic acid functions across a double bond (Cook *et al.*, 1974) or via replacement of an aromatic Cl atom (Goodrow *et al.*, 1990). Phenols will react relatively cleanly and efficiently with 2-halo acids in the presence of a base (Williamson reaction) to give a carboxy derivative. The highly reactive iodoacetic acid ethyl ester has been used in one of our laboratories (Law, unpublished data). This reagent reacts cleanly and rapidly, and, following removal of the ethyl ester under mild basic conditions, gives an *O*-carboxymethyl derivative in high yield. An *O*-carboxymethyl derivative of phenytoin was also prepared using 2-chloroacetic acid (Tigelaar *et al.*, 1973). Diazotised 4-aminobenzoic acid can be employed to introduce a carboxylic acid group into an antigen having an aromatic ring such as a phenol or an imidazole (Wring *et al.*, 1994b).

In addition to providing a functional group for subsequent conjugation, the formation of these derivatives effectively introduces a bridge or spacer-arm between the hapten and the protein. It is thought that the spacer group, by reducing the steric hindrance effect of the protein molecule on the hapten allows the hapten to be more easily recognised by the circulating lymphocytes. It has been shown, by affinity chromatography (Bermudez *et al.*, 1975), that spacer groups of four to six carbon atoms are necessary for full antigen–antibody interaction, with a four-carbon bridge (hemisuccinate) resulting in maximum immunogenicity (Robinson *et al.*, 1975).

The synthesis of a derivative may also allow the simple incorporation of ^{3}H or ^{14}C into the molecule. For example, where a derivative has been prepared using ^{14}C-succinic anhydride, the presence of the ^{14}C atom in the resulting conjugate can be used for the determination of the hapten–protein conjugation ratio. This point is discussed in greater detail under conjugate characterisation below.

Irrespective of the approach used, care must be taken to ensure that the hapten is as pure as possible to avoid the generation of antibodies to impurities which could result in reduced assay specificity. Whilst it may seem obvious, it is important to be sure that the hapten is stable to the conditions used for conjugation.

Carrier protein

The only proviso in the selection of a carrier protein is that it must be of a high molecular weight (typically greater than 20 000), and phylogenically unrelated to the animal species in which the antisera are to be raised. As a consequence of these fairly loose restrictions a wide variety of proteins have been employed in the synthesis of immunogens. These include serum albumins (particularly bovine and human serum albumin, BSA and HSA respectively), ovalbumin, thyroglobulin, gamma globulins, keyhole limpet haemocyanin (KLH), fibrinogen and the synthetic polypeptides poly-L-lysine and polyglutamic acid. The first of these, BSA, despite not being particularly immunogenic (at least in rabbits and sheep) is probably the most commonly used carrier protein. This choice stems from the fact that the material is widely available in relatively pure form, it is inexpensive and well characterised (molecular weight of around 64 000 with 60 primary amino groups for conjugation). It is also relatively resistant to denaturation which can be useful in some of the conjugation procedures which involve organic solvents, such as the mixed anhydride reaction. BSA conjugates have the added advantage that they are usually readily soluble which makes isolation and characterisation easier.

Although less well characterised, the immunogenic protein KLH (molecular weight approximately 1 000 000 Dalton) is increasingly used as a carrier protein along with thyroglobulin and is the second choice after BSA in the authors' laboratories. The use of repetitive carriers such as poly-L-lysine is not recommended since this can lead to antisera with low affinities as a result of T-cell independent responses (see Chapter 4). In a discussion by Erlanger (1980) it was claimed that poly-L-lysine is a poor carrier protein in comparison to BSA.

Most proteins have a range of functional groups that can be used for conjugation. In addition to the N-terminal amino group, the lysine residues offer a rich source of primary amino functions. Glutamic and aspartic acids are a source of carboxylic acid moieties in addition to the terminal carboxylic acid. Although generally less useful, phenolic, sulphydryl, and imidazole groups in proteins have been used on occasions. The potentially reactive functional groups on common carrier proteins are shown in Figure 3.4.

Immunogen incorporation ratios

Opinion is divided on the extent of substitution necessary to produce good reagent antisera to haptens. Some workers consider it desirable to obtain high degrees of substitution (Niswender and Midgley, 1970; Niswender, 1975). In an effort to obtain high levels of incorporation a massive excess (up to 100-fold) of hapten over protein functional groups is often employed in the conjugation reaction. Other workers claim that the fewer the number of haptenic residues per molecule of carrier the better. There is little unequivocal data, and that reported may only apply to the specific examples studied. For example there is data to suggest that very high incorporation levels on BSA (50 : 1) give a poor IgG response (Erlanger, 1980), with between 5 : 1 and 19 : 1 giving good responses. However, it is clear that satisfactory responses can usually be obtained, using BSA as the carrier protein, with substitution ratios anywhere between 5 and 30. The latter figure approaches the maximum number of lysine residues present in BSA which are accessible for coupling, the remainder are buried in the centre of the protein and consequently inaccessible. It is important to be aware that it is not the molar substitution ratio, but the packing density, that is important in the hapten–protein conjugate. Thus, a large carrier protein such as thyroglobulin (molecular mass 680 000 Dalton) should have a molar

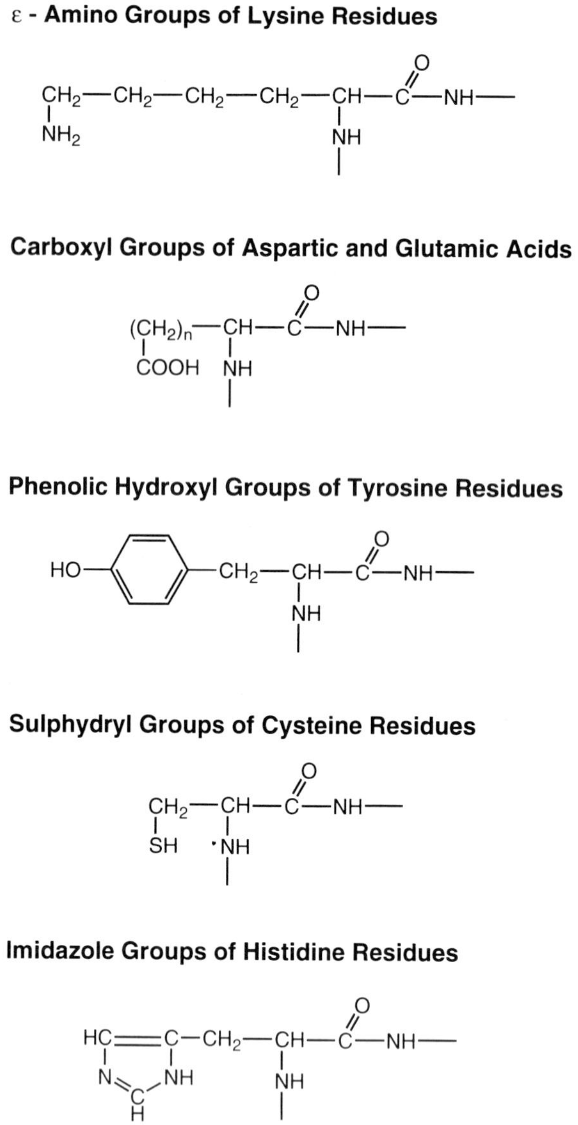

ε - Amino Groups of Lysine Residues

$$\underset{NH_2}{CH_2}-CH_2-CH_2-CH_2-\underset{NH}{CH}-\overset{O}{\overset{\|}{C}}-NH-$$

Carboxyl Groups of Aspartic and Glutamic Acids

$$\underset{COOH}{(CH_2)_n}-\underset{NH}{CH}-\overset{O}{\overset{\|}{C}}-NH-$$

Phenolic Hydroxyl Groups of Tyrosine Residues

$$HO-C_6H_4-CH_2-\underset{NH}{CH}-\overset{O}{\overset{\|}{C}}-NH-$$

Sulphydryl Groups of Cysteine Residues

$$\underset{SH}{CH_2}-\underset{NH}{CH}-\overset{O}{\overset{\|}{C}}-NH-$$

Imidazole Groups of Histidine Residues

$$HC{=}C(-N{=}CH-NH-)-CH_2-\underset{NH}{CH}-\overset{O}{\overset{\|}{C}}-NH-$$

Figure 3.4 Functional groups in proteins suitable for conjugation.

substitution ratio at least 10 times greater than for BSA to maintain the same packing density.

The approaches outlined below are based on our own experience and that in the literature (e.g. Erlanger, 1980) and have been designed to give, where possible, a hapten–BSA incorporation ratio of around 15 : 1.

Conjugation reactions

After considering the point of attachment and the possible use of analogues or derivatives, equal care should be taken in the selection of an appropriate reaction and in the conditions used for the conjugation. The reactions available may not necessarily be specific for the targeted functional groups in the molecule and side reactions could occur. It is also possible that the hapten may not be stable under the conditions used and it may be insoluble or precipitate during the course of the reaction. If there is any doubt about the suitability of the reaction conditions these should be assessed before embarking on the synthesis of the immunogen. Small scale pilot experiments can be set up which can be monitored by HPLC or TLC to confirm the stability of the hapten under the proposed reaction conditions.

If the chosen reaction involves conjugation of a carboxylic acid moiety on the hapten with a primary amino group in the protein, the pilot reaction could be set up with *n*-propylamine or a similar simple model amine instead of the protein (Lauer *et al.*, 1974). If the analysis of this reaction mixture indicates the presence of a single product in good yield (the propylamide derivative of the hapten in this case) then one could proceed with the protein conjugation with some confidence. If necessary, the reaction product from the pilot reaction could be isolated and its structure identified to provide absolute confirmation of the suitability of the chemistry.

The conjugation methods described below have been widely used to effect the covalent linkage between hapten and carrier, the reactive groups necessary for the linkage are shown in brackets. A typical practical schedule (PROCEDURE) is provided in some cases where the methods have been well tested in the authors' laboratories, or extensive literature is available. Although representing a good starting point these conditions may not be optimal for every hapten and some modification may be necessary. In the reported PROCEDURES it is assumed that the molecular mass of the hapten is 500 Dalton, and the reagent quality is assumed to be AnalaR grade or equivalent, unless stated otherwise.

Carbodiimide reaction (-*COOH* + NH_2-)

The use of carbodiimides to facilitate conjugation of a carboxylic acid and amine (Goodfriend *et al.*, 1964) is one of the most widely used conjugation methods. The carbodiimide activates the carboxylic acid function for subsequent attack by the amine. A variety of different carbodiimides can be employed (Bauminger and Wilchek, 1980), such as dicyclohexylcarbodiimide (DCC) which is used in non-aqueous media with non-polar, poorly water-soluble haptens. When these reagents are employed, the carrier protein in aqueous solution is usually added to the reaction mixture after the carbodiimide activation of the hapten (see PROCEDURE 2 below). More commonly, the water soluble derivatives of this reagent, e.g. 1-ethyl-3-(3-dimethylaminopropyl)carbodiimide (EDC) or 1-cyclohexyl-3-(2-morpholino-ethyl)carbodiimide metho-*p*-toluenesulphonate (CMC or Morpho CDI), are used. These reagents allow the reaction to be carried out in a single step (PROCEDURE 1).

A generalised reaction scheme for carbodiimide coupling is shown in Figure 3.5. The formation of the active *O*-acylurea intermediate is acid catalysed. The protein carrier however is most reactive at higher pH, where the lysine amino groups are unprotonated. A compromise is therefore necessary to provide the most favourable conditions: a pH near 6 is usually chosen. The formation of the unwanted *N*-acyl urea is claimed to be temperature dependent and it is recommended that the reaction is carried out near 0°C (Bauminger and Wilchek, 1980). It is important to use non-reactive buffer species with the water soluble reagents; for example acetate buffer which will react with the carbodiimide should be avoided.

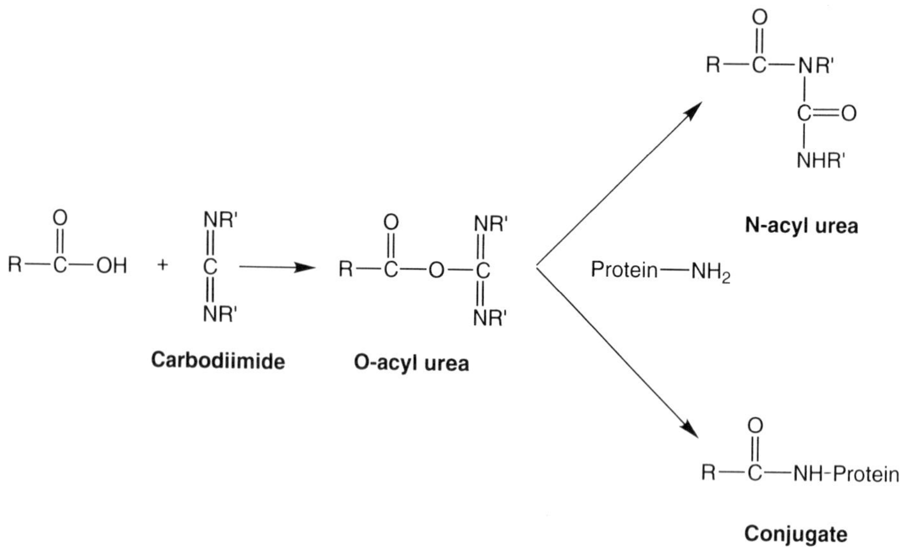

Figure 3.5 Conjugation of an amine and a carboxylic acid using a carbodiimide reagent.

The reaction with the water-soluble reagents is straightforward, although the duration of reaction is uncertain with reaction times from 3 hours (Cheng *et al.*, 1973) to 30 days! (Bermudez *et al.*, 1975) being reported. It is recommended therefore that the reaction is monitored using some chromatographic procedure to ensure it goes to completion. A typical method is given in PROCEDURE 1.

PROCEDURE 1 Conjugation of a carboxy bearing hapten to BSA using EDC

Reagents

- 1-Ethyl-3-(3-dimethylaminopropyl)carbodiimide HCl (EDC)
- Hapten
- BSA (Sigma, Fraction V or similar)
- Phosphate buffer (pH 6, 0.1 M) prepared from KH_2PO_4 (1.21 g), Na_2HPO_4 (0.156 g) and water (100 ml)

Method

Dissolve the hapten (40 mg, 0.08 mmol) in phosphate buffer pH 6 and add BSA (100 mg, 0.0016 mmol) followed by EDC (300 mg, 1.56 mmol). Stir the mixture at room temperature to ensure all the reagents have dissolved and then leave the reaction mixture at room temperature for at least 24 h. If possible monitor the reaction for disappearance of starting materials. When the reaction is considered complete (the relative proportions of the reactant(s) and product(s) are relatively constant) the mixture should be purified by gel filtration chromatography.

The use of the water-soluble carbodiimide reaction is not always successful as extensive cross-linking or alteration of the carrier can occur. Nevertheless, this highly water-soluble reagent is a widely used and successful method of preparing conjugates. Where the hapten has poor aqueous solubility the indirect method can be employed as discussed below.

N-Hydroxysuccinimide ester mediated conjugation (-COOH + NH_2-)

Activated *N*-hydroxysuccinimide esters of carboxylic acid moieties can be prepared by reacting the carboxy containing hapten with *N*-hydroxysuccinimide in the presence of dicylohexylcarbodiimide (DCC) (Figure 3.6). These esters are quite stable if kept dry, but they react quickly and in good yield with amino groups to form amide bonds (Lauer *et al.*, 1974). A typical reaction procedure is given below.

PROCEDURE 2 Conjugation of a carboxy bearing hapten to BSA using DCC via an *N*-hydroxysuccinimide ester

Reagents

- *N,N'*-dicyclohexylcarbodiimide (DCC)
- *N*-Hydroxysuccinimide (NHS)
- Dimethylformamide (DMF) 99+ % grade from Aldrich, Dorset, UK
- Hapten
- BSA (Sigma Fraction V or similar)
- Phosphate buffer (pH 7.4, 0.1 M) prepared from Na_2HPO_4 (0.114 g), KH_2PO_4 (0.268 g) and distilled water (100 ml)

Method

Dissolve the hapten (40 mg, 0.08 mmol) in DMF (1 ml) and add DCC (30 mg, 0.15 mmol) followed by NHS (40 mg, 0.34 mmol). The reaction is maintained at room temperature for 2 h then cooled to 4°C overnight. The side product, dicyclohexyl urea, that precipitates is removed by centrifugation and the supernatant added to BSA (100 mg, 0.0016 mmol) in phosphate buffer (approximately 5 ml). The reaction mixture is maintained at room temperature for a further 2 h and then the conjugate is purified by gel filtration chromatography.

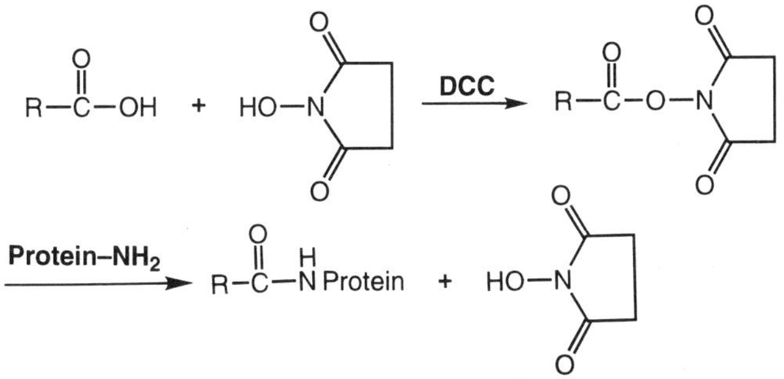

Figure 3.6 Conjugation of an amine and a carboxylic acid via an *N*-hydoxysuccinimide derivative.

Mixed anhydride procedure (-COOH + NH_2-)

This method was introduced for hapten protein conjugation by Erlanger and co-workers (Erlanger *et al.*, 1957, 1959) and has been used for many years with steroids. As with the carbodiimide method this reaction also results in the formation of an amide bond between the hapten and carrier (Figure 3.7). In this case however a two-step procedure is used and, if necessary, the activated mixed anhydride, which shows reasonable chemical stability can be isolated and characterised.

Unlike the carbodiimide reaction, in this process the carboxylic acid must be present on the hapten which is dissolved in an inert dipolar aprotic solvent such as dioxane. The chloroformate reagent is then added along with an amine catalyst. The reaction occurs readily under anhydrous conditions to form the mixed anhydride and is usually complete in 60 min. An aqueous solution of the carrier protein is then added to the activated carboxylic acid in dioxane, and the pH maintained at around 8.5. The reaction is usually carried out at low temperature (approximately 10°C) as this is believed to minimise side reactions. Typical reaction conditions for conjugation of a hapten of molecular weight 500 Dalton are given in PROCEDURE 3.

PROCEDURE 3 Conjugation of a carboxy bearing hapten to BSA using the mixed anhydride procedure

Reagents

- 1,4-Dioxane (99 + %, Gold Label, Aldrich, Dorset, UK)
- Hapten
- BSA (Sigma Fraction V or similar) (130 mg, 0.002 mmol) dissolved in distilled water (5 ml) adjusted to pH 9 with NaOH solution
- Isobutyl chloroformate
- Tributylamine (99%, Gold Label from Aldrich, Dorset, UK)

Method

Dissolve the hapten (40 mg, 0.08 mmol) in dioxane (5 ml) in a small tube and cool to around 10°C. To this solution add tributylamine (21 µl, 0.088 mmol) followed by isobutyl chloroformate (11.5 µl, 0.088 mmol). Maintain the reaction mixture at around 10°C for 60 min to allow activation of the carboxylic acid through mixed anhydride formation. The solution of BSA is then added and the reaction mixture is stirred for a further 4 h. The pH should be monitored over this period and maintained at around 8.5 by the addition of dilute NaOH solution. The conjugate can be purified by dialysis or gel filtration chromatography.

Because of the need to work in non-aqueous media the reaction is not as universally applicable as the water-soluble carbodiimide procedure. However it has been used extensively for the production of conjugates of non-polar haptens, particularly steroids. It is also a common reaction employed in the synthesis of radioiodinated tracers (see Chapter 5).

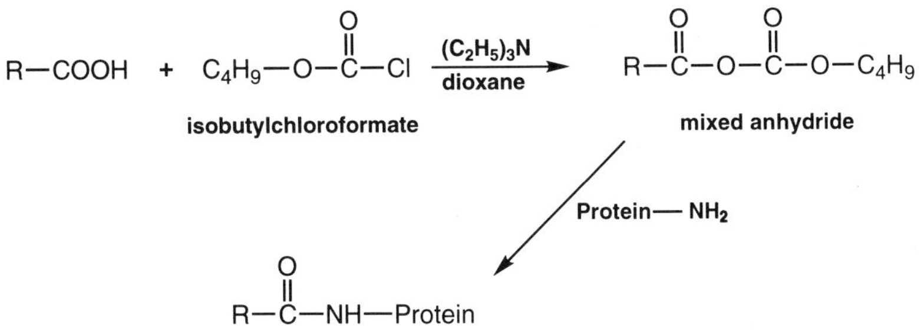

$$R{-}COOH \; + \; C_4H_9{-}O{-}\overset{\overset{\displaystyle O}{\|}}{C}{-}Cl \xrightarrow[\text{dioxane}]{(C_2H_5)_3N} R{-}\overset{\overset{\displaystyle O}{\|}}{C}{-}O{-}\overset{\overset{\displaystyle O}{\|}}{C}{-}O{-}C_4H_9$$

isobutylchloroformate **mixed anhydride**

Protein— NH_2

$$R{-}\overset{\overset{\displaystyle O}{\|}}{C}{-}NH{-}Protein$$

Figure 3.7 Conjugation of an amine and a carboxylic acid via a mixed anhydride derivative.

Glutaraldehyde condensation (-NH_2 + NH_2-)

This method of conjugation has been used for many years in the production of protein–protein conjugates and its use in the production of immunogens is a logical extension of this. The exact reaction mechanism and the structure of the resulting conjugate (which is believed to involve four molecules of glutaraldehyde per linkage) is still unclear (Reichlin, 1980). Despite this, glutaraldehyde has found extensive use in one of the authors' (BL) laboratories for the generation of hapten–protein conjugates.

It is important that the glutaraldehyde is fresh and has not undergone polymerisation, this may be checked by adding a few drops of water to the stock solution; a white cloudiness or precipitate is indicative of polymerisation – a fresh preparation gives a clear solution. A recommended method for the conjugation of an amino containing hapten to BSA is given in PROCEDURE 4 below.

PROCEDURE 4 Conjugation of an amino bearing hapten to BSA using the glutaraldehyde method

Reagents

- Phosphate buffer (0.1 M, pH 7.0) prepared from KH_2PO_4 (5.62 g), Na_2HPO_4 (8.34 g) and water (1 litre)
- Glutaraldehyde solution (0.2%, 0.02 M) in buffer
- Lysine monohydrochloride (18 mg/ml, approx. 1 M) in water
- Hapten (molecular weight 500 Dalton)
- BSA (Sigma Fraction V or similar)

Method

Dissolve the BSA (20 mg, 0.3 µmol) and the hapten (7.5 mg, 15 µmol) in buffer (2 ml). Add the glutaraldehyde solution (1 ml) dropwise over a period of 30 min with stirring and then continue to stir for a further 90 min. During this period the reaction mixture should turn yellow. Add the lysine solution (0.1 ml) to quench the reaction and continue to stir for a further 60 min. After this time the reaction mixture is ready for purification either by dialysis or gel filtration chromatography.

If KLH is the carrier protein then it may be difficult to solubilise the protein in pH 7 buffer. Under these circumstances the pH of the reaction medium buffer can be increased to 8.5 without undue effect on the outcome.

The main perceived disadvantage of this reaction is that besides conjugating hapten to carrier, it can also result in the production of dimers of the hapten and polymers of the carrier. In practice this does not seem to be a problem although it can be reduced to some extent by limiting the conjugation period to 2 to 3 hours, by stopping the reaction either by gel filtration of the reaction mixture or by the addition of an excess of an amine-containing compound, e.g. lysine or cysteamine hydrochloride. A two-stage approach has also been recommended (Zegers *et al.*, 1990) to overcome the problem of dimerisation which can be particularly problematical in the preparation of antigen–enzyme conjugates. However, the use of the one-stage procedure as outlined above has proved highly successful. In one of our authors' (BL) laboratories we have regularly obtained good quality antisera which can be used with a tracer generated from the same precursor conjugated to Bolton–Hunter reagent.

DFDNB (-NH_2 + NH_2-)

1,5-Difluoro-2,4-dinitrobenzene was introduced for the conjugation of peptides to proteins by Tager (1976) and has seen limited use in the production of conjugates for immunoassay work (Visser *et al.*, 1977; Young *et al.*, 1983; Eckert *et al.*, 1985). The aromatic nature of this reagent would appear to complement the properties of many of the other reagents which involve an aliphatic linking group. The strong UV characteristics of the reagent both in the free and conjugated form allows the coupling to be followed and the incorporation ratio to be easily determined.

Mannich reaction ('active' H + primary or secondary amine)

This procedure involves a condensation between formaldehyde, a primary or secondary amine (usually on the protein) and a compound containing an active hydrogen. The reaction results in the formation of a -CH_2- bridge between the hapten and the carrier protein (Figure 3.8). An active hydrogen is exemplified by that attached to the nitrogen atom in an indole moiety (Ranadive and Sehon, 1967), or in the case of a phenol, the hydrogen atom attached to the carbon atom *ortho* to the phenolic OH (Diener *et al.*, 1981). This method is not widely used and there are few literature reports in addition to those listed above (Taunton-Rigby *et al.*, 1973; Grota and Brown, 1976; Collignon and Pradelles, 1984). However the method has been successfully used in one of the authors' (WNJ) laboratories.

Diazotisation (-NH_2 *+ aromatic ring*)

Aromatic amines can be converted to diazonium salts with ice-cold nitrous acid. These salts can then react with a protein at alkaline pH (approximately 9) where electrophilic attack occurs primarily at histidine, tyrosine and tryptophan residues of the protein carrier (e.g. Yamamoto and Iwata, 1982).

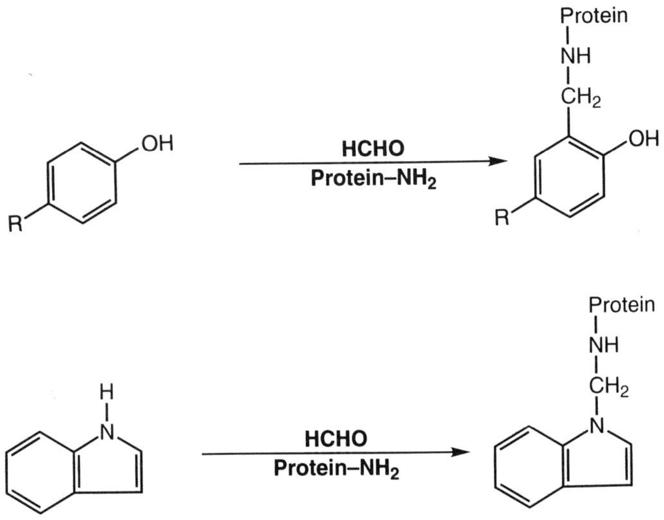

Figure 3.8 Conjugation of a phenol and an indole to an amino compound by the Mannich reaction.

Other reactions

There are a number of other reactions that can also be used under certain circumstances for coupling haptens to protein carriers. These include periodate oxidation which is suitable for compounds possessing a sugar moiety with two vicinal hydroxyl groups. *Meta*-maleimidobenzoyl-*N*-hydroxysuccinimide ester (MBS) has seen increasing use for the production of conjugates. This reagent and its more water-soluble analogue, sulfo-MBS, are heterobifunctional reagents which cross link molecules having a free amino on one hand and a free thiol group on the other. Where the molecules of interest contain thiols in the oxidised form (i.e. -S-S-) they can be reduced with Cleland's reagent (dithiothreitol). Alternatively Traut's reagent (2-iminothiolane HCl) can be used to convert amino groups to thiols for subsequent conjugation.

For a more complete discussion on many of the newer cross-linking and conjugation reagents the reader is referred to the *Pierce Handbook and Catalogue of Life Science and Analytical Research Products.*

Purification of conjugates

Purification of the crude immunogen is necessary for a number of reasons. It removes unreacted hapten and reagents, any of which could be toxic when injected into the animal. It also ensures specificity of the resultant antiserum to the targeted epitope or antigenic determinant on the hapten. Purification is also essential prior to characterisation of the immunogen and determination of the degree of hapten incorporation.

The usual method of purification involves dialysis. The reaction mixture is transferred to visking tubing and the solution is dialysed against a large excess (5 to 10 litres) of cold water or saline. Initial stages of dialysis may be performed at a slightly alkaline pH (2% sodium bicarbonate in dialysis fluid) to discourage precipitation of the protein (Jenner, unpublished data). Dialysis is normally carried out at 4°C with several changes of water or saline over a period of at least 48 h. A faster and somewhat more efficient process is pressure dialysis. In this procedure the reaction mixture is held in a continuously stirred container and the small-molecular-weight species are forced through a filtration membrane under pressure. The necessary equipment is available from Amicon, Stonehouse, Gloucestershire, UK. Neither dialysis procedure however will remove all the non-covalently linked hapten molecules, particularly when these are lipophilic. Removal of non-covalently bound hapten is important as this may be adsorbed to the carrier in a way which presents an epitope very different to that of the chemically conjugated material. The net result of injecting an immunogen containing both covalently linked and adsorbed hapten could be the generation of a mixed population of antibodies of differing specificity. For this reason the recommended final purification stage is gel filtration chromatography (GFC) which is very efficient at removing non-covalently linked material. For an excellent guide to GFC the reader is referred to the recently published book *Gel Filtration Theory and Practice*, 6th Edition, from Pharmacia (ISBN 91-97-0490-2-6).

GFC is normally carried out using Sephadex G-25 (either medium or fine grade) which has a molecular weight cut-off of around 1000. A column of 20 cm × 2.5 cm (I.D.) is commonly employed and once packed the column can be re-used many times (providing it is stored in buffer containing azide) and, with care, should be useable for 1 to 2 years. A column of this size will accept a sample volume of up to 5 ml without loss of resolution. The eluent from the column can be monitored using a UV detector, allowing precise identification of the eluent portion containing the immunogen, and the fraction of interest collected using a fraction collector.

Sephadex particles expand to different degrees in aqueous and organic solvents such as dimethylformamide. Where the conjugation reaction is carried out in organic solvents some dilution of the reaction mixture may be necessary before application to the column. Alternatively the sample can be dialysed prior to gel filtration. To minimise secondary interactions on the column a salt can be included in the eluent at a concentration of approximately 0.1 M. If the immunogen is to be stored in solution, NaCl can be used, or if it is to be freeze-dried then a volatile buffer such as ammonium acetate or ammonium formate should be used.

Compared with dialysis, GFC is very fast, most separations take only 20 min. The immunogen and the unreacted hapten are recovered in relatively small volumes (approximately 1.5 × the sample volume in the case of the immunogen) which can be advantageous.

Characterisation of conjugates

It is strongly recommended that the extent of incorporation of hapten into the conjugate is determined. Whilst on one occasion we successfully produced antisera from a conjugate where the degree of incorporation was too low to measure (M. J. Warwick, unpublished data), injecting immunogens into animals where there is no evidence of incorporation is usually a waste of time. Failure to make such measurements could result in months of delay if new conjugates have to be produced.

In some cases the hapten may be coloured or the reaction used to produce the conjugate could yield a coloured product which is a useful qualitative indicator that the hapten has been incorporated. However, in all cases it is desirable to determine the extent of substitution quantitatively. Most of the procedures outlined below depend on the conjugates being soluble and available in a pure state, i.e. all non-covalently attached hapten molecules have been removed during the purification and isolation procedures.

Radiolabelled methods

The most convenient method of determining incorporation is to include a small amount of radiolabelled hapten (typically ^{14}C) of known specific activity in the conjugation reaction. A direct estimation of the extent of substitution can then be made by determining the specific activity of small purified aliquots of the conjugate. This approach is generally employed when the analyte or a simple derivative is used as the hapten. If necessary a ^{14}C cross-linking agent can be used such as ^{14}C-succinic anhydride. If the hapten has to be synthesised *de novo*, then this approach is more costly and less applicable.

A worked example showing the calculation of incorporation ratio using the radiolabelled method is given below.

A hapten (99 mg) was mixed with a small amount (1 mg) of ^{14}C-labelled hapten (specific activity 850 MBq/mmole) to give a final specific activity of 8.5 MBq/mmole. This material was then reacted with BSA (80 mg) and the soluble conjugate was purified by gel filtration chromatography and the eluent fraction containing the conjugate was freeze-dried. An aliquot of this conjugate (10 mg) was then dissolved in water (1 ml) and the radioactivity in 0.1 ml aliquots was determined by scintillation counting and found to be 54 000 cpm/0.1 ml, equivalent to 10 580 dps/10 mg, or 1058 dps/mg.

Given that the molecular mass of the hapten is 750 Dalton, and that 1 dps = 1 Bq, then 1 milligram of conjugate contains

$$1058\ (\text{Bq})/8.5\ (\text{MBq/mmol}) = 1.24 \times 10^{-4}\ \text{mmol} \equiv 0.0933\ \text{mg of hapten}$$

Each milligram of conjugate therefore contains 0.906 mg of BSA (molecular weight 68 000) and 0.0933 mg hapten

$$0.906\ \text{mg BSA} = 0.906/68\,000 = 1.33 \times 10^{-5}\ \text{mmol}$$
$$0.933\ \text{mg hapten} = 0.0933/750 = 1.24 = 10^{-4}\ \text{mmol}$$

The incorporation ratio is therefore

$$1.24 \times 10^{-4}/1.33 \times 10^{-5} = 9\ \text{mol/mol}$$

UV and visible spectroscopic methods

If the hapten has a characteristic UV (or visible) absorbance spectrum that distinguishes it from the carrier protein then this property can be readily used to determine the degree of incorporation into the conjugate. Even when the hapten has a similar λ_{max} to the protein the extent of incorporation can still be determined providing the concentration of the protein and the spectral characteristics of the hapten and protein are known. The difference in absorbance between the conjugate and the starting protein is proportional to the amount of hapten conjugated. A typical example involving the 3-*O*-(carboxymethyloxime) hapten of beclomethasone dipropionate (3-CMO-BDP) is shown in Figure 3.9 (Jenner and Kirkham, 1988). The degree of conjugation was based on the difference in absorbance at 276 nm between the conjugate and the starting protein.

Indirect methods

In conjugates produced by reaction of lysine ε-amino groups, the extent of incorporation can be determined indirectly, by measuring the number of free amino groups remaining in the conjugate. The method of Habeeb (1966) involves the reaction of

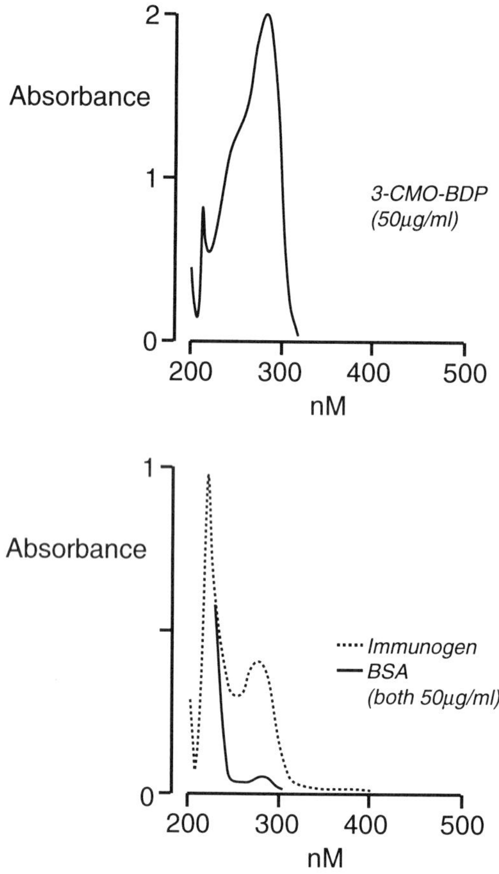

Figure 3.9 The UV spectra used in the assessment of conjugation ratio. The spectra are shown for the 3-*O*-(carboxymethyloxime) of beclomethasone dipropionate (3-CMO-BDP), BSA and the immunogen, 3-CMO-BDP-BSA.

trinitrobenzene sulphonic acid with the residual primary amino groups. The number of amino groups in the conjugate and the starting protein are then determined spectrophotometrically. The difference between these two measurements gives the number of hapten groups conjugated. This technique may give higher values than the other methods because some of the lysine residues may be involved in protein–protein cross-linking. The technique is also unsuitable for use with immunogens produced by the glutaraldehyde method since lysine amino groups may be derivatised with glutaraldehyde but not be linked to a hapten.

Other methods

Two methods which have been recently reported are ^{19}F NMR (Wring *et al.*, 1994c) and matrix assisted laser desorption time of flight mass spectrometry (MALD TOF MS) (Wengatz *et al.*, 1992; Wring *et al.*, 1994c). These highly sophisticated techniques are both capable of unequivocally demonstrating conjugation of the hapten to the protein. MALD TOF MS also has the added advantage that it can give quantitative information on conjugation ratios. In addition, the NMR technique can discriminate between covalently and non-covalently bound hapten.

Storage of immunogens

With regard to storage, the process of freeze-drying may lead to denaturation of the hapten–protein complex and consequently lyophilised immunogens can become less soluble with time. Since particulate immunogens are considered to be more immunogenic than soluble materials (see Chapter 4) this in itself is no great problem. However, during denaturation the hapten molecules may become occluded with resulting loss of immunogenicity. It is therefore preferable, in most cases, to store immunogens in aqueous solution at 4°C. Sodium azide (0.1 per cent) can be added as a preservative or the solution can be sterilised by passing through a 0.22 μm filter. If the immunogen solution is filtered into and stored in a plastic syringe this can facilitate preparation of the emulsion for immunisation using the double syringe technique (see Chapter 4). Under these conditions the immunogen should be stable indefinitely.

References

BAUMINGER, S. & WILCHEK, M. (1980) *Methods in Enzymology*, **70**, 151.

BEISER, S. M., BUTLER, V. P. & ERLANGER, B. F. (1968) In: MIERCHER, P. A. & MULLER, E. H. J. (eds) *Textbook of Immunopathology*. Grune and Stratton, New York, USA, pp. 15.

BERMUDEZ, J. A., CORONADO, V., MIJARES, A., LEON, C., VELAZQUEZ, A., NOBLE, P. & MATEOS, J. L. (1975) *J. Steroid Biochem*, **6**, 283.

BRINKLEY, M. (1992) *Bioconjugate Chem.*, **3**, 2.

BRUNSWICK, D. J., NEEDELMAN, B. & MENDELS, J. (1978) *Life Sci.*, **22**, 137.

CHENG, L. T., KIM, S. Y., CHUNG, A. & CASTRO, A. (1973). *Febs Lett.*, **36**, 339.

COLLIGNON, F. & PRADELLES, P. (1984) *Eur. J. Nucl. Med.*, **9**, 23.

COOK, C. E., TALLENT, C. R. & CHRISTENSEN, H. D. (1974) *Life Sci.*, **14**, 1075.

DIENER, U., KNOLL, E. & WISSER, H. (1981) *Clin. Chim. Acta.*, **109**, 1.

ECKERT, H. G., MUENSCHER, G., OEKONOMOPULOS, R., STRECKER, H., URBACH, H. & WISSMANN, H. (1985) *Drug Res.*, **35**, 1251.

ERLANGER, B. F. (1980) *Methods in Enzymology*, **70**, 85.

ERLANGER, B. F., BOREK, F., BEISER, S. M. & LIEBERMAN, S. (1957) *J. Biol. Chem.*, **228**, 713.

(1959) *J. Biol. Chem.*, **234**, 1090.

GOODFRIEND, T. L., LEVINE, L. & FASMAN, G. D. (1964) *Science*, **144**, 1344.

GOODROW, M. H., HARRISON, R. O. & HAMMOCK, B. D. (1990) *J. Agric. Food Chem.*, **38**, 990.

GROTA, L. J. & BROWN, G. M. (1976) *Endocrinology*, **98**, 615.

HABEEB, A. F. S. A. (1966) *Anal. Biochem.*, **14**, 328.

JENNER, W. N. & KIRKHAM, D. J. (1988) In: REID, E., ROBINSON, J. D. & WILSON, I. D. (eds) *Bioanalysis of Drugs and Metabolites.* Plenum, New York, pp. 77.

JENNER, W. N., MARTIN, L. E., WILLOUGHBY, B. A. & FELLOWS, I. (1981) *Life Sci.*, **28**, 1323.

KAWASHIMA, K., LEVY, A. & SPECTOR, S. (1976) *J. Pharmacol. Exp. Ther.*, **196**, 517.

LANDSTEINER, K. (1945) *The Specificity of Serological Reactions.* Harvard University Press, Boston, USA.

LAUER, R. C., SOLOMON, P. H., NAKANISHI, K. & ERLANGER, B. F. (1974) *Experientia*, **30**, 558.

MICHIELS, M., HENDRIKS, R. & HEYKANTS, J. (1977) *Eur. J. Clin. Pharmacol.*, **12**, 153.

MOULD, G. P., CLOUGH, J., MORRIS, B. A., STOUT, G. & MARKS, V. (1981) *Biopharmaceutics Drug Disp.*, **2**, 49.

MOUNT, M. E., KURTH, M. J. & JACKSON, D. Y. (1988) *J. Immunoassay*, **9**, 69.

NISWENDER, G. D. (1975) In: CAMERON, E. H. D., HILLIER, S. G. & GRIFFITHS, K. (eds) *Steroid Immunoassay: Proceedings of the Fifth Tenovus Workshop.* Alpha Omega Publishing Ltd., Cardiff, UK, pp. 47.

NISWENDER, G. D. & MIDGLEY, A. R. (1970) In: PERON, F. G. & CALDWELL, B. V. (eds) *Immunological Methods in Steroid Determination.* Plenum, New York, pp. 149.

PONTIKIS, R., SCHERRMANN, J. M., NAM, N-H., BOUDET, L. & PICHAT, L. (1980) *J. Immunoassay*, **1**, 449.

RANADIVE, N. S. & SEHON, A. H. (1967) *Can. J. Biochem.*, **45**, 1701.

REICHLIN, M. (1980) *Methods in Enzymology*, **70**, 159.

ROBINSON, J. D., MORRIS, B. A., PIALL, E. M., AHERNE, G. W. & MARKS, V. (1975) In: PASTERNAK, C. A. (ed.) *Radioimmunoassay in Clinical Biochemistry.* Heyden, London, pp. 101.

TAGER, H. S. (1976) *Anal. Biochem.*, **71**, 367.

TAUNTON-RIGBY, A., SHER, S. E. & KELLEY, P. R. (1973) *Science*, **181**, 165.

TIGELAAR, R. E., RAPPORT, R. L., INMAN, J. K. & KUPFERBERG, H. J. (1973) *Clin. Chim. Acta.*, **43**, 231.

VISSER, T. J., KLOOTWIJK, W., DOCTER, R. & HENNEMANN, G. (1977) *Febs Lett.*, **83**, 37.

WENGATZ, I., SCHMID, R. D., KREISSBIG, S., WITTMANN, C., HOCK, B., INGENDOH, A. & HILLENKAMP, F. (1992) *Anal. Lett.*, **25**, 1983.

WONG, S. S. (1993) *Chemistry of Protein Conjugation and Cross-linking.* CRC Press, Florida, USA.

WRING, S. A., ROONEY, R. M., GODDARD, C. P., WATERHOUSE, I. & JENNER, W. N. (1994a) *J. Pharm. Biomed. Anal.*, **12**, 361.

WRING, S. A., O'NIEL, R. M., WILLIAMS, J. L., BIRCH, H. L., GODDARD, C. P., ANDREW, P. D. & JENNER, W. N. (1994b) *Analyst*, **119**, 2395.

WRING, S. A., ROONEY, R. M., WILLIAMS, J. L., JENNER, W. N., BLACKSTOCK, W. P., OXFORD, J., HUGHES, S., ISMAIL, I. M., PARKHOUSE, A. & PANCHAL, T. A.

(1994c) In: Reid, E., Hill, H. M. & Wilson, I. D. (eds) *Biofluid and Tissue Analysis for Drugs*. The Royal Society of Chemistry, Cambridge, UK, pp. 33.

Yamamoto, I. & Iwata, K. (1982) *J. Immunoassay*, **3**, 155.

Young, R. N., Kakushima, M. & Rokach, J. (1983) *Biochem. Biophys. Res. Commun.*, **117**, 574.

Zegers, N., Gerritse, K., Deen, C., Boersma, W. & Claassen, E. (1990) *J. Immunol. Methods*, **130**, 195.

4

Immunology and the production of reagent antibodies

C. G. COPLEY and B. LAW

Zeneca Pharmaceuticals, Macclesfield

W. N. JENNER

GlaxoWellcome Research and Development, Ware

Introduction

Whilst it is eminently possible to produce an inadequate assay from excellent antibodies, the converse is not true. This book should assist the inexperienced worker in producing useful assays from good sera, but neither it, nor any other work, can assist in producing useful assays from poor sera. Unfortunately, it is impossible to be prescriptive about exactly what one should do when faced with the task of generating suitable antisera against a novel molecule. Optimising the production of antibodies for one chemical entity is no guarantee that the same method can be successfully applied to a second target. There are, perhaps, as many detailed methods as there are workers in the field, each based on previous success and current pragmatism. However, the underlying principles remain the same, and it is these that this chapter will attempt to explain. Sometimes the theory described below may appear somewhat esoteric; however, it should help explain why some of the protocols have been developed and help the newcomer to the field develop his own. Furthermore, it should help provide a framework of what is possible and what is not.

When one tries to hijack the immune system for the generation of immunoassay reagents, it is worth bearing in mind that its principal function is to protect animals from infectious organisms or the toxins that they produce. The immune system has many mechanisms and weapons it can deploy against the invading foreigner, but here discussion will be limited to the so-called humoral response. That is the system by which animals produce antibodies which are exquisitely tailored to be capable of tightly binding specific foreign molecules.

The following discussion will start by first considering the structure of the antibody and then examine how the protein sequences of the polypeptides, which make up this antibody, are encoded in the animal's genetic material. Consideration will then be given to how the generation of antibodies is controlled. To the immunologist this description will seem overly simplistic, but, we trust, not inaccurate. To the average reader it is hoped that it is comprehensible. Finally, the practical consequences of this theory will be considered in relation to the production of antibodies for immunoassays.

The meaning of some of immunology's more prosaic language will be explained in the text, for other unfamiliar terms the reader is referred to the glossary.

Antibody structure

The basic antibody unit consists of four polypeptide chains: two identical heavy chains, which are linked by one or more disulphide bridges, and two identical light chains, each of which is paired with a heavy chain to form two identical antigen binding sites (Figure 4.1a) (Edelman *et al.*, 1969). In some classes of antibody further polymers are formed from this basic four-chain unit and other polypeptide chain(s).

Heavy chains

All heavy chains can be thought of as comprising two regions: one part, which is variable in sequence, contributes to the antibody's antigen binding characteristics;

(a) The basic antibody unit

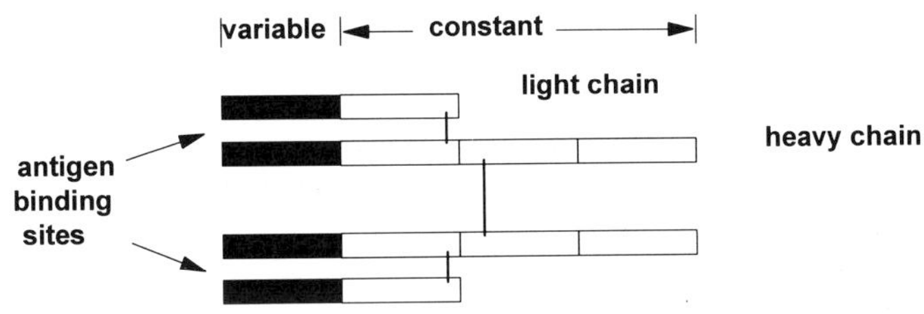

(b) Enzyme derived fragments of IgG

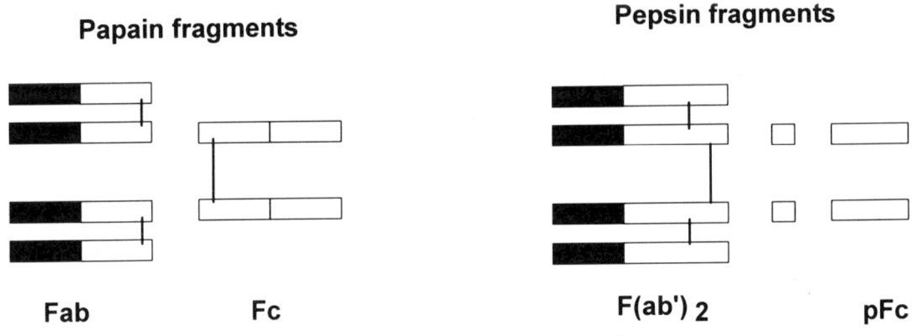

(c) Fragments derived through molecular biology

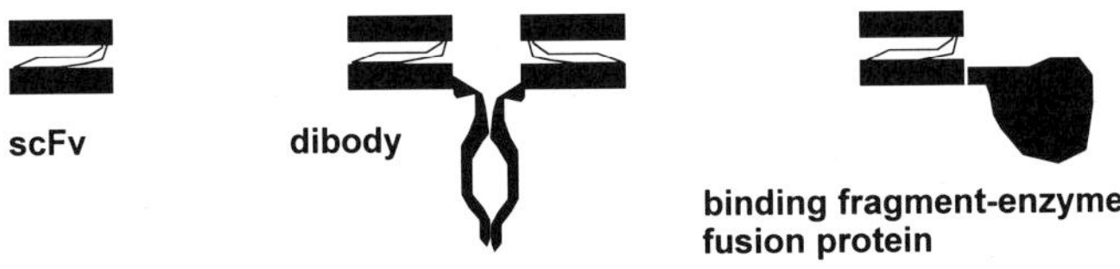

Figure 4.1 The basic antibody unit and fragments of IgG.

the other part, which is constant for a given class of antibody, determines biological characteristics such as the ability to cross the placenta and the ability to react with other components of the host's defence systems. Five major variants of heavy chain have been detected in mammals: γ, α, δ, ε, μ. These determine the five major classes of immunoglobulin: IgG, IgA, IgD, IgE, IgM, which fulfil different functions in the body's defensive armoury. All heavy chains are glycosylated.

Light chains

Like heavy chains, light chains may be thought of as comprising two regions, one variable, which together with its corresponding heavy chain variable region determines the antigen binding characteristics of the antibody, and the other, constant for a particular class of light chain. Two classes of light chain exist: κ and λ. A given antibody will only contain one type of heavy chain and one type of light chain. All classes of antibody may contain either κ or λ chains. The proportion of κ to λ containing antibodies varies with species, for instance it is about 60 : 40 in man but 95 : 5 in mice and rats.

Classes of antibody

The properties of the different antibody classes are summarised in Table 4.1. For the immunoassayist, IgG is the most important class of antibody, and will form the basis of most of the subsequent discussion. IgG comprises two light chains and two γ heavy chains. This class of antibody predominates in the later stages of the immune response and, by virtue of its potentially higher affinity, is the class of immunoglobulin on which most, if not all, successful immunoassays are based. However, IgM will be encountered early in an immunisation schedule, and may persistently predominate the response to some antigens (see T-cell independent responses).

The amino acid sequence of the constant regions of particular classes of heavy chain and classes of light chain vary between species. Thus it is possible to raise antibodies in species 'B' against antibodies from species 'A'. These anti-IgG antibodies are used by the immunoassayist to allow efficient separation of bound and free analyte in the so-called second antibody methods (see Chapter 6).

Fragments of IgG antibodies

Historically enzymatic cleavage of IgG molecules has been used to produce a number of fragments (Figure 4.1b). Treatment with papain produces three fragments, two of which are monovalent antigen binding proteins, called Fab fragments. These comprise one light chain and approximately half a heavy chain. The third fragment obtained during papain cleavage is the Fc fragment which is part of the constant region of the two heavy chains still linked through disulphide bridges.

Treatment with pepsin cuts the molecule in more than one position at the other side of the inter-heavy-chain disulphide bridge to produce a single divalent antigen binding molecule, called $F(ab')_2$ and a pFc fragment which comprises the terminal portion of the two heavy chains.

Table 4.1 Classes of immunoglobulin and their characteristics

Characteristics	IgG	IgM	IgA	IgD	IgE
Heavy chain	γ	μ	α	δ	ε
Mass (kDa)	50	70	65	70	72.5
Light chain	κ or λ	κ or λ	κ or λ	κ or λ	κ or λ
Molecular formula	$\gamma 2\kappa 2$ or $\gamma 2\lambda 2$	$(\mu 2\kappa 2)5$ or $(\mu 2\lambda 2)5$	$(\alpha 2\kappa 2)1$–2 or $(\alpha 2\lambda 2)1$–2	$\delta 2\kappa 2$ or $\delta 2\lambda 2$	$\varepsilon 2\kappa 2$ or $\varepsilon 2\lambda 2$
Concentration in serum	8–16 mg/ml	0.5–2 mg/ml	1–4 mg/ml	10–400 ng/ml	0–0.4 mg/ml
Function	Secondary response	Primary response	Protects mucous membranes	?	Anti-parasite

The introduction of molecular biology to the study and production of antibodies (Marks *et al.*, 1991) has produced a new range of possible antigen binding fragments (Figure 4.1c), the most widely quoted of which is the single chain Fv (scFv). This engineered fragment consists of the variable part of the heavy chain linked to the variable part of the light chain via a linker peptide. By addition of suitable peptide sequences to the end of the scFv it can be encouraged to dimerise to form a divalent 'dibody'. Alternatively, the sequence coding for an enzyme may be spliced onto the scFv sequence to produce a single chain binding fragment–enzyme molecule. Whilst, at present, these engineered fragments play little part in immunoassays, they are likely to become increasingly important as the recombinant technology develops.

Sub-classes of immunoglobulin G

Various subclasses of this type of immunoglobulin have been identified based on subtle differences in the constant regions of the γ heavy chain. The number of subtypes and their nomenclature varies with species. For instance, four subtypes have been identified in the mouse and human (G1, G2, G3 and G4 in human; G1, G2a, G2b and G3 in mouse), whereas only two subtypes are found in the pig, cow and guinea pig. Only a single subtype of IgG is found in the rabbit and goat.

Different batches of anti-IgG (i.e. second antibody reagents) vary in their relative binding to different subclasses of IgG. Figure 4.2 shows how the ability of five anti-

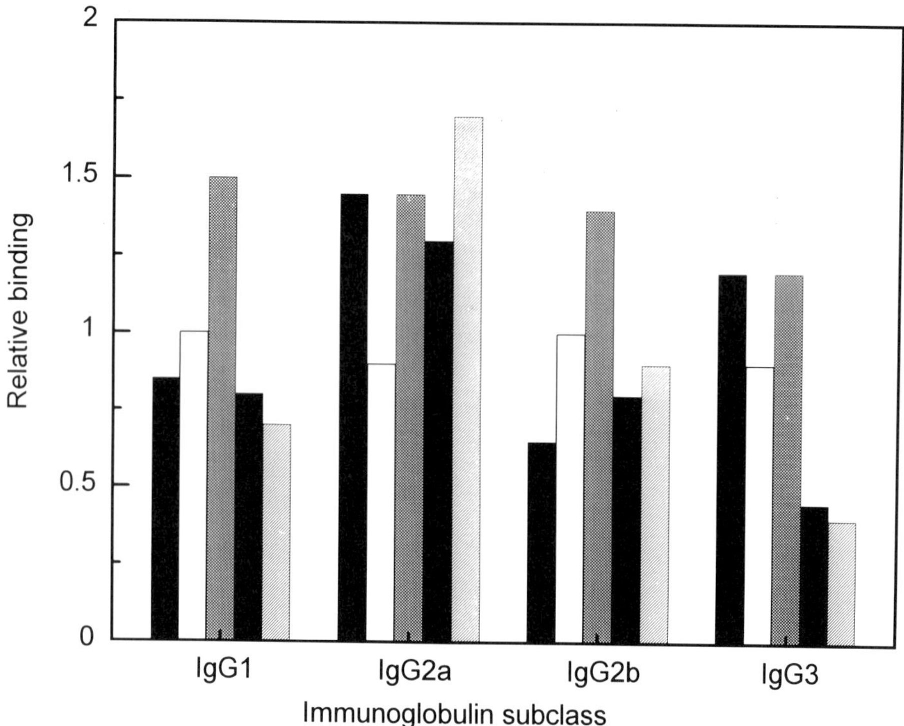

Figure 4.2 The ability of five different anti-mouse IgG (represented by different shading) to recognise subclasses of murine IgG.

mouse IgG sera to react with the different mouse IgG subclasses can vary. This can have implications in the use of second antibody reagents in separation of bound and free since it necessitates the reoptimisation of each new batch of second antibody reagent.

Variable regions and antigen binding

The variable part of the heavy chain can be subdivided into four framework regions, which are moderately conserved between immunoglobulins from the same species, and three hypervariable regions (Kehoe and Capra, 1971). As their name would suggest, the hypervariable regions show great variability, even between different antibodies which apparently react with the same antigen. The light chain is similarly arranged with its variable region comprising four framework regions surrounding three hypervariable regions.

The antigen binding site is formed from the hypervariable regions of both heavy and light chains. Because of this, these hypervariable regions are also known as Complementary Determining Regions or CDRs. Figure 4.3 illustrates the relation-

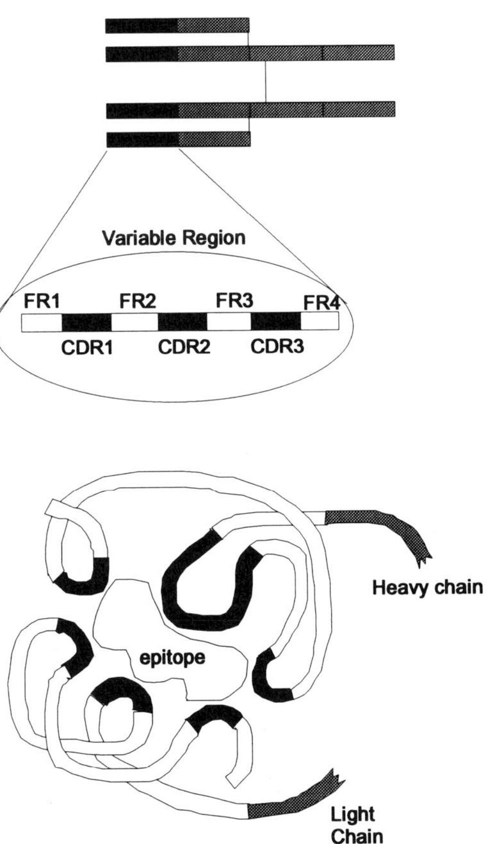

Figure 4.3 Structure of the variable regions and antigen binding. The three hypervariable regions (CDR1, 2, 3) of each chain are shown with heavy shading.

ship between the linear arrangement of the CDRs in the schematic representation of the variable regions and their role in antigen binding.

The forces involved in antibody–antigen interactions are a combination of weak non-covalent forces, all of which can only operate over short distances: (i) electrostatic interactions; (ii) Van der Waals forces; (iii) hydrogen bonding and (iv) hydrophobic interactions. A lack of fit between the antigen and the surface presented by the CDRs countervails by preventing the close approach of the two molecules, which is necessary for the weak attractive forces to be effective.

It is difficult to predict which of the above forces will predominate in any given antibody–antigen interaction. However, the relative balance can impart different characteristics to the reaction and can be important in determining the conditions under which an immunoassay should be performed. For instance, hydrogen bonding is essentially an exothermic reaction and thus is favoured by lower temperatures. Interactions in which these bonds dominate are more stable at lower temperatures, i.e. 4°C or room temperature as opposed to 37°C. Electrostatic interactions are sensitive to changes in pH and ionic strength. Organic solvents may also disrupt antibody–antigen interactions (Chan-Shu and Blair, 1979).

Affinity, avidity, titre and specificity

These terms have assumed monumental importance in the field of immunoassay. Not only do they contribute to the confusion of the neophyte, but, as their absolute values are a function of the precise method of measurement, they can be a source of conflict between experienced workers in the field. Each is related to the other.

Affinity is a measure of the strength with which a monovalent antigen binds to one of the antibody binding sites. For the reaction:

$$Ag + Ab \leftrightharpoons AgAb$$

At equilibrium the affinity constant (K) is given by:

$$K = [AgAb]/[Ag][Ab] = k_1/k_2$$

where [AgAb] is the concentration of the antibody–antigen complex, [Ag] is the concentration of free antigen, [Ab] is concentration of free antibody and k_1 and k_2 are the rate constants for the forward and back reaction respectively. Values in the region of 10^6 to 10^{12} litre moles^{-1} are commonly encountered, although for a sensitive and robust immunoassay, affinity constants of at least 10^{10} are probably necessary.

As mentioned above, the binding of an antigen can be severely influenced by pH, ionic strength, temperature and non-polar solvents, thus only under precise conditions can absolute figures be generated. Furthermore, as polyclonal sera will contain several species of antibody, each with different binding characteristics for a given antigen, accurate and meaningful affinity figures can only be generated for monoclonal preparations. It is frequently, and rightly, asserted that high affinity antibodies are needed for sensitive immunoassays. However, it is a misconception that immune sera ranked by affinity under one set of conditions will show the same order of performance when included in an assay performed under other conditions.

Thus, it is recommended that a panel of immune sera are assessed in the methods and under the conditions in which they are ultimately to be used.

Avidity is a measure of the strength with which an antigen may react with the antibody molecule as a whole. Thus the avidity of an antibody for a multivalent antigen such as a highly substituted hapten–carrier conjugate will be higher than its avidity for a monovalent hapten. Similarly, if we consider the reaction of a multivalent antigen with two antibodies, one IgG and one IgM, each with identical variable regions, the IgM will have greater avidity for the antigen by virtue of its higher valency. The importance for the immunoassayist lies in assay design, as displacement in a divalent interaction, such as between IgG antibody and a $(hapten)_n$–carrier conjugate with monovalent hapten will require a high concentration of the free hapten, and thus produce an insensitive assay.

Titre is a characteristic of antisera that is relatively easy to measure and thus frequently quoted. It is determined by assessing the ability of dilutions of the test sera to bind antigen. The dilution which binds half the antigen is usually recorded as the titre. This is dependent on three factors: the mass of tracer; affinity of the antibody for the hapten; and the quantity of specific antibody present in the serum. It is common practice to quote the working dilution of the antiserum rather than the actual dilution in the assay tube. The latter is more correct since it allows titre to be compared in absolute terms without reference to the volumes of reagents used in the assay. A frequent mistake, made by workers new to immunoassay, is to assume that high titre is synonymous with a good (high affinity) antibody. As shown in Table 4.2, titre is not predictive of quality. Since the serum with the highest titre (No. 4) is not the one with the best affinity (or sensitivity), which is No. 5. Titre is actually a measure of quantity.

Specificity, if the discussion is limited to small molecules, is a measure of the relative affinities the antibody shows for a range of compounds under defined conditions. If the discussion is broadened to include multivalent antigens then it is a measure of their relative avidities. Specificity is probably the one area where immunoassays often fail in relation to the physicochemically based counterparts, e.g. chromatographic methods. Obtaining the desired specificity is therefore one of the greatest challenges for the practising immunoassayist.

Table 4.2 Titre and ED_{50} (an indirect measure of affinity) for antisera from six rabbits immunised with a hapten–BSA conjugate

Rabbit no.	Titre	ED_{50} (ng/ml)
1	1500	5.8
2	4500	1.6
3	<200	ND
4	6000	4.3
5	3000	0.4
6	3000	1.7

ND = not determined.

Basis of antibody diversity and the immune response

Cell types involved

A number of different cell types within the animal must interact in order to produce an appropriate antibody response.

B-lymphocytes (B-cells) form approximately 30 per cent of the blood lymphocytes and arise continuously from progenitor stem cells in the bone marrow. They have specific antibody molecules bound to their surface and, after antigen stimulation, can develop into antibody-secreting plasma cells.

T-lymphocytes (T-cells) form approximately 70 per cent of the blood lymphocytes and are derived from bone marrow precursors after development and selection in the thymus. Unlike B-cells, which recognise native antigen, T-cells recognise short peptides derived from intracellular proteolytic digestion of antigens, which are subsequently complexed with Major Histocompatability Complex (MHC) molecules expressed on the cell surface of Antigen Presenting Cells (see below). We are concerned with a subpopulation of T-cells called T-helper cells, which provide the cytokines required for the B-cell maturation into antibody-secreting plasma cells.

Antigen Presenting Cells (APCs) is the general term used to describe all cells that take up antigen non-specifically by phagocytosis and, after processing it, present part of the antigen on their surface in association with MHC proteins. They include macrophages, Langerhans cells in the skin and dendritic cells of the spleen and lymph nodes.

Genetic structure of the germ line

The first clue to how the wide diversity of antibodies arises can be gleaned by examining how the variable regions of both heavy and light chains are coded for in germ-line DNA. We have seen how the variable regions of both heavy and light chains can be subdivided into framework regions and hypervariable regions or CDRs (Figure 4.3). In the germ line (that is pre-B-cells) the variable region of the heavy chain is coded for by three different DNA regions (Figure 4.4) (Early *et al.*, 1980). The first of these is a germ-line gene V_H (rather confusingly the V also stands for variable) which covers a region encoding CDRs 1 and 2. For the mouse heavy chain there are thought to be 500 different versions of this region (Roitt, 1991). The remaining CDR is encoded in two separate DNA regions called the D, or diversity region, and the J, or joining region. In the mouse there are thought to be 15 D regions and 4 J regions. The V, D and J regions associate randomly as the B-cell develops, leading to 3×10^4 ($15D \times 4J \times 500V_H$) possible heavy chains.

The mouse kappa light chain variable region is only coded for by two DNA regions: V_K of which there are 200 variants in the mouse and J of which there are four variants, leading to a possible 800 variants of mouse kappa chain. By random association of the mouse heavy and kappa light chains we could expect 2.4×10^7 different antibody molecules to be generated. This is undoubtedly an underestimation, as some D genes found in differentiated B-cells have been found to be

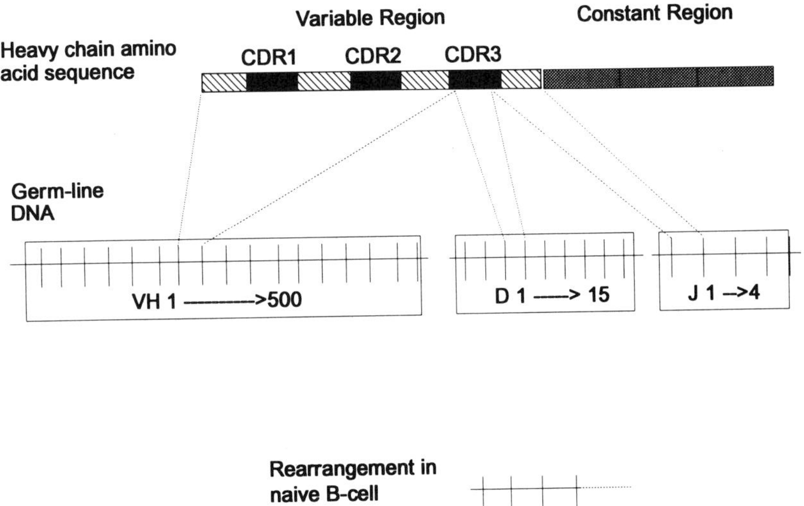

Figure 4.4 Relationship of heavy chain strucure to germ-line genes and subsequent gene rearrangement.

longer than their germ-line counterparts suggesting unusual joining into D–D segments. Also there is a variable boundary, where joining between these regions occurs at different points producing hybrid codons (and thus different amino acids) as well as insertions and deletions.

A given animal will have two sets of germ lines, one inherited from each parent. Thus it can be expected that an outbred animal will have a wider range of V_H, J and D regions from which to select than will an inbred animal. After rearrangement one of the two sets will be ignored through a mechanism called allelic exclusion (Early and Hood, 1981). Whilst the range of diversity present even in an inbred animal should ensure that the pool of germ-line V_H, J and D regions do not limit an animal's ability to mount some kind of response to an antigen, it may limit its ability to produce the perfect antibody. For this and other reasons presented below (see tolerance), the use of outbred strains of animals is strongly recommended for the production of immunoassay reagents.

Clonal selection

Each lymphocyte carries a receptor which is capable of recognising a single antigen. However, different lymphocytes carry different receptors, thus a population of lymphocytes is capable of recognising a wide range of antigens. The receptors on the B-lymphocytes are membrane bound versions of antibodies derived from the germ-line genetic material, as described in the section above.

When an antigen enters the immune system, it is exposed to a vast array of different lymphocytes but it is only bound to those which have a receptor capable of recognising it (Burnet, 1959). Such cells usually respond by proliferation and further differentiation (Figure 4.5). During this antigen-induced proliferation and differentiation, lymphocytes develop down one of two alternate routes: either they may terminally differentiate into short-lived immune effector cells capable of secreting antibodies; or they may form the expanded pool of long-lived 'memory' cells, which lie in wait for a second invasion of the same antigen. When the immune system first encounters an antigen very few cells will carry a receptor capable of recognising it. However, during the initial response this population will proliferate, so that on a second encounter with the same antigen a larger number of cells will carry the necessary recognising receptors. Thus the response to a second dose of antigen will be quicker and more effective.

Control mechanisms

The mechanism whereby antibodies are produced is frequently more complex than simply antigen encountering a B-cell that expresses the relevant surface-bound antibody. A schematic diagram which covers the main events, is presented in Figure 4.6. When an antigen enters the immune system it is first engulfed by APCs, which then process the antigen so that it is degraded into peptides. These in turn are presented on the surface of the APC in association with MHC molecules (Unanue, 1984). Antigens can be engulfed by phagocytosis and the process need not involve specific recognition of the antigen. When presented in this manner, T-helper cells, via

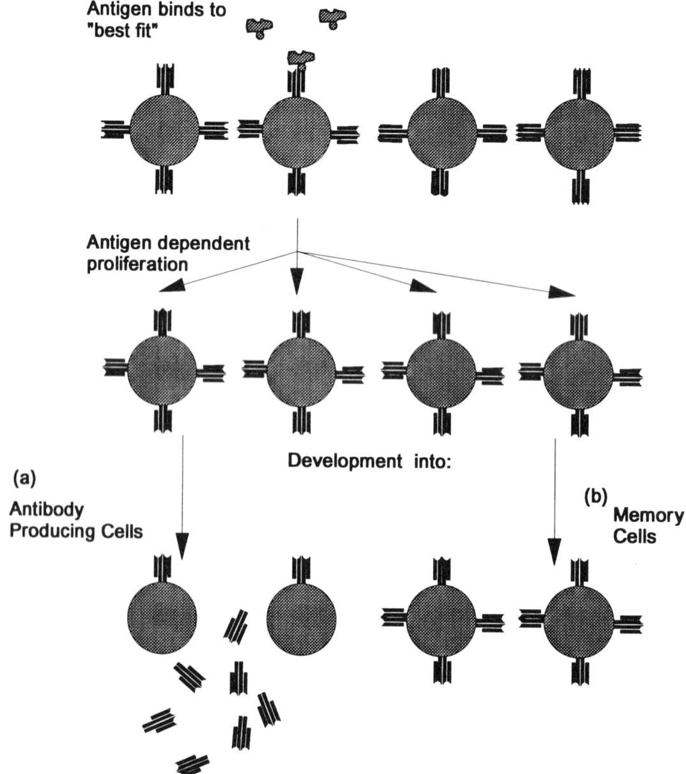

Figure 4.5 Clonal selection.

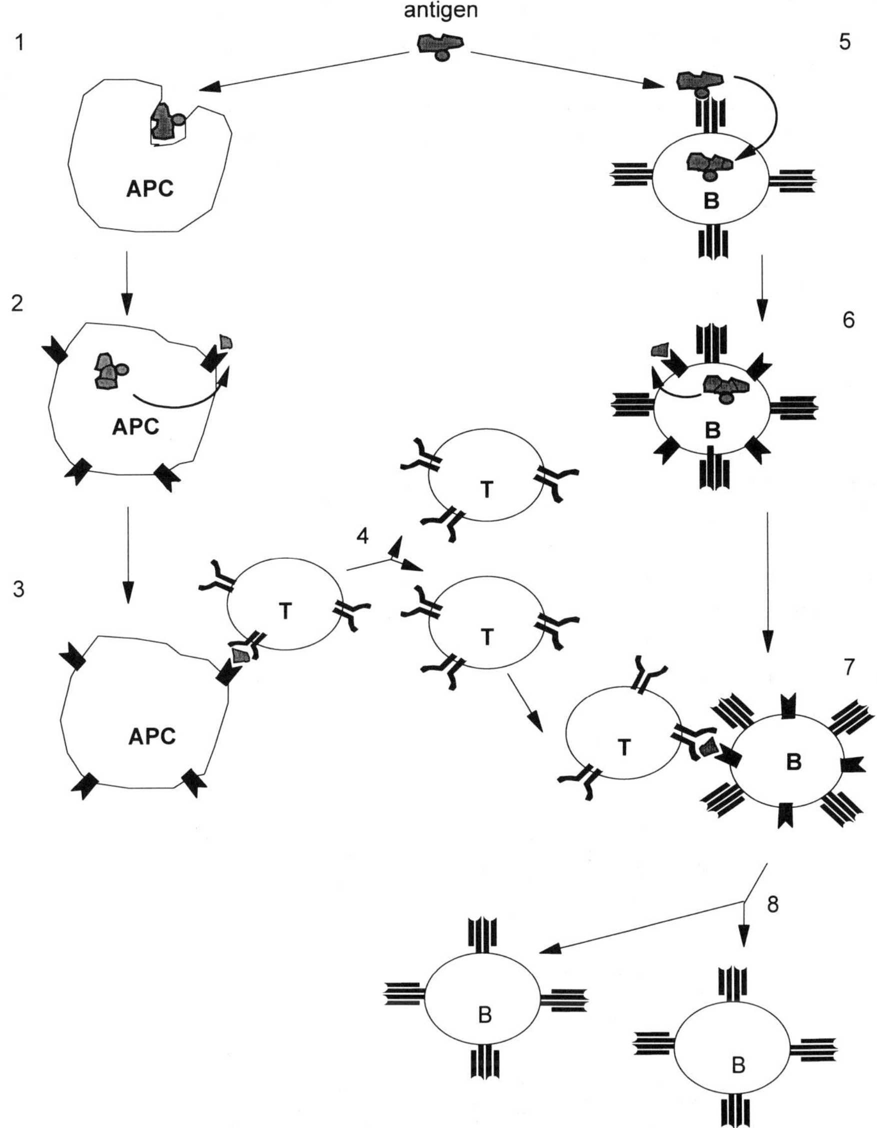

Figure 4.6 The interaction of APCs, T-cells and B-cells. (1) APC phagocytoses antigen. (2) Antigen processed, and peptide from the antigen displayed on APC surface in association with MHC protein. (3) Combination of peptide and MHC protein bound by receptor on T-cell surface. (4) T-cells proliferate in response to recognising peptide/MHC complex. (5) Antibody molecule on surface of B-cell specifically binds native antigen. Antigen taken up by B-cell. (6) Antigen 'processed' and peptide from the antigen displayed on B-cell surface in association with MHC protein. (7) Combination of peptide and MHC protein bound by receptor on T-cell surface. (8) B-cells proliferate and differentiate (see Figure 4.5).

specific receptors on their surface, can recognise the combination of MHC and peptide (although either peptide or MHC alone will not be recognised). This leads to proliferation and secretion of B-cell activating cytokines by this particular T-helper cell population.

Concurrently with APC antigen uptake, specific B-cells also take up and process the antigen, then present the same part-antigen in combination with the same protein on their surface (Kakiuchi *et al.*, 1983). Unlike uptake by the APCs, B-cell uptake relies on specific recognition between the antigen and membrane bound antibody molecules. The specific sub-population of T-cells, which was expanded through interaction with the APCs, now interacts with the specific B-cells which have taken up, processed and presented the same antigen. This interaction leads to the proliferation and differentiation of the specific B-cell population, as described in the section above.

The determinants (or parts of the molecule) recognised by the receptors on T-cells and the surface bound antibody on B-cells are separate and distinct. The need for two separate epitopes may, in part, explain why small molecules on their own do not elicit an antibody response.

The requirement for two separate determinants, one recognised by B-cells and one recognised by T-cells, has further relevance for the immunoassayist. For example, if a group of animals, which have been previously immunised with a hapten linked to one carrier (for instance BSA), are divided into two subgroups, then one subgroup is re-immunised with the same preparation and the other subgroup with the same hapten linked to a second carrier (for instance ovalbumin), the first subgroup mount a strong secondary response to the hapten whereas the second subgroup do not. This, so-called carrier effect (Mitchison, 1971) demonstrates the role of determinants recognised by T-cells, and stresses the importance of not switching carriers during an immunisation schedule. We would go further and recommend the preparation, distribution in aliquots and storage of sufficient hapten–carrier conjugate to complete an immunisation schedule.

Class switching

The initial antibody response is predominantly IgM. However, during the development of the immune response and B-cell differentiation the genes undergo a further rearrangement. This time the genes encoding for the constant part of the antibody are affected. The μ-gene which encodes the constant part of the IgM heavy chain, is replaced by a γ-gene and the protein predominantly produced becomes IgG (Rabbitts *et al.*, 1980). This switch is driven mainly in response to the production of T-cell derived differentiation factors.

Somatic mutation and affinity maturation

It is well known to experienced immunoassayists that the affinity of the antisera they obtain improves with the length of immunisation. A practical example of this is given in Figure 4.7, where it is shown that the ED_{50}, or mid-point of the standard curve, for an enzyme-based inhibition assay, becomes less as the immunisation proceeds, i.e. affinity improves with time. Consequently, the sensitivity obtainable using the sera of a particular animal improves as the immunisation of that animal proceeds. The mechanism by which this occurs is thought to be through somatic mutation of the DNA encoding for the variable region of the antibody. Studies have shown that the genes which encode for antibodies produced later in the immune

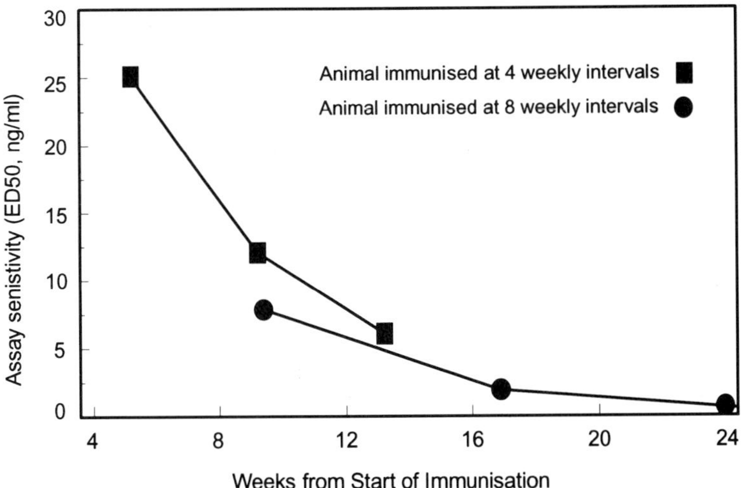

Figure 4.7 Improvements in assay sensitivity (decreasing ED_{50}) with increased length of immunisation period.

response have single nucleotide substitutions in the variable portion of the gene compared with their germ-line counterparts. These point mutations lead to changes in the amino acid sequence of the variable region and so can result in antibodies of higher affinity (Kim *et al.*, 1981). The mutation rate for V_H genes is estimated at 2 to 4 per cent as opposed to less than 0.0001 per cent for non-immunological lymphocyte genes. This mutation of the variable regions is in some way bound with class-switching, as mutations are more frequent in IgG molecules than IgM molecules (Gearhart *et al.*, 1981). This may explain why higher affinity antibodies are found in the IgG class rather than the IgM class. It is thought that the mutations occur during the generation of memory cells, and thus do not add to the repertoire of antibodies available in the primary response.

Once further diversity in the memory cells has been generated through somatic mutation, clonal selection operates to select the highest affinity variants on subsequent administration of a further dose of antigen. If large doses of booster immunisations are administered, B-cells carrying relatively low affinity antibodies will be stimulated in addition to the low number of B-cells carrying mutated, higher affinity antibodies. The overall effect may be to produce a relatively low affinity response. Thus, more does not mean better, and low doses of antigen may produce higher affinity sera (Siskind and Benacerraf, 1969; Werblin and Siskind, 1972 and references therein). The need to pass through the formation, then subsequent selection by antigen stimulation, of memory cells may explain why it takes time to generate high affinity sera.

T-cell independent responses

Whereas the majority of protein antigens require T-cell involvement, some antigens elicit an antibody response without the involvement of T-cells. Many of these so-called T-independent antigens are large polymeric molecules with multiple identical antigenic determinants. It is thought they may short circuit the normal T-cell involvement by cross linking the membrane bound antibodies on the surface of B-cells. T-dependency for a particular antigen may vary with species (Galanaud, 1979). T-independent antigens may present problems for the immunoassayist because the response they elicit does not develop in the same way as the response to T-dependent antigens. It remains predominantly IgM, and the affinity for the antigen does not mature above the initial levels. Whilst such problems are infrequently encountered, choice of a repetitive carrier (e.g. polylysine) and/or oversubstitution of the hapten may inadvertently generate a novel T-independent antigen. Feldmann *et al.* (1974) have shown that T-dependent hapten–carrier conjugates can be made T-independent by coupling them to inert beads.

Tolerance

Tolerance for a particular antigen means that the animal in question fails to produce an immune response to it. From Figure 4.6 it should be apparent that tolerance can be achieved by interference with either T-cell recognition of the processed antigen in association with MHC proteins or with B-cell recognition of the native antigen. Natural immunological tolerance ensures that the animal does not produce antibodies to its own body components. If this mechanism fails autoimmune disease develops. Natural tolerance is thought to be learned and not acquired at birth. Billingham *et al.* (1953) have shown that an injection of antigen into a neonate can make that animal tolerant of that antigen. When raising antisera therefore, should the antigen of interest bear a close relationship to molecules in the animal's make up, it may be seen by the animal's immune system as 'self'. If this is suspected a different species should be used.

As well as ability to recognise self, the genetic background of an animal can influence its ability to respond to foreign antigens. It has been known for some time that strains of a particular species vary in their ability to respond to particular antigens. Furthermore in breeding experiments over 20 generations Biozzi *et al.* (1979) were able to derive two groups of mice from a wild-type population; one of which consistently produced a high antibody response to particular antigens, and the other group which produced a low response. Whilst it is impractical to adopt such a breeding programme for every antigen for which antibodies are needed, it is reasonable to use several wild-type animals rather than inbred strains, in order to improve one's chance of success.

Acquired immunological tolerance arises through some manipulation which renders the animal incapable of recognising a particular antigen. In the field of transplant surgery, suppression of a patient's response to donor tissue is a major and continuing goal. For the immunoassayist, suppression of a response to the antigen of interest is a pitfall to be avoided. Experiments in which animals were administered various concentrations of BSA, prior to challenge with BSA in Freund's Complete Adjuvant, demonstrated that both repeated low doses (1 μg) and repeated high doses (10 mg) could induce tolerance (Mitchison, 1968). The tolerance induced by high doses has been shown to be the result of effects on the B-lymphocytes, whereas the tolerance induced by low doses was caused by effects on the T-lymphocytes (Weigle, 1971).

It must be said that we have not experienced any instance where we have inadvertently made animals tolerant to an antigen of interest. We have, however, experienced difficulties when trying to elicit an immune response to some mouse proteins by immunising the closely related rat. This we attributed to the close relationship between the mouse and rat proteins, and the natural tolerance of the rat for self. Tolerance is usually manifested at the T-helper cell level, and so the problem can often be overcome by conjugation to a totally unrelated carrier protein (Green *et al.*, 1966).

Polyclonal immune serum or monoclonal antibody?

A polyclonal serum will contain a variety of antibodies. Even in a highly immune animal only about 10 per cent of the circulating IgG will be directed against the immunogen of interest. Within this 10 per cent some antibody species will be against the carrier and some against the hapten; even within the fraction of antibodies capable of binding the hapten, a range of antibodies of different affinities and specificities will be found (Klinman and Press, 1975; Kohler, 1976). This mixture will vary from animal to animal, and even from the same animal at different times (Murphy, 1980). Thus, it is difficult, if not impossible, to reproduce polyclonal preparations precisely.

Kohler and Milstein (1975) developed a method of immortalising single-antibody producing cells by fusion to a tumour line. The resulting hybridoma produces just one species of antibody (a monoclonal antibody) which can be grown indefinitely. Thus this technology offers a means to achieve a consistent product in unlimited quantities. However, the work needed to produce a stable hybridoma, secreting suitable high affinity antibodies can be considerable and specialist facilities and techniques are required which are not available to everyone. There is a feeling among some immunoassayists that monoclonal preparations do not exhibit as high an affinity as polyclonal preparations. This may reflect the random nature by which cell fusion occurs and the relatively low number of B-cells secreting high affinity antibodies. There are also reports, possibly apocryphal, that to obtain the necessary specificity some workers had to mix several monoclonal antibodies.

The main advantage of monoclonal antibodies is in two-site assays for large molecules, where one monoclonal antibody is used to capture the molecule of interest and a second against a separate and non-overlapping epitope is used to detect it. In these assays which are only applicable to large molecules, reagents need to be used in excess and this is facilitated by the unlimited supply of monoclonal antibodies.

For small molecule immunoassays we usually rely on the generation of suitable polyclonal sera, and the remainder of this chapter will be devoted to methods for their successful production.

Practical considerations

It is impossible and dangerous to be too prescriptive about what one must do to generate good antibodies against a given antigen. However, some guidance, especially for the novice is required. Much of what is reported in the literature on antibody raising is based around a successful outcome, there are few if any reports of failed attempts at raising antibodies. Since it is not difficult to generate an antibody response, providing some basic rules are followed, the literature abounds with what is often presented as 'the method' for raising antibodies. Whilst it is difficult not to fall into this trap, the following guidelines are based on a distillation of what is seen as best in the collective experience of all the authors, backed up by literature reports. The methods presented have been used successfully in our laboratories and are by and large in accord with the preceding discussion on the theory of immunology. The fact that some of the recommendations may appear contradictory merely serves to show the diversity of (successful) approaches that can be taken, and the lack of firm science in this important area. Where possible however, some justification will be given for the recommended approaches in relation to the preceding theory and the practice of others.

Choice of species

Apart from the general recommendation that the species to be immunised is phylogenically distinct from that providing the immunogen carrier, this choice is usually constrained by pragmatic considerations, such as what is available and how much antisera is required. Some groups favour sheep, rabbits or goats; if monoclonal antibodies are needed one is practically constrained to rodents, particularly mice. It is important to remember that all animal experimentation work, including immunisation, is controlled by law. In the UK the Home Office can place restrictions on the procedures used and the volumes of blood (and thus volumes of sera) that can be taken, these are discussed in detail below for the two most commonly used species, rabbits and sheep.

Rabbits

For practical reasons, rabbits may represent a good choice for the routine production of polyclonal antisera. They are easy to keep and handle, they can be safely and repeatedly bled, and the antibodies they produce are well characterised and easily purified. With careful management, at least 300 ml of serum can be obtained from one rabbit through the course of an immunisation regime (see below).

Rabbits reach immune maturity at 12 weeks and a large breed should be used to maximise the volume of blood that can be taken. A recommended strain is the F_1-hybrid half-lop from Ranch Rabbits Ltd, Crawley Down, Sussex. Because of the relative cost and convenience of using rabbits, relatively large numbers of animals and several haptens or immunogens for the given analyte can easily be investigated to increase the probability of producing a good antiserum.

Sheep

It is often claimed that sheep in comparison to rabbits produce superior antisera to haptens in terms of titre and affinity. In addition, much larger volumes of blood can be taken on any one occasion. This can be a major advantage in terms of long-term assay viability, especially when the antiserum titre is low.

The initial cost of a sheep is certainly higher than that for a rabbit, around £60 per animal. Providing some fairly basic facilities are available however, such as a field, shelter against inclement weather and penning to hold the animals when they are being immunised and bled, the running costs can be as low as 25 pence per week. This is in contrast to the elaborate air-conditioned facilities (with the consequence of high overheads) that most companies would provide for rabbits. If at least two experienced animal handling staff are available, the immunisation and bleeding of sheep is no more difficult than that for rabbits.

Although several different breeds of sheep have been used for the production of reagent antibodies, different workers tend to have their own favourites. Soay sheep are recommended by a number of workers, although their claimed advantages have not been clearly established. The important factor however is to use an outbred strain to maximise the genetic pool.

Blood volumes

As mentioned above, experimentation on animals including taking of blood samples is a licensed activity, at least in the UK. The scientist in charge should ensure that animals are humanely treated and that any suffering is kept to a minimum. This includes the physiological distress and discomfort brought on by blood loss through the withdrawal of blood.

Some laboratories may have their own local rules controlling the withdrawal of blood, but as a rule of thumb, 15 per cent of the animal's blood volume can be removed on a single occasion per month without causing undue distress. Larger volumes can be taken if fluid replacement is given. The data in Table 4.3 gives general guidelines on blood withdrawal volumes for the common species.

Number of animals

Even in genetically identical animals, a single preparation of antigen will elicit different antibodies. When an outbred animal strain is used, these differences are heightened. If the amount of antigen is not limiting, as many animals as practicable should be used for immunisation, irrespective of the species. This view is borne out by experience in the authors' laboratories. In one immunisation programme, of 24 animals immunised with four different conjugates only two gave antisera with the requisite specificity. With other compounds wide variations in titre and assay sensitivity have also been observed using the same immunogen. For example, Table 4.2 shows the variety of responses obtained from six rabbits immunised in the same manner. From these six, the titre varied considerably and only one serum generated an assay with the desired sensitivity (ED_{50}) of less than 1 ng/ml.

To maximise the chances of obtaining the optimum antiserum, it is strongly recommended that at least four animals should be used with each immunogen, and if only one immunogen is used this minimum should be increased to at least six

Table 4.3 General guidelines for blood withdrawal volumes in animal species commonly used for antibody raising

Species	Weight (kg)	Blood volume (ml/kg)	Recommended volumes (ml)		
			15%* volume	10%** volume	7.5%*** volume
Sheep	40.0	60	360	240	180
Rabbit	4.0	56–70	30–40	22–28	17–21
Guinea pig	0.25	75	4	2.6	2
Mouse	0.015	78	0.15	0.1	0.09

* A single sample with 30 days recovery.
** Limited to once every two weeks.
*** Limited to once every week.

animals. The approach adopted by some workers of using one animal per immunogen (e.g. Peskar *et al.*, 1972; Hoebeke *et al.*, 1978) is to be strongly discouraged.

Form of the antigen

Although soluble immunogens are easier to characterise and more convenient to use, it is generally recognised that particulate or insoluble immunogens can be more effective in stimulating an antibody response. One of the reasons for this is the rapid phagocytosis of particulate antigens compared with soluble material. Some soluble immunogens can be made more immunogenic by coupling them chemically to beads or cells (commonly erythrocytes) but these procedures are not widely used in the generation of reagent antibodies to low-molecular-weight analytes. From a practical point of view, immunogens that precipitate on storage or that are poorly soluble should not be discarded since these may well give an enhanced immune response.

Adjuvants

Adjuvants can be considered as immunopotentiators which act to enhance the humoral response to weakly immunogenic molecules, such as many of the hapten–protein conjugates used to generate reagent antibodies. It is difficult to postulate a single and simple mode of action since a wide variety of materials possess adjuvant properties. A wide range of adjuvants have been used, although discussion here will be limited to those commonly employed in immunoassay work and a number of recommendations will be made.

By forming depots, the repository adjuvants provide a long-lived reservoir of antigen, avoiding the need for repeated and frequent injections. The most commonly used agents to achieve this effect are the aluminium compounds (phosphate and hydroxide) and water-in-oil emulsions (e.g. Freund's). Other materials are also added to help improve the immune response. For example, *Bordetella pertussis* has been used in conjunction with alum to stimulate B-cell production. Mycobacteria, which are a component of Freund's Complete Adjuvant (FCA), expand T-cell populations. Freund's Complete Adjuvant also leads to the local formation of granulomata, which are rich in macrophages (APCs).

In an effort to minimise granulomas and consequent skin ulcers some workers dilute FCA one-to-one with Freund's Incomplete Adjuvant (FIA). Alternatively a modified non-ulcerative form of Freund's adjuvant can be used. This adjuvant is commercially available from Guildhay Antisera, University of Surrey, England, but only in the incomplete form. BCG vaccine (intradermal, Evans Medical) should be added to produce the complete form.

Various newer adjuvant preparations have been introduced using only components of the mycobacteria or synthetic peptides, e.g. muramyl dipeptide. Whilst relatively expensive compared with the Freund's or Alum, it is important that these are evaluated and compared with the more traditional methods. However, experience from one of our laboratories and of other workers (Pratt, 1978) indicates that when faced with a new antigen, the use of Freund's Complete Adjuvant for the first administration, and Freund's Incomplete Adjuvant for subsequent boosters, produces the most consistent response. The use of Freund's adjuvants is strongly recommended therefore. It must be stressed however that the complete version of

Freund's adjuvant should only be used once per animal, as second injections can often result in excessive ulceration.

Dose of immunogen

In immunising an animal much of the injected material will be catabolised and cleared before reaching an appropriate target cell. The efficiency of this process will vary with host factors, the route of injection, the use of adjuvants, and the intrinsic nature of the antigen itself. Thus, the effective dose delivered to the immune system may bear little relationship to the injected dose, and so descriptions of dose requirements are inevitably empirical.

There is a generally held view (Pratt, 1978; Tijssen, 1985) that immunisations have been overdone with too much, too often. This is supported by a number of literature reports which indicate that much smaller doses of immunogen (less than 1 mg) than is typically employed leads to higher antibody affinities (Siskind and Benacerraf, 1969; Werblin and Siskind, 1972 and references therein) ultimately giving more sensitive assays. This view is also reflected in work from our own laboratories.

Traditionally for rabbits, where a pure and soluble immunogen is being used, then a dose of 0.5 to 1 mg has been employed for primary immunisation with about half this amount for booster immunisations. In view of the above reported findings the primary immunisation can be safely reduced to 0.1 to 0.5 mg with a concomitant reduction for the boosters.

In the sheep primary doses of about 0.5 to 5 mg have generally been employed with about half this amount for booster immunizations. In one of our laboratories we have carried out many successful immunisation programmes in sheep using as little as 0.1 to 0.25 mg of immunogen for primary immunisations and 0.050 to 0.1 mg for booster immunisations.

The use of lower doses as well as giving higher antibody affinities also means that less immunogen needs to be prepared, an important factor when the hapten is in short supply.

Preparation of emulsions

For dosing, the aqueous solution or suspension of the immunogen (usually in buffer or saline) is mixed with the oil based adjuvant (either FCA or FIA) to give a water-in-oil emulsion. Insoluble immunogens should first be finely divided into a stable suspension by use of a small hand-held glass homogeniser or a pestle and mortar.

The emulsion should be prepared a short time before use by mixing the aqueous immunogen and adjuvant (each cooled to 4°C). The ratio of immunogen to adjuvant can vary from 1 : 1 to 1 : 3. The latter is claimed to be more effective (Hurn and Chantler, 1980) and it has the advantage that it is less viscous making the preparation and immunisation easier. If complete non-ulcerative Freund's is required 50 μl of BCG vaccine should be added to the aqueous immunogen for every 2 ml of oil to be used.

Vigorous and prolonged mixing is necessary to form the emulsion, which ideally should have the consistency of clotted cream. This can be prepared in one of three ways depending on the amount of emulsion required:

1 Constant vigorous agitation in a small conical centrifuge tube using a rotary mixer (small volumes only).
2 For larger volumes an electrically powered emulsifier or tissue homogeniser is appropriate. The adjuvant should be added to the homogeniser first. After running the homogeniser for a short period to coat the tube and blades with the adjuvant, the aqueous solution should be added slowly.
3 For intermediate volumes (2 to 15 ml) a modification of the procedure of Hurn and Chantler (1980) is recommended and this is described in PROCEDURE 1. This method has the advantages that the process is totally enclosed, loss of immunogen is minimal (a problem with method 2) and the procedure is simple and efficient.

PROCEDURE 1 Preparation of emulsions for immunisation

Materials

- Two glass syringes, with luer lock fittings each capable of holding the total emulsion volume
- Two 1.5″ 17 gauge blunt needles
- A short length (approx. 5 cm) of PVC autoanalyser tubing (1.14 mm I.D.), e.g. type 116-0549-10 from Gradko International Ltd, Winchester, Hants, UK
- Disposable plastic syringes for immunisation (1 ml)

Reagents

- Immunogen dissolved in saline, buffer, or sterile water
- Adjuvant (FCA or FIA)

Equipment

- A face visor and thick leather gloves

Method

Attach a blunt needle to each glass syringe and load one with the immunogen solution and one with the adjuvant, taking care to remove as much air as possible from both syringes. Carefully connect the two syringes via the needles and the length of tubing which should fit tightly over the needles. Because the rest of the procedure involves the handling of liquids under pressure in glass syringes the use of a visor and thick leather gloves is recommended. Grasp a syringe in each hand with thumb over the plunger and rapidly force the aqueous phase into the oil. Continue the mixing process by passing the mixture between the two syringes around 15 to 20 times by applying pressure to each plunger in turn. After a few transfer operations the action of the syringe plungers will become stiff and it is important to use as much force as possible. When an emulsion of the correct consistency has been obtained it can be tested by carefully adding a drop to the surface of a saline solution or water. A stable water-in-oil emulsion should remain as a distinct blob and not disperse over the surface.

Once the emulsion has been formed transfer it all to one syringe and remove the other syringe from its needle. Plastic immunisation syringes can then be connected in turn to the glass syringe containing the immunogen and easily loaded by depressing the plunger of the glass syringe.

If a 1 : 1 ratio is required then the aqueous phase should be added in three separate aliquots, with thorough mixing after each addition, starting initially with a 1 : 3 aqueous to oil mixture.

Routes of injection

There are five possible routes that can be used for immunisation. These are, in general order of increasing efficacy:

- intravenous (iv)
- intraperitoneal (ip)
- subcutaneous (sc)
- intramuscular (im)
- intradermal (id)

The intravenous route is not recommended and cannot be used for particulate antigens or adjuvants. Intraperitoneal injections are not a practical proposition for rabbits and sheep. If large volumes of emulsion are to be given the subcutaneous route is useful, but the intramuscular route is considered to be the most effective for rabbits and sheep, presumably because the inoculum is released slowly from the sites of injection.

The use of multiple intradermal injections in rabbits (Vaitukaitis, 1981) is claimed to be highly effective, with the response to the primary injection being greater than that by other routes such that only one booster is required. A comparison with inoculation by the intramuscular route (Lader *et al.*, 1974) showed the two procedures to be of similar efficacy although the intradermal method gave a more rapid production of sera.

Immunisation by id, im or sc injection in several sites is better than a single large injection at one site.

Immunisation schedules

There are three stages to an immunisation procedure: the primary injection, the booster injections and withdrawal of blood. Although the last two of these may be repeated many times over in an immunisation schedule, careful control, particularly of the relative timing is essential to ensure the best antiserum is produced.

Frequency of injecting

Following the initial or primary injection, some delay is necessary prior to boosting. Since animals will remain primed for up to 1 year after a primary immunisation this delay can range up to this time. In many cases effective priming can take place in the absence of a detectable antibody response which may have implications for the monitoring of antibody production (see below). Immunisation schedules involving frequent immunisations (less than 4 week intervals) should be avoided as they could ruin a potentially good antiserum through induction of tolerance. Some workers consider it advantageous to leave the animal for an interval of several months before boosting, particularly if a route with slow-release characteristics (id or im) has been used for the primary immunisation. These workers would argue that the animal should not be boosted while it is still responding to the initial exposure of immunogen. To obtain the maximum secondary response, boosting should not be carried out until the antiserum titre has decreased to a low level, or at least plateaued (Herbert, 1968). Under such circumstances a response similar to that observed in the production of an antiserum for ranitidine (Figure 4.8) would be expected.

As many immunoassay development projects are run to tight deadlines, especially in the pharmaceuticals industry, it may be impractical to wait months for the production of the 'ultimate' antiserum, so more frequent boosters are generally used. In rabbits and sheep the first booster injection is commonly given 6 to 8 weeks after the primary, with subsequent boosters at 4 to 6 week intervals.

Blood withdrawal

Prior to starting the immunisation it is useful to take a small blood sample (around 5 ml) from each animal to act as a control for the subsequent antiserum evaluation. Once the immunisation programme has begun small test bleeds should also be taken before each booster injection and at a defined period after each booster injection. Antibody is usually detected in the serum within a month of the primary immunisation although the primary response is often very weak, particularly for readily catabolised, soluble antigens.

For maximum antibody yield the time between boosting and sampling should be 7 to 14 days. Ten days after a boost is generally considered optimal for the collection of sera and this is confirmed by the data for an antibacterial metabolite shown in Figure 4.9 (Ballard *et al.*, 1996). In this instance, antisera titres were relatively poor, even after several boosters and there was concern that the time of sampling, in relation to the time of boosting was inappropriate. To confirm that blood samples

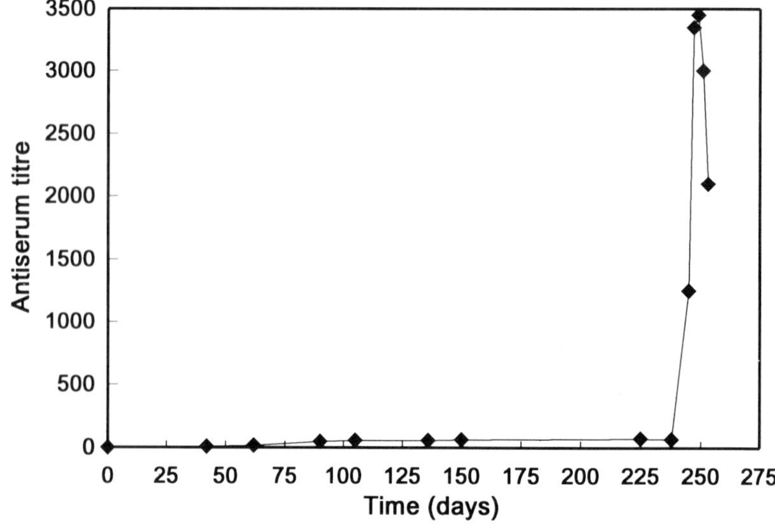

Figure 4.8 Variation in sheep antiserum titre following a simple immunisation programme with a ranitidine immunogen. The animal received a primary immunisation on day 0 and a single boost on day 237.

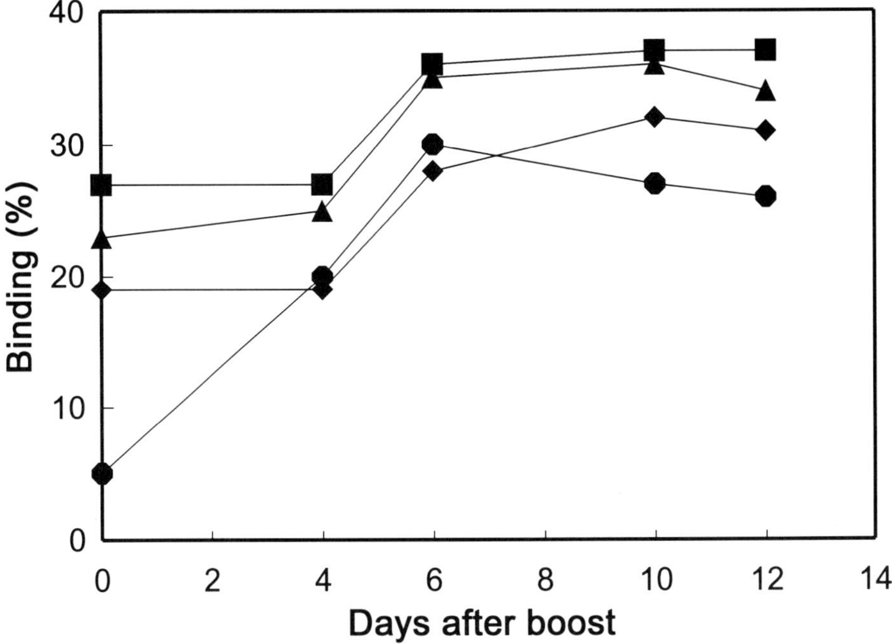

Figure 4.9 The variation in antiserum titre with time for four different sheep, showing the optimum blood withdrawal point at around 10 days after boosting.

were being taken at the appropriate time, frequent sampling of the animals was undertaken after the third booster. The data in Figure 4.9 clearly shows that 10 days after boosting was the optimal time to take blood samples with maximal (although in this instance relatively low) titres. If antibody response appears to be poor then more frequent sampling as described above will help define the point at which large bleeds should be taken.

It is important to note that the nature and quality of the antibodies present in the serum changes with time particularly after further boosting. These changes are the result of maturation of the immune response and have considerable practical importance. It is well known that antibody affinity increases throughout the course of an immunisation programme (Siskind and Benacerraf, 1969; Werblin and Siskind, 1972 and references therein). Thus sera taken following the 3rd or 4th boost would be expected to give a more sensitive assay than that taken after the 1st or 2nd boost. This point is clearly shown in Figure 4.7.

Specificity is also claimed to change, decreasing throughout the course of the immunisation programme (Tijssen, 1985). If this is so then the optimum time for sampling is very much a compromise. However this view is possibly derived from one literature report (Hooker and Boyd, 1941) which over the years has become accepted fact. Where specificity has been observed to change then this may have been the result of the development of antibodies to impurities in the immunogen. This would be especially true with protein and peptide immunogens on which much of the early immunoassay work was carried out.

The monitoring of the sera for specific antibody production is carried out as discussed in Chapters 6 and 7 on immunoassay development. A poor response or no response at all after the second booster would probably lead us to prepare fresh immunising conjugates, probably with different carrier proteins or it may even lead us to re-initiate the synthesis of the hapten.

In practice test bleeds would be taken via syringe using a 20 G needle, from the ear vein of rabbits (1 to 2 ml) and from the jugular vein of sheep (5 to 10 ml) by experienced animal technicians. Once acceptable antisera have been produced large blood samples can be taken (see below) or the animals can be sacrified and exsanguinated.

Harvesting of antiserum

When the antiserum shows the required characteristics in terms of sensitivity, specificity and titre it should be harvested to give adequate supplies for the intended use. Table 4.3 gives the recommended volumes that can be taken from animals over a defined time period without causing undue distress.

For rabbits, up to 20 to 40 ml should be taken at peak titre following each booster or the animal should be sacrificed and exsanguinated, which would produce around 200 ml. In the case of sheep around 300 ml can be taken on any one occasion. The most convenient method of taking large volumes of blood from a sheep is to pierce the jugular vein with a large gauge needle (14 G × 25 mm) and allow the blood to flow into a suitable container.

Recommended immunisation procedures

Practical details of a number of recommended immunisation procedures in each species are given below:

PROCEDURE 2 The multiple intradermal method of immunisation in rabbits

Materials

- Fine-cut veterinary clippers
- Immunogen in a 2 : 1 or 3 : 1 adjuvant : aqueous emulsion, the concentration of immunogen should be 1 mg/2.5 ml for the primary and 0.5 mg/2.5 ml for the boosts. The adjuvant should be complete for the primary inoculation and incomplete for boosts, with non-ulcerative preferred over Freund's
- Disposable plastic syringes (1 or 2 ml volume) fitted with 1″ 25 G needles for intradermal injections and 1.5″ 25 G needles for intramuscular and subcutaneous injections

Methods

The rabbit should be shaved with the veterinary clippers as close to the skin as possible. A large area of the back and flanks should be exposed. The animal should be restrained as appropriate and injected intradermally into about 50 sites with a freshly prepared emulsion, approximately 50 μl should be injected at each site. As wide an area as possible on the back and flanks should be used with at least 2 cm between injection sites.

The needles should be secured tightly to the syringe and slightly bent towards the bevel. The animal's skin should be stretched between thumb and forefinger and the needle inserted almost horizontally into the skin layers for at least 0.5 cm. The inoculum should form a tight and distinct blister under the skin. The needle should be withdrawn whilst holding the needle track with the thumb and forefinger. The disposable plastic syringes used for injection may need to be discarded after a few injections because the Freund's adjuvant can attack the rubber seals of the syringe making dispensing difficult.

If complete Freund's adjuvant is used small sores will appear at the sites of injection but these will clear within a few weeks. Since the only reaction will be a few raised lumps if the non-ulcerative Freund's is used this latter adjuvant is recommended.

Booster immunisation should be given by a combination of the intramuscular and subcutaneous routes. A second worker may be required to immobilise the rabbit for im injections but wrapping the animal in a towel is often sufficient.

Two injections (25 G long needle) of 200 μl each should be given into the thigh muscle on each back leg near the hip. Gently withdraw the plunger when in position to ensure that the needle has not found one of the small veins or arteries of the leg. The inoculum should be added slowly with a steady motion. Withdraw the needle whilst gently massaging the site of injection.

A further 1.2 ml of the emulsion should be injected subcutaneously over six sites between the shoulder blades. For each injection the skin should be pinched between the thumb and forefinger and pulled away from the body, and the needle (25 G long) inserted into the space that has been created. After withdrawing the needle, the hole should be gently rubbed between the forefinger and thumb to stop any of the inoculum from escaping.

An immunisation procedure for sheep is given in PROCEDURE 3 below. This approach is designed to give high titre and high affinity antisera through careful monitoring of the antibody response and immunising at the optimum time. The disadvantage of this approach is that antibody production can take many months.

PROCEDURE 3 Immunisation of sheep

Materials

- Plastic disposable syringes (5 ml) fitted with a 20 G × 25 mm needle
- There should be 1 syringe per animal, loaded with the immunogen emulsified in Freund's (FCA for primary immunisations and FIA for booster immunisations)
- The immunogen concentration should be 0.2 to 1.0 mg/ml of emulsion for primary injections and 0.1 to 0.5 mg/ml for booster injections in a total volume of 4 ml
- A minimum of six sheep per immunogen

Methods

A total of seven to eight injections of the inoculum are made per animal. Each animal receives 0.5 ml in two sites in each inner thigh (inguinal region) and a further 0.5 ml into the muscle of each front leg. The remaining 1 ml should be injected in one or two sites subcutaneously, between the shoulder blades.

A small test bleed should be taken from each animal at approximately monthly intervals over the next 6 to 8 months and the antibody response monitored (see Chapters 6 and 7). If there is no response after 2 to 3 months the animals are reprimed using 5 mg of immunogen in FCA. Once the antibody titre is seen to plateau or begin to fall, a booster should be given and the animal bled 10 to 14 days after this. If the antibody response in terms of titre or affinity is inadequate for the intended use then levels of circulating antibody should be allowed to fall back to a low and/or steady level before further boosts are given.

A typical immunisation procedure for sheep designed to give rapid production of high quality antisera is described in PROCEDURE 4 below. This method has been widely used at Zeneca Pharmaceuticals with considerable success. Good antisera are normally obtained by the second booster (typically 18 weeks into the immunisation programme). Because a standard procedure is used, real-time monitoring of antibody response is not essential and so the immunisation programme can be started without the need for a tracer to monitor antibody production.

PROCEDURE 4 Immunisation of sheep, the 'fast track' method

Materials

- Plastic disposable syringes (1 ml) fitted with a 20 G × 25 mm needles
- There should be 1 syringe per animal, loaded with the immunogen emulsified in Freund's (FCA for primary immunisations and FIA for booster immunisations)
- The immunogen concentration should be approximately 0.1 mg/ml of emulsion for primary injections and 0.05 mg/ml for booster injections.
- A minimum of six sheep per immunogen

Method

The sc route is used for all injections. For the primary immunisation inject each sheep with 5 × 0.2 ml of inoculum (0.1 mg/ml) on each of the hind limbs and at three points on the flank. The immunisation and bleeding schedule presented in Figure 4.10 should be followed. After 6 to 8 weeks take a small test bleed (approximately 5 ml) and boost each animal using the same procedure as for the primary immunisation except with the immunogen concentration reduced by a factor of 2. Take a test bleed 7 to 14 days after the injection. Further boosters should be given every 4 to 6 weeks until a suitable serum is obtained.

Serum preparation

Serum should be separated from cells as soon as possible after collection of blood; otherwise the red cells can lyse and release contaminating proteins, including proteolytic enzymes which will degrade the antibodies. After collection, preferably into glass tubes, blood should be allowed to clot for approximately 1 h at room temperature or preferably 37°C. The tubes should then be transferred to 4°C to facilitate clot contraction. After a period of 2 to 16 h in the cold the clot should then be

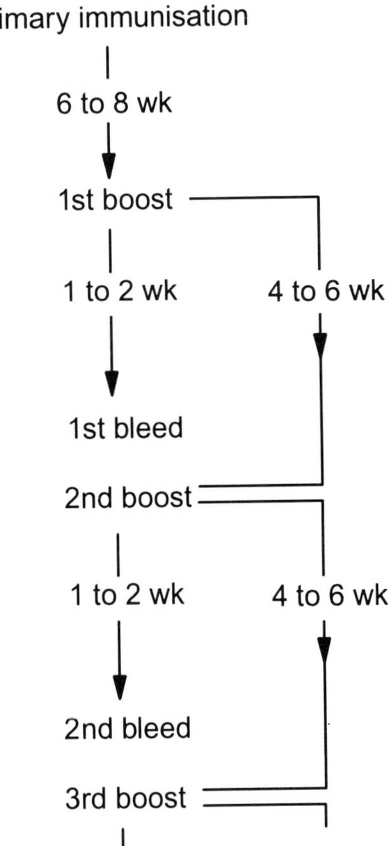

Figure 4.10 A recommended immunisation schedule for sheep.

separated from the sides of the collection vessel using a Pasteur pipette or similar instrument in a process known as 'rimming'. At this stage the serum can be carefully poured into a clean tube. The clot can then be cut up and centrifuged to release further serum which is then combined with the initial collection. Finally the bulked sera may need to be centrifuged to remove any trace of red cells and then transferred to a clean and preferably sterile container. Sodium azide is normally added as a preservative at a concentration between 0.01 to 0.1 per cent.

Storage and stability of antiserum

There has been little systematic study on the storage of antisera (Middleton *et al.*, 1988) although the general view is, that given a number of basic precautions, neat antiserum is quite stable. Antisera can be stored for many years at −20°C, or preferably at −70°C or even at 4°C following addition of a preservative, providing precautions have been taken to avoid contamination with red cell lysates. The last of these storage conditions is much underrated despite its obvious simplicity.

Lyophilisation is also a convenient storage method, albeit the process requires some specialised equipment, especially if the recommendation that the vials are sealed *in vacuo* is followed. Since sera stored in this way are dry it is a particularly useful method where there is a necessity to send sera out to other laboratories and transportation of 'wet' sera is difficult. Where lyophilisation is being carried out on dilutions of the sera the addition of a bulking agent such as bovine gamma globulins is recommended. Sugars such as lactose or trehalose or even glycerol can also be used to prevent denaturation. The hydroxy groups of these materials are believed to replace the water of hydration around proteins which helps maintain the tertiary structure and hence activity.

Stock antisera and antibody solutions should not be repeatedly frozen and thawed as this can lead to aggregation of the immunoglobulins. This can cause loss of activity by steric interference of the antigen combining site or by generating insoluble material that is lost during centrifugation or filtration. To avoid the need for frequent thawing and freezing the antibody should be stored in small aliquots. It is convenient to store antisera in small tubes partly diluted in assay diluent: one tube would then supply just enough material for one day's immunoassay requirements.

Molecular biology

Recent advances in molecular biology have led to the prospect of generating antibodies without the use of animals (Marks *et al.*, 1991; Hoogenboom and Winter, 1992; Lerner *et al.*, 1992). These approaches hold great promise but at the time of writing have not seriously displaced the role of animals in the preparation of immune serum for immunoassay.

Conclusions

Workers in the field of antibody generation sometimes seem polarised between those who believe that it is an extension of scientific endeavour, and those who feel that it is a black art; more influenced by talisman and ritual than logic. For our part, we fully acknowledge luck can play a large part, but believe that, by the rationalisation of successes and failures in the light of the most appropriate immunological theories, the odds can be shortened in our favour. Nevertheless . . . GOOD LUCK.

References

Ballard, P., Stafford, L. E. & Law, B. (1996) *J. Pharm. Biomed. Anal.*, **14**, 409.

Billingham, R. E., Brent, L. & Medawar, P. B. (1953) *Nature*, **172**, 603.

Biozzi, G., Mouton, D., Sant'Anna, O. A., Passos, H. C., Gennari, M., Reis, M. H., Ferreira, V. C., Heumann, A. M., Bouthilier, V., Ibanez, O. M., Stiffel, C. & Siqueira, M. (1979) *Curr. Top. Microbiol. Immunol.*, **85**, 31.

Burnet, F. M. (1959) *The Clonal Selection Theory of Acquired Immunity*. Cambridge University Press, London.

Chan-Shu, S. A. & Blair, O. (1979) *Transfusion*, **19**, 182.

Early, P. & Hood, L. (1981) *Cell*, **24**, 1.

EARLY, P., HUANG, H., DAVIS, M., CALAME, K. & HOOD, L. (1980) *Cell*, **19**, 981.

EDELMAN, G. M., CUNNINGHAM, B. A., GALL, W. E., GOTTLIEB, P. D., RUTISHAUSER, U. & WAXDAL, M. J. (1969) *Proc. Natl. Acad. Sci.*, **63**, 78.

FELDMANN, M., GREAVES, M. F., PARKER, D. C. & RITTENBERG, M. B. (1974) *Eur. J. Immunol.*, **4**, 591.

GALANAUD, P. (1979) *Immunol. Rev.*, **45**, 141.

GEARHART, P. J., JOHNSON, N. D., DOUGLAS, R. & HOOD, L. (1981) *Nature*, **291**, 29.

GREEN, I., PAUL, W. E. & BENACERRAF, B. (1966) *J. Exp. Med.*, **123**, 859.

HERBERT, W. J. (1968) *Immunology*, **14**, 301.

HOEBEKE, J., VAUQUELIN G. & STROSBERG, A. D. (1978) *Biochem. Pharmacol.*, **27**, 1527.

HOOGENBOOM, H. R. & WINTER, G. (1992) *J. Mol. Biol.*, **227**, 381.

HOOKER, S. B. & BOYD, W. C. (1941) *Proc. Soc. Exptl. Biol. Med.*, **47**, 187.

HURN, B. A. L. & CHANTLER, S. M. (1980) *Methods in Enzymology*, **70**, 104.

KAKIUCHI, T., CHESTNUT, R. W. & GREY, H. M. (1983) *J. Immunol.*, **131**, 109.

KEHOE, J. M. & CAPRA, J. D. (1971) *Proc. Natl. Acad. Sci.*, **68**, 2019.

KIM, S., DAVIS, M., SINN, E., PATTEN, P. & HOOD, L. (1981) *Cell*, **27**, 573.

KLINMAN, N. R. & PRESS, J. L. (1975) *J. Exp. Med.*, **141**, 1133.

KOHLER, G. (1976) *Eur. J. Immunol.*, **6**, 340.

KOHLER, G. & MILSTEIN, C. (1975) *Nature*, **256**, 495.

LADER, S., HURN, B. A. L. & COURT, G. (1974) *Radioimmunoassay and Related Procedures in Medicine.* International Atomic Energy Agency, Vienna, pp. 31.

LERNER, R. A., KANG, A. S., BAIN, J. D., BURTON, D. R. & BARBAS, C. F. (1992) *Science*, **258**, 1313.

MARKS, J. D., HOOGENBOOM, H. R., BONNERT, T. P., MCCAFFERTY, J., GRIFFITHS, A. D. & WINTER, G. (1991) *J. Mol. Biol.*, **222**, 581.

MIDDLETON, B. A., MORGAN, L. M., AHERNE, G. W. & MARKS, V. (1988) *Ann. Clin. Biochem.*, **25**, 89.

MITCHISON, N. A. (1968) *Immunology*, **15**, 509.

MITCHISON, N. A. (1971) *Eur. J. Immunol.*, **1**, 10.

MURPHY, J. E. P. (1980) *J. Immunoassay*, **1**, 413.

PESKAR, B. A., PESKAR, B. M. & LEVINE, L. (1972) *Eur. J. Biochem.*, **26**, 191.

PRATT, J. J. (1978) *Clin. Chem.*, **24**, 1869.

RABBITTS, T. H., FORSTER, A., DUNNICK, W. & BENTLEY, D. L. (1980) *Nature*, **283**, 351.

ROITT, I. (1991) *Essential Immunology.* Blackwell Scientific Publications, UK.

SISKIND, G. W. & BENACERRAF, B. (1969) *Adv. Immunol.*, **10**, 1.

TIJSSEN, P. (1985) *Practice and Theory of Enzyme Immunoassays.* Elsevier, Amsterdam.

UNANUE, E. R. (1984) *Annu. Rev. Immunol.*, **2**, 395.

VAITUKAITIS, J. L. (1981) *Methods in Enzymology*, **73**, 46.

WEIGLE, W. O. (1971) *Clin. Exp. Immunol.*, **9**, 437.

WERBLIN, T. P. & SISKIND, G. W. (1972) *Transplant Rev.*, **8**, 104.

5

Radiolabelling procedures for radioimmunoassay

B. LAW

Zeneca Pharmaceuticals, Macclesfield

Introduction

A radiotracer was at the heart of the first reported immunoassay (Yalow and Berson, 1960), yet over 30 years later radioimmunoassay is still in widespread use and accounts for around 20 per cent of all publications in the field of immunoassay methods. Although initially surprising there are a number of good reasons for this. In many respects radiotracers still offer a number of significant advantages over the competition which, in the short term at least, are unlikely to be superceded. The most important of these is the fact that the measurement of the end point, i.e. radioactivity detection, is totally specific for the labelled tracer. This is in contrast to the position in fluoro- and enzymeimmunoassays where the samples themselves may contain background fluorescence or enzyme activity. The sensitivity of detection is also very good such that as little as 0.3 fmoles of labelled material can be reliably detected in one minute. Unlike chemiluminescent or enzymeimmunoassays the end point measurement in RIA can, if necessary, be repeated many times over.

The tracer is at the heart of every immunoassay, however it should never be considered alone, but always together with the antisera with which it can be considered a close partner. The closeness and importance of this partnership is particularly apparent when using heterologous tracers, that is tracers which are structurally different to the analyte which is being measured. This is always the case in enzymeimmunoassays and is also generally true for most RIAs using ^{125}I tracers, but not when ^{3}H or ^{14}C tracers are used. With a heterologous tracer, bridge recognition effects can seriously reduce assay sensitivity. This can only be avoided or ameliorated if the structure of both the immunogen and tracer are known and understood.

In any immunoassay the sensitivity (and to a degree the specificity) are ultimately determined by the affinity of the antisera for the analyte. The definition, determination and control of affinity has been discussed previously (Chapter 4). The sensitivity of an assay is generally taken to be of the same order of magnitude as the reciprocal of the antibody affinity constant (K). Thus an assay with an affinity constant of 10^{10} litre/mol would be expected to give a limit of detection of around

10^{-10} mol/litre. However to be able to achieve this, it is necessary to have a tracer of sufficient specific activity that 10^{-10} mol/litre or typically 10^{-13} mol/assay tube can be detected. Therefore to realise the sensitivity afforded by the antisera in an immunoassay it is necessary to use tracers with very high specific activities.

Confusion often arises in the literature with regard to affinity and its affect on assay sensitivity. It is the analyte itself that is required to bind avidly to the antiserum and not necessarily the tracer. In fact, by reducing the antisera affinity for the tracer (through some structural change to the latter) it may actually be possible to improve sensitivity. A side effect of this however may be a concomitant drop in assay specificity or robustness.

The remainder of this section will deal with the selection, production and purification of radiotracers to afford the most sensitive, specific and robust methods.

Choice of radiotracer

There are several radioisotopes that can be used as tracers in radioimmunoassay procedures and these are shown in Table 5.1, along with relevant data such as half-life and maximum specific activity etc. Although on the face of it there are several isotopes to choose from, in practice the choice is somewhat limited. There are few drugs or small biochemical molecules of interest that possess sulphur or phosphorus, although these atoms occur more frequently in agrochemical agents. The relatively short half-life of phosphorus is also obviously a limiting factor to its general use. The three commonly used isotopes are discussed below.

Carbon-14

All analyte molecules contain carbon, at least one atom of which can be replaced by the radioisotope ^{14}C. However the specific activity that is typically achieved is relatively low, only 62 mCi/mmol for a single atom of ^{14}C per molecule. This seriously constrains the potential assay sensitivity and consequently ^{14}C is rarely used in immunoassay work.

Tritium

All molecules of interest contain hydrogen and replacement of one or more of these atoms with tritium (^{3}H) to give a radiotracer is a more viable proposition, both in terms of synthetic simplicity and in giving a more sensitive immunoassay procedure.

Table 5.1 Physical properties of some common radioisotopes

Radionuclide	$t_{1/2}$	Maximum specific activity (Ci/mmol)
^{3}H	12.6 y	29.2
^{14}C	5730.0 y	0.0624
^{125}I	60.0 d	2180
^{35}S	82.7 d	1500
^{32}P	14.3 d	9200

The specific activities that can be obtained whilst retaining reasonable stability are generally high. Replacement of one atom of hydrogen in a molecule with tritium would give a specific activity of 29 Ci/mmol and as a consequence the literature abounds with reports of sensitive assays employing ^{3}H tracers. The major limitations on the use of this isotope relate to problems associated with the separation and counting stages of the assay procedure, in particular: quenching, long counting times and counter technology. The recent introduction of multi-head beta counters and scintillation proximity assays however (see Chapter 6), may have given a new lease of life to assays employing tritiated tracers.

Iodine-125

The advantages associated with ^{125}I make it ideally suited as a radiotracer for immunoassay work, and the content of this chapter very much reflects this view.

Iodine-125 (^{125}I) can be used to label a wide range of drugs, pesticides, herbicides, environmental pollutants and molecules of biochemical interest. Relative to ^{3}H for example, very high specific activities are easily achievable (e.g. 2200 Ci/mmol), which can result in very sensitive assay techniques and short counting times. The highly penetrating radiation of the gamma emission allows great flexibility at the assay separation stage and the use of simpler and direct, solid scintillation counting. The widespread availability of multi-head gamma counters also results in relatively short overall processing times. The relatively short half-life of ^{125}I (60 d) compared with ^{3}H for example, necessitates the regular repeat synthesis of the iodinated tracer. However, in the author's experience most ^{125}I labelled compounds are stable and usable for at least 3 months and frequently longer. A point often overlooked but which is very important in the context of assay development is the simplicity, low cost and ease of iodination procedures, especially when compared with tritiation. Labelling with ^{125}I using any of the common approaches can be carried out within a few hours, including purification. The techniques used are well within the capabilities of anyone involved in immunoassay development and the cost per iodination is relatively cheap, often less than £100. The latter point means it is well suited to laboratories with budgetary constraints.

Radioactive decay processes

Radiochemical decay can be considered in two ways. First, it involves a transfer of energy from the decaying atom or molecule to the emitted particle and second it involves a change in chemical identity of the radioactive atom in question. The first of these points is generally well accepted but the second is worthy of some discussion.

When an atom of tritium (^{3}H) undergoes radioactive decay it produces a beta particle and an atom of ^{3}He. Similarly when ^{125}I undergoes radioactive decay it emits a gamma ray and is converted to non-radioactive ^{125}Te; a stable metal. Thus on radioactive decay there is a change in chemical identity, not the conversion of a radioactive molecule into its non-radioactive analogue. Since tellurium (Te) does not readily form bonds with carbon, any organic molecule which has undergone radioactive decay will also have rearranged to accommodate the effective disappearance of one of its atoms. This new chemical entity may still be antigenic and hence affect the specific activity of the remaining tracer. The decay process also releases energy which can further disrupt the original molecule, or it can be passed on to other molecules (either radioactive or non-radioactive) which may then break down resulting in secondary radiation damage.

The relatively short half-life of 60 days for ^{125}I means that even with minimal radiation damage and ideal chemical stability the tracer will need to be prepared at regular intervals. For compounds labelled with ^{14}C and ^{3}H the longer half-lives (Table 5.1) would be expected to result in these compounds having a good shelf life. In practice, however, the interaction of the decay particle with other molecules and the consequences of the secondary radiation damage necessitates regular synthesis or repurification even with these long half-life isotopes.

Site of labelling

In tritiated or ^{14}C labelled molecules, the replacement of the naturally occurring isotope by the radioactive isotope is a facile change which is considered to have no effect on antibody binding. The location of the radioactive atom in the molecule is therefore dictated by synthetic chemistry considerations.

The site of labelling however is especially important in the preparation of radioiodinated tracers where a hydrogen atom in the molecule is replaced by an iodine atom or a relatively bulky tag molecule such as iodohistamine. This chemical modification will inevitably result in significant changes in the stereochemistry, shape and size of the labelled molecule (it should be remembered that an iodine atom is approximately the size of a benzene ring). If the iodine atom or iodo-tag is attached in the wrong position then the antibody may fail to recognise the tracer and no binding will be obtained. Careful siting of the iodine atom or tag is therefore essential if this type of problem is to be avoided. The best site for labelling is generally the point of attachment used in the synthesis of the immunogen. Because of steric hindrance by the protein carrier in the conjugate, this part of the molecule is inaccessible to the T-helper cells which initiate antibody formation. The antibodies which result are therefore blind to changes at this site of the molecule, and hence it is possible to make major chemical changes to the molecule, whilst still retaining antibody binding.

Tracer synthesis

^{14}C labelling

The synthesis of compounds labelled with ^{14}C usually involves the use of relatively simple starting materials such as barium ^{14}C-carbonate, potassium ^{14}C-cyanide or possibly simple organic molecules such as ^{14}C-phenol. As the molecule is built up from such simple materials every synthesis is different, and it is difficult therefore to discuss this subject in a general manner. The cost of such work is also high, time consuming and requires considerable synthetic expertise. Given their poor characteristics it is unlikely that anyone would synthesis ^{14}C-labelled molecules purely for immunoassay purposes, therefore this subject will not be discussed further.

^{3}H labelling (tritiation)

Synthesis of ^{3}H labelled materials usually involves one of a number of standard procedures. These include: reduction of an unsaturated compound using tritium gas and a metal catalyst; catalytic replacement of a halogen atom with tritium; reduction of a ketone, aldehyde, ester or aldamine with a tritiated metal hydride; or replacement of acidic or other labile hydrogens by tritium using tritiated solvents and metal catalysts. Should the molecule of interest have a methoxy or an *N*-methyl group then a suitable derivative can be labelled using tritiated methyl iodide. An example of one reaction (catalytic replacement of halogen) for the β_1-partial agonist xamoterol is shown in Figure 5.1. In this procedure a bromo analogue of the drug compound is used and the sensitive phenol group is protected as a benzyl ether. The benzyl group is also replaced by ^{3}H during the tritiation procedure but the resulting O^3H, being weakly acidic and labile, exchanges with the protons from water during the subsequent work-up procedure.

The example described above is typical of most methods in that a precursor molecule is required to obtain the labelled molecule of interest. In the above example this is a brominated and benzyl-protected analogue. This obviously necessitates some chemical support for the labelling project. Furthermore the tritiation procedures frequently require the handling of large quantities (typically greater than 25 Ci) of tritium gas or tritiated solvents and the use of specialist facilities such as vacuum handling apparatus. The incorporation of tritium into the final tracer is often inefficient, around one per cent, making waste disposal a significant problem. Taken together these factors mean that tritiation is usually outside the capabilities of most people involved in the development of immunoassays.

Many large organisations such as pharmaceutical and agrochemical companies employ radiochemists, who, given the appropriate facilities should be able to synthesise the necessary precursor and carry out the tritiation and subsequent chemical clean-up. Alternatively the major suppliers of radiochemicals offer a tritiation service. Although the cost of the tritiation itself is relatively cheap, the work involved in cleaning up the crude material and characterising the final product raises the overall cost to around £4000 per synthesis. This could be a serious disadvantage when the work is speculative or when there are financial constraints.

Although the half-life for tritium is relatively long, many compounds with the high specific activity necessary for RIA show poor stability. As a consequence the synthesis may need to be repeated every few years or the tracer preparation regularly repurified.

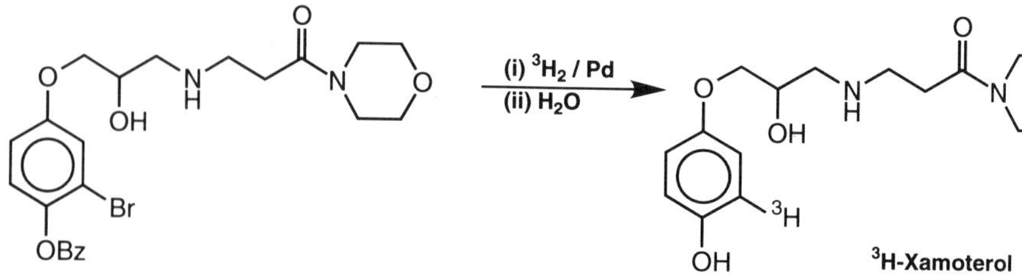

Figure 5.1 Reaction scheme showing the tritiation of xamoterol using a benzyl protected brominated analogue and tritium gas with a palladium catalyst.

^{125}I labelling

Iodinated tracers can be produced in a number of different ways and this gives a flexible approach to labelling which can be necessary in overcoming bridge recognition problems (see below). Basically iodination procedures can be divided into two types: direct and indirect. Each of these will be considered in turn and examples given of the most important methods used. For a broader account of radioiodination methods the reader is directed to the reviews of Seevers and Counsell (1982) and Grassi *et al.* (1987).

Direct iodination

In the direct procedure the analyte or a suitable analogue is labelled by replacing an atom of hydrogen with ^{125}I. The most commonly used direct iodination procedure is that of Hunter and Greenwood (1962), often referred to as the chloramine-T method. This procedure involves mixing the compound of interest with sodium ^{125}I-iodide and then adding chloramine-T (*N*-chloro-*p*-toluene sulphonamide sodium salt). Chloramine-T is a mild oxidising agent which reacts with the sodium ^{125}I-iodide to release the electrophile I^+. This electrophilic species then attacks an electron-rich site such as a phenol or a histidine group in the molecule to be labelled. A typical reaction scheme for the radioiodination of the drug morphine is shown in Figure 5.2.

The electrophilic attack of I^+ on the phenol or histidine is very rapid and the reaction is terminated usually after about 15 s by the addition of a reducing agent. Sodium metabisulphite is commonly used, which converts any unreacted $^{125}I^+$ back to sodium ^{125}I-iodide and reduces any residual chloramine-T. More recently the milder reducing agent cysteine has also been used (Corrie *et al.*, 1981). Prior to further handling or purification, unlabelled sodium iodide is sometimes added to the reaction mixture. This acts as a diluent or carrier for the residual sodium ^{125}I-iodide, thus minimising any potential contamination during the work-up procedure.

The literature contains many references to the use of the chloramine-T and a wide range of variants of the original method have been reported. What makes this particularly confusing is that changes to the original procedure have often been made without any justification or reasons given. The reported ratio of reactants are

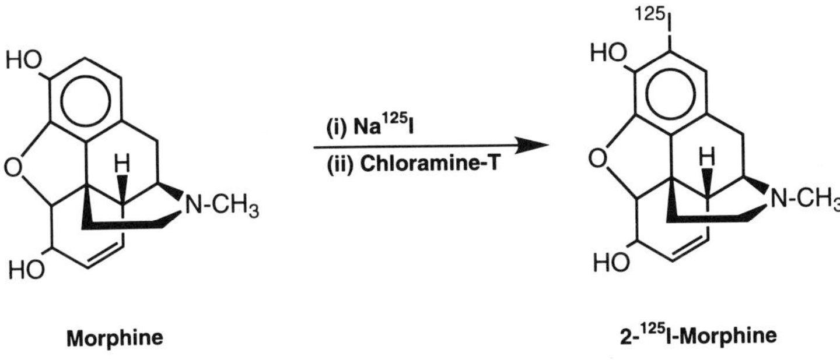

Figure 5.2 Radioiodination of morphine using the chloramine-T procedure.

found to vary dramatically. For example in the iodination of simple phenolic compounds the ratio of substrate to radioiodine varies from 16 : 1 to 111 : 1, and the ratio of chloramine-T to radioiodine varies from 115 : 1 to 704 : 1. This reported variability obviously makes the selection of starting conditions difficult, especially for someone new to this area.

The molar ratio of substrate to radioiodine in the examples presented in this chapter are set very high (100 : 1) in favour of the compound to be labelled. This ratio has been selected to ensure maximal utilisation of the radioiodine, and as a consequence it is assumed that the compound to be labelled is freely available and of minimum cost. Whilst this generally holds true for most standard industrial-type chemicals it may not be the case for some peptides or other molecules of biological interest and adjustments to the ratio may be necessary.

Although high incorporation of the radioiodine is important from a cost point of view other factors reinforce this strategy. Any radioiodine not incorporated into the final tracer must be disposed of. For a synthesis with a relatively low yield (less than 50 per cent), this may necessitate the disposal of a large amount of radioiodine at one time. This could pose a significant waste management and possibly environmental problem. The high ratio also favours the formation of mono-iodo derivatives which are generally considered to be more stable than the di-iodo analogues.

The ratio of chloramine-T to substrate has also been reduced to minimise any oxidative damage to the substrate. Some adjustment to the concentration of the substance to be iodinated may be necessary where its aqueous solubility is low. In these circumstances the use of co-solvents or detergents is permissible. Following these guidelines the reagents and conditions for a typical iodination of a phenol-containing molecule are given in PROCEDURE 1 below.

PROCEDURE 1 Labelling of a phenol-containing molecule using the chloramine-T method

Reagents

- Phosphate buffer (0.25 M, pH 7.4) prepared from KH_2PO_4 (anhydrous, 6.70 g), Na_2HPO_4 (anhydrous, 28.50 g) and water (1 litre)
- Chloramine-T solution (5 mg/ml) prepared from chloramine-T trihydrate (50 mg) and phosphate buffer (10 ml)
- Sodium metabisulphite solution (6 mg/ml) prepared from sodium metabisulphite (60 mg) and distilled water (10 ml)
- Sodium ^{125}I-iodide (1 mCi, 37 MBq ≡ 0.45 nmol) in 10 μl sodium hydroxide solution (e.g. IMS.30 from Amersham International, UK)

Note: the chloramine-T and sodium metabisulphite solutions are prepared fresh daily

Equipment

- Two air displacement pipettes capable of delivering 10 μl and 20 μl
- A vortex mixer
- A stopcock or other timing device
- A reaction vessel such as a 1.5 ml polypropylene microcentrifuge tube

Method

This procedure and the others involving radioactive materials should be carried out in a well-ventilated fume cupboard and the operator should be wearing an overgarment and two pairs of disposable gloves. Further safety precautions are discussed in Chapter 2.

The compound to be iodinated is dissolved in phosphate buffer to give a final concentration of around 5 μmol/ml (≡1.5 mg/ml for a compound with molecular mass of 300 Dalton). An aliquot (10 μl) of this solution is transferred to a plastic microcentrifuge tube (1.5 ml capacity). To this is added the sodium ^{125}I solution (10 μl). An aliquot (10 *μ*l) of the chloramine-T solution is then placed in the tube, as a small drop on the side, separate from the other reagents, and the tube carefully capped. The surface tension holds this drop of liquid separate from the other reagents. The stopcock is started and the reagents rapidly mixed using a vortex mixer. After 15 s the vial is uncapped and sodium metabisulphite solution (20 μl) is added rapidly from a prefilled pipette, and the vial again capped and vortex mixed.

The solution (total volume 50 μl) is then ready for any necessary purification and evaluation.

Where the molecule of interest does not possess the necessary phenolic functional group to facilitate direct iodination, it is sometimes possible to use a drug metabolite, as in the case of phenobarbitone (Mason and Law, 1982). Although phenobarbitone itself did not contain the necessary activated ring for direct iodination the major metabolite, 4-hydroxyphenobarbitone, which was commercially available did. Since the position of linkage for preparation of the immunogen was the 4-position of the aromatic ring, i.e. the same site as oxidative metabolic attack, the metabolite was successfully iodinated using the above procedure to give a radiotracer for a phenobarbitone RIA.

A number of alternatives to the chloramine-T procedure have been developed over the years mainly to address specific problems. For example, although only a mild oxidising agent, chloramine-T is powerful enough in certain instances to cause chemical damage to the molecule that is being labelled. In the case of peptides this damage could result in reduced binding of the tracer, or at the extreme, total loss of biological activity. In the iodination of 4-hydroxyphenobarbitone (Mason and Law, 1982), the chloramine-T actually oxidised this precursor. It was therefore necessary to employ a large excess of this compound to overcome the problem.

A more general approach to the problem of side reactions has been the use of other methods of oxidation, such as electrochemical or enzymic procedures. These however, have not proved as popular because of their more specialised and technically demanding nature.

A more recent practical alternative is Iodo-gen (glycoluril) which is claimed to be a milder oxidising agent than chloramine-T (Fraker and Speck, 1978; Pillai *et al.*, 1987). This reagent also has the advantage that it has very poor aqueous solubility, and it can therefore be used in a solid-phase reaction system. This avoids the necessity of stopping the reaction with an additional reagent; instead the reaction mixture is merely pipetted off the solid-state oxidising agent which is usually coated onto the wall of the reaction tube. The milder properties of this reagent are claimed to be particularly useful in the iodination of redox-sensitive peptides containing disulphide bridges. For the iodination of most drug compounds, Iodo-gen does not offer any significant advantage over chloramine-T (Woltanski *et al.*, 1990). A procedure for the iodination of a phenolic molecule using the Iodo-gen method is given in PROCEDURE 2.

PROCEDURE 2 Iodination of a phenol-containing compound using the Iodo-gen method

Reagents

- Iodo-gen
- Chloroform
- Sodium ^{125}I-iodide
- Gas source, e.g. oxygen-free nitrogen
- Phosphate buffer (0.25 M, pH 7.4) prepared from KH_2PO_4 (anhydrous, 6.70 g), Na_2HPO_4 (anhydrous, 28.50 g) and water (1 litre).
- Silica gel, self-indicating (6–16 mesh, 1–3 mm)

Equipment

- Blowing down apparatus
- Polypropylene microcentrifuge tube, 1.5 ml volume

Method

Preparation of coated tubes – prepare a solution of Iodo-gen in chloroform at a concentration of 100 µg/ml. Transfer aliquots (20 µl) to a series of microcentrifuge tubes and gently evaporate the solvent to dryness with a stream of gas at room temperature. Each tube is now coated with a thin layer of Iodo-gen (2 µg). These tubes can be stored desiccated (over silica gel) either at room temperature or -20°C where they remain stable for at least 6 months.

Iodination – rinse a coated reaction tube with buffer (0.1 ml) to remove any loose flakes of Iodo-gen which could cause variable incorporation of iodine. The compound to be iodinated is then dissolved in phosphate buffer to give a final concentration of around 2.5 µmol/ml ($\equiv$0.75 mg/ml for a compound with molecular mass of 300 Dalton). Add the compound solution (50 nmol is 20 µl of buffer) followed by sodium ^{125}I-iodide (1 mCi, 10 µl, as supplied). Mix gently by vortexing and allow to stand for around 10 min with occasional mixing. The reaction is stopped by removing the reaction solution from the tube.

The above procedure does offer one small advantage over the chloramine-T iodination procedure in that once the coated tubes have been prepared no additional reagents apart from the buffer are required to carry out the iodination.

Indirect iodination

If there are no suitable ring systems present in the molecule to allow direct radioiodination then an indirect method employing a radio-tag can be used. Radio-tags are pre-iodinated molecules synthesised in the laboratory or bought commercially which can be linked to the analyte of interest under simple conditions. The resultant radiotracer is usually formed in high yield and of high specific activity. The two common iodo-tags are Bolton–Hunter reagent (Bolton and Hunter, 1973) and iodohistamine (Nars and Hunter, 1973; Tantchou and Slaunwhite, 1979). These can be attached to molecules bearing amino (primary or secondary) or carboxylic acid groups respectively. If the molecule of interest does not possess the necessary functional group then it can be derivatised in a similar manner to that used for immunogen synthesis (Chapter 3).

Bolton–Hunter reagent

A typical reaction scheme for the labelling of the stimulant amphetamine with Bolton–Hunter reagent is shown in Figure 5.3.

The *N*-hydroxysuccinamide moiety of the Bolton–Hunter reagent activates the carboxyl function towards nucleophilic attack by an amine; the ensuing reaction results in the formation of an amide linkage in the final molecule. The reaction is generally rapid taking approximately 15 min, although careful control of the pH is necessary for optimal conjugation. To maintain the amine in an unprotonated state, a high pH is indicated; however, the competitive base catalysed hydrolysis of the *N*-hydroxysuccinamide ester would suggest use of a low pH. The optimum appears to be around pH 8.6, and borate buffer at this pH is commonly used as the reaction medium. Typical reaction conditions and reagents for an iodination using Bolton–Hunter reagent are given in PROCEDURE 3.

PROCEDURE 3 Labelling of a primary-amine-containing drug with Bolton–Hunter reagent

Reagents

- Sodium hydroxide solution (1 M) prepared from sodium hydroxide (4 g) and water (100 ml)
- Borate buffer (0.1 M, pH 8.6) prepared from boric acid (6.18 g) and sodium hydroxide solution (1 M, 29 ml) and water (970 ml)
- Bolton–Hunter reagent (1 mCi, 37 MBq ≡ 0.45 nmol) in benzene/dimethylformamide solvent (0.2 ml) contained in a septum-sealed vial (Amersham International), supplied with a charcoal trap
- Granulated charcoal (ca. 10–18 mesh)
- $CaCl_2$ (anhydrous), granular (ca. 20 mesh)
- Compound to be iodinated dissolved in borate buffer at a concentration of 90 nmol/50 μl (≡ 0.54 mg/ml for a compound with a molecular mass of 300 Dalton)

Equipment

- Hypodermic needles 22 G and 18 G
- A vortex mixer
- Cotton wool
- A glass syringe (50 or 100 μl) with a sharp needle
- A Pasteur pipette
- Rubber tubing
- A source of compressed gas such as Ar, He or N_2

Method

First prepare a gas drying tube by cutting the tapered end from a Pasteur pipette and plugging the narrow end lightly with a small ball of cotton wool. Fill the pipette body with $CaCl_2$ (anhydrous) and pack the open end lightly with cotton wool also. The wide end of this drying tube is then connected to the gas supply and a further section of rubber tubing is connected to the narrow end. A 22 G hypodermic needle is then connected to the loose end of the tubing.

The rubber septum of the vial containing the Bolton–Hunter reagent is pierced with the wide bore (18 G) needle to which is attached the charcoal trap. The gas regulator is adjusted to give a gentle stream of gas through the drying tube and the 22 G hypodermic needle. The septum seal is then pierced with this needle. The position of the 22 G needle is adjusted so that the gas stream plays gently on the surface of the liquid. Excessive gas flow should be avoided as this can result in the reagent being spread over the inner walls of the vial or even lost to the charcoal trap. After approximately 5 min at room temperature the solvent (benzene/dimethylformamide) will have evaporated.

The solution of compound to be iodinated (50 μl containing 90 nmol of compound) is then added through the septum, using a glass syringe. The vial is vortexed thoroughly to ensure effective dissolution of the dried reagent. After 15 to 20 min at room temperature the reaction can be considered complete and tracer ready for purification.

The use of the charcoal trap is essential since volatile or nebulised iodinated material can be expelled in the gas stream. The use of the drying tube serves to prevent hydrolysis of the Bolton–Hunter reagent by moisture in the gas. When necessary, alternatives to borate buffer can be used as the reaction medium. For one particular compound which was sensitive to borate we successfully used *N*-methylmorpholine (1.0% v/v in water, pH 9.9) which is a non-nucleophilic base used widely in organic synthesis. In aqueous alkaline solution, pH 8.4 to 9, Bolton–Hunter reagent is relatively unstable and is completely hydrolysed within 30 min in the absence of a suitable base with which to react. In practice reaction times of between

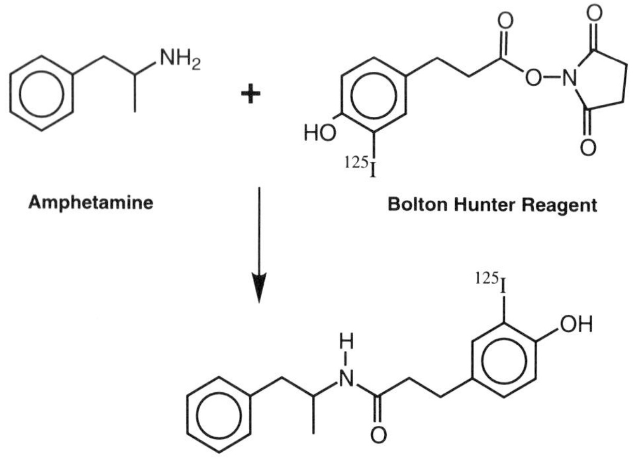

Figure 5.3 Iodination of the stimulant amphetamine by reaction with Bolton–Hunter reagent.

15 to 30 min have been found to be optimal. On occasions we have found that the use of prolonged reaction times (over lunch or overnight) actually reduced the yield. Using the procedures outlined above we have regularly obtained high radiochemical yields, typically 80 per cent.

Where the compound to be labelled has poor aqueous solubility or aqueous conditions are required to be avoided, the reaction can be carried out in a dipolar aprotic solvent such as dimethylformamide (DMF). In this instance we have used as catalyst non-nucleophilic organic bases such as Proton Sponge (Aldrich Chemical Co., Dorset, UK) or tri-*N*-butylamine. Experiments have shown that in non-aqueous conditions Bolton–Hunter reagent has better stability and the reaction with an amine is much slower, typically taking around 3 hours (Law, unpublished data). The yield however can be higher presumably because of a lack of competing hydrolysis. The rate of reaction, as well as being dependent on the solvent and reaction conditions is also dependent on the structure and pK_a of the solute, with weak bases such as aniline being much slower than simple aliphatic bases of much higher pK_a.

Bolton–Hunter reagent which will react with both primary and secondary amines probably represents the ideal method of radioiodination when direct methods are not possible. Furthermore, given the mild conditions used, the high yields and specific activities obtained and the relative simplicity of clean-up, it is probably superior to the direct techniques. The reagent is commercially available at high specific activity (2200 Ci/mmol) and a di-iodinated analogue is also available at twice this activity, although this is not widely used. The conjugation reaction is carried out under very mild conditions making it particularly suited to protein or peptide labelling, the purpose for which it was originally introduced (Bolton and Hunter, 1973). Although many analytes possess primary or secondary amino groups necessary for labelling with an iodo-tag, when they do not it is possible to use a metabolite or analogue. For example, the *N*-desalkyl metabolites of compounds such as the phenothiazines or tricyclic antidepressants (Mason *et al.*, 1984) have proved particularly useful in allowing iodination when the tertiary amine parent compounds were unreactive. If functionalisation of the molecule is necessary, then methods similar to those for the production of immunogens can be used (Chapter 3).

Conjugation with Bolton–Hunter reagent not only changes the acid/base character of the molecule: an amine is converted to a neutral amide, but the molecular weight and consequently the lipophilicity are increased. Both these factors lead to the tracer having very different physicochemical properties to the precursor, allowing simpler purification techniques to be used than with direct iodination methods.

Benzimidate reagent

The only major disadvantage associated with Bolton–Hunter reagent is the change in acid/base character mentioned above. Examination of Figure 5.3 shows that on conjugation, a basic amino function in the amphetamine molecule has been converted to a non-basic amide. The amino function has a pK_a of 10 and hence it would be fully ionised at physiological pH (7.4). The labelled molecule in contrast is neutral having lost the amino group and hence it would be uncharged. Although in the radioiodination of small molecules this change in acid/base character is rarely a problem, it can be a major concern in the labelling of proteins where the positive charge of a basic amino acid may be necessary for maintaining tertiary structure

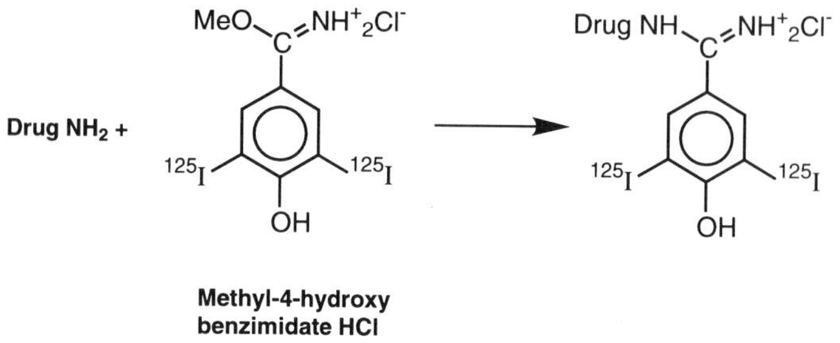

Figure 5.4 An example of the labelling of a primary amine with methyl-4-hydroxy-benzimidate HCl.

and possibly antigenicity. A compound which overcomes this problem in the labelling of peptides is the iodinated amidation reagent, methyl-3,5-di-iodo-*p*-hydroxybenzimidate (Wood *et al.*, 1975). This reagent reacts under similar simple conditions to Bolton–Hunter reagent, however, it is claimed to be more specific for amino groups and to be more stable in aqueous conditions, even at high pH. The tracer resulting from the reaction with the benzimidate reagent (Figure 5.4) still retains an amine capable of protonation. Consequently a peptide or protein labelled with this reagent would be expected to retain its tertiary structure. Although originally developed for labelling of proteins there is no reason why this reagent cannot be used to label small molecules. However, the fact that this material is no longer commercially available has probably contributed to its lack of use in this area.

Iodohistamine

The other commonly used iodo-tag is ^{125}I-iodohistamine (Nars and Hunter, 1973; Tantchou and Slaunwhite, 1979), again this is a reagent which can be purchased commercially or synthesised in the laboratory at high specific activity. Alternative tags which also possess primary amine groups, such as tyramine and tyrosine

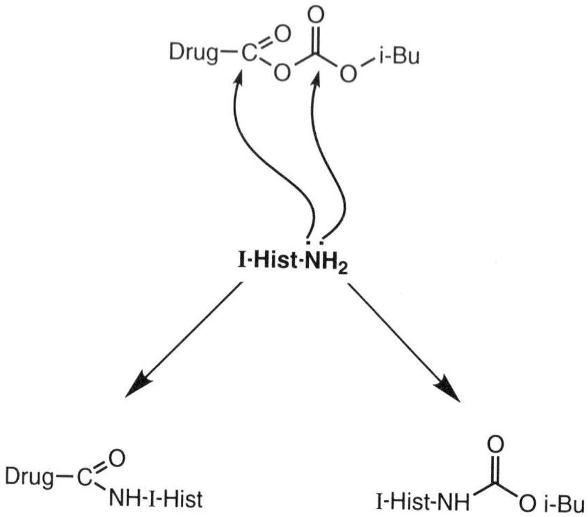

Figure 5.5 Attack of iodohistamine (I-Hist-NH$_2$) on a mixed anhydride derivative of a drug molecule showing the formation of the desired tracer and a by-product.

Table 5.2 Antigenic and radioactive materials present in the reaction mixture following iodination of histamine and its conjugation to THC-11-oic acid using the mixed anhydride procedure

Compound	Antigenic	Radioactive
THC-11-oic acid mixed anhydride	yes	no
THC-11-oic acid	yes	no
THC-11-oic acid-(2-^{125}I-iodohistamide)	yes	yes
Isobutyl-2-(2-^{125}I-iodoimidazo)-4-yl ethylcarbamate	no	yes
THC-11-oic acid histamide	yes	no
2-^{125}I-iodohistamine	no	yes
Na^{125}I-iodide	no	yes

methyl ester (TME), have also been evaluated. However, these compounds are more difficult to prepare or have poor stability (Gilby *et al.*, 1973) and consequently have seen little use.

Unlike the situation with Bolton–Hunter reagent, iodohistamine itself is not activated. It is necessary therefore to activate the acid functional group on the analyte molecule to facilitate reaction. Once again the necessary chemistry is identical to that used in the preparation of immunogens. Tantchou and Slaunwhite (1980) recommended the use of the *N*-hydroxysuccinamide esters of carboxylic acids which are formed using the carbodiimide method. The acid so activated could be stored in aliquots for future iodination. Alternatively the acid can be activated as a mixed anhydride by reaction with isobutylchloroformate (Law *et al.*, 1982). This derivative although considered unacceptable by Tantchou and Slaunwhite (1980) is simple to prepare and as it possesses good stability it can be prepared in bulk and stored, preferrably in small aliquots for future use. Using ^{125}I-iodohistamine with the mixed anhydride method does have the disadvantage that a significant amount of a radioactive by-product is produced, Figure 5.5.

Furthermore if the iodohistamine is prepared in the laboratory and conjugated to the acid without purification the resulting reaction mixture is complex, containing a number of components with a wide range of properties (Table 5.2), (Law *et al.*, 1982). This necessitates powerful separation procedures such as HPLC to ensure high specific activity and radiochemical purity.

A method for the iodination of iodohistamine and its subsequent conjugation to an acid using the mixed anhydride method are given in PROCEDURES 4 and 5 respectively. The reaction of iodine with histamine is somewhat slower than that with phenols and a reaction time of 1 to 2 min is normally used. The pH optimum for the iodination of histamine is 8.0 compared with 7.4 for the iodination of phenols. This pH gives mainly monoiodohistamine which has improved stability compared with the di-iodo analogue (Tantchou and Slaunwhite, 1979).

PROCEDURE 4 Iodination of histamine using the chloramine-T procedure

Reagents

- Phosphate buffer (0.1 M, pH 8.0) prepared from KH_2PO_4 (anhydrous 0.504 g), Na_2HPO_4 (anhydrous 13.67 g) and water (1 litre)

- Histamine dihydrochloride solution (6.3 mg/100 ml) in phosphate buffer
- Chloramine-T trihydrate (6 mg/ml) in phosphate buffer
- Sodium metabisulphite (10 mg/ml) in phosphate buffer
- Sodium ^{125}I-iodide (1 mCi, 37 MBq ≡ 0.45 nmol) in 10 μl sodium hydroxide solution (e.g. IMS.30 from Amersham International plc).

Equipment

- Two air displacement pipettes capable of delivering 10 μl and 20 μl
- A vortex mixer
- A stopclock or other timing device
- A reaction vessel such as a 1.5 ml polypropylene microcentrifuge tube

Method

An aliquot (10 μl) of the iodohistamine solution (4.5 nmol) is mixed with sodium ^{125}I-iodide (10 μl, 0.45 nmol) in a reaction tube. An aliquot of chloramine-T solution (10 μl) is placed in the tube as a small drop on the side, separate from the other reagents. The tube is carefully capped and the reaction initiated by vortex mixing. The stopclock is started and the reaction is allowed to proceed at room temperature for 2 min. The vial is then uncapped and sodium metabisulphite solution (20 μl) is rapidly added from a prefilled pipette and the vial again capped and vortexed.

Using the iodohistamine prepared above, conjugation to a drug molecule can be effected as described in PROCEDURE 5.

PROCEDURE 5 Coupling of ^{125}I-iodohistamine to a carboxylic-acid-containing drug using the mixed anhydride method

Reagents

- ^{125}I-iodohistamine (1 mCi (0.45 nmol)/50 μl phosphate buffer, pH 8.0) as prepared above
- Dioxane
- Isobutylchloroformate
- Tri-*N*-butylamine
- Alumina (basic, Brockman grade I)

Method

The dioxane is first purified and made peroxide-free by passage through a small column of aluminium oxide. The latter is conveniently prepared by plugging a Pasteur pipette with cotton wool and filling with approximately 40 mm height of alumina. The dioxane is passed through the column and the first millilitre or so discarded and up to a further 5 ml collected. The dioxane should be prepared fresh for use.

The molecule to be iodinated (10 mg, ca. 30 μmol) is dissolved in dioxane (0.6 ml) to which is added tri-*N*-butylamine (7.5 μl, 31.6 μmol) followed by isobutylchloroformate (4.2 μl,

32 μmol). The reaction is maintained at room temperature for approximately 90 min, to allow the reaction to go to completion. The reaction mixture can be stored in this form at −20°C where the mixed anhydride derivative shows good stability.

The conjugation is carried out by adding dioxane (50 μl) to the ^{125}I-iodohistamine solution, followed by an aliquot (1 μl, 50 nmol) of the mixed anhydride reaction solution. The reaction is allowed to proceed to completion at room temperature, for 60–90 min, prior to any separation procedure.

Other methods of iodination

In the two sections above the major and most commonly used methods of introducing radioiodine into an organic molecule have been described. Although less well known, other methods have been employed and these will be discussed briefly here. Because they have been used only occasionally no recommended methods can be given for their use, although reference will be made to the original work.

Molecules containing an aniline function can be iodinated using the chloramine-T method. There are few reports in the literature using this procedure which probably reflects the infrequent occurrence of this functional group, at least in biochemicals and pharmaceuticals. One method presented in the literature (Langone, 1980) would appear to be incorrect as the conditions used, i.e. low pH, actually deactivate the aniline molecule towards iodination. Limited experiments in the author's laboratory (Law, unpublished data) indicates that aniline and *N,N*-dialkyl substituted anilines can be iodinated under the conditions described in PROCEDURE 1 to give exclusively the 4-^{125}I-iodo derivative, when the ring is unsubstituted.

An alternative procedure for the labelling of anilines involves the replacement of the amino function by radioiodine using a Sandmeyer-type reaction (Foster *et al.*, 1981; Goddard *et al.*, 1986). In this procedure the amino group is first converted into a diazonium compound which is then reacted with sodium ^{125}I-iodide. The latter stage can be carried out directly or via a stable pyrrolidine triazine which is claimed to give higher yields and a cleaner reaction. Such a reaction scheme is shown in Figure 5.6 where the drug clonazepam was iodinated. In this instance the drug itself did not have the necessary amino function but this was produced by simple reduction of the aromatic nitro group, using tin and hydrochloric acid. Following a clean-up of the reaction mixture by TLC a radiotracer of high purity and high specific activity was produced (Goddard *et al.*, 1986).

Bridge recognition

One of the problems associated with the use of iodo-tags is that of bridge recognition. Examination of the reaction schemes in Figures 5.3 and 5.5 shows that the drugs are linked to the iodo-tag via an amide bond. The common linking procedures used in the production of immunogens also results in the compound being linked (in this instance to a protein carrier) via an amide bond (see Chapter 3). A consequence of this is that the tracer, by virtue of this amide bond, may possess an extra antigenic determinant compared with the native analyte and hence show

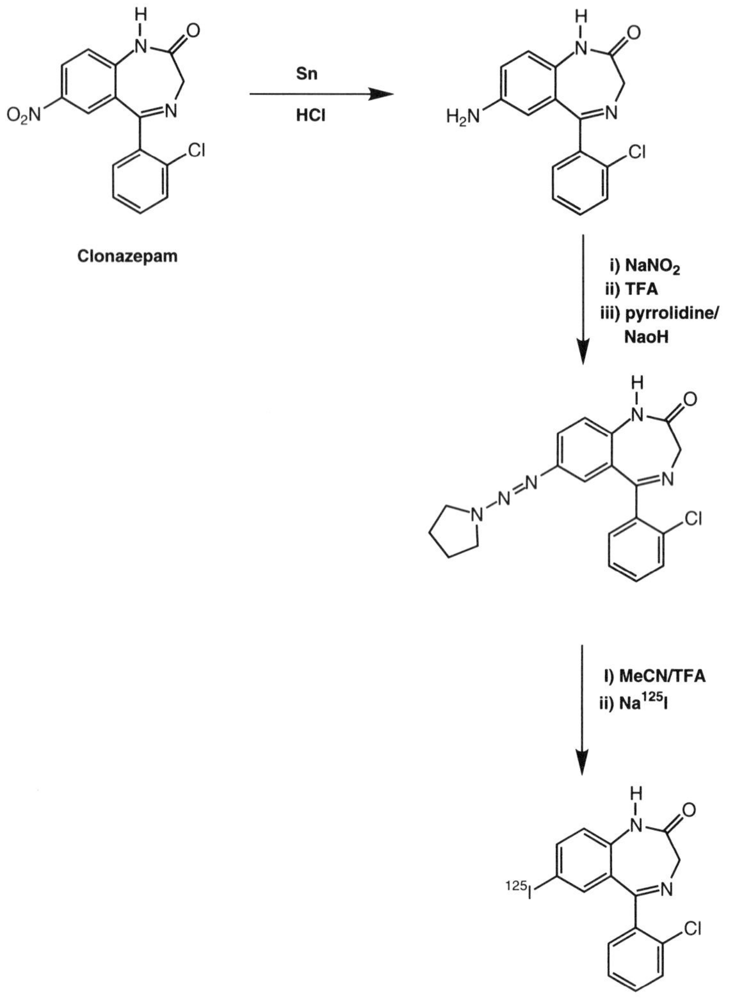

Figure 5.6 Iodination of the benzodiazepine drug clonazepam via reduction of the nitro group to an amine and subsequent diazotisation with formation of a stable pyrrolidine derivative and displacement by iodine.

greater affinity for the antiserum. If this occurs then the tracer can be difficult to displace from the antiserum and an insensitive assay results.

The problem of bridge recognition can be ameliorated by the use of different precursors for synthesis of the immunogen and the radiotracer, although this obviously involves extra resource in terms of synthetic chemistry. A simpler solution involves the use of the same precursor, but with different linking procedures for conjugation to the iodo-tag and the protein carrier. For example, a drug bearing a primary amine could be linked to the carrier protein using a carbodiimide procedure (giving an amide linkage) and the same amine linked to an iodo-tag via an *N*-alkyl linkage as shown in Figure 5.7 (Mason *et al.*, 1983). Using this approach the structure and stereochemistry of the immunogen and tracer were quite different and bridge recognition was avoided. A further interesting example is described in detail below.

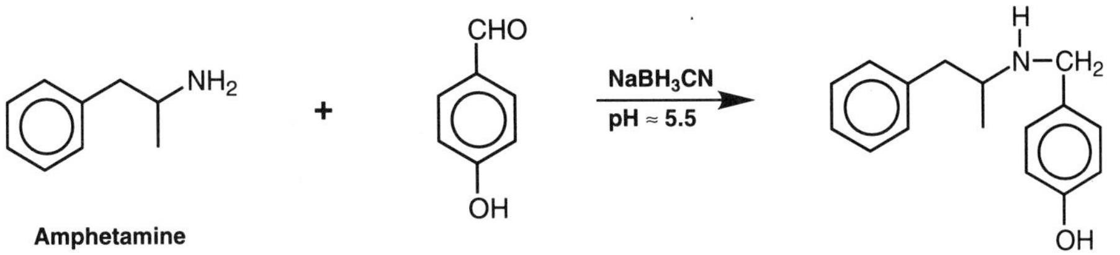

Amphetamine

Figure 5.7 Derivatisation of amphetamine via an *N*-alkyl linkage for subsequent radiolabelling.

Figure 5.8a shows ICI 160181, a β_2-blocker for which an immunoassay was developed using the hapten ICI 193833 (Figure 5.8b) which was used for preparation of both the immunogens and tracers. Two immunogens were produced for this compound and these are shown in Figures 5.8c and 5.8d. The first of these involved conjugation to bovine serum albumin (BSA) through the primary amine using hemisuccinate (Figure 5.8c). The second involved the same functional group on the analogue and the same protein but linking via glutaraldehyde (Figure 5.8d). These two conjugates were used to immunise sheep, all of which responded well.

For use with the resultant antisera two tracers were prepared, these are shown in Figures 5.8e and f. The first of these was prepared by reacting ICI 193833 with Bolton–Hunter reagent (Figure 5.8e) and the second was prepared by reductive amination of ICI 193833 using 4-(4-hydroxyphenyl)-2-butanone and subsequent iodination of the product (Figure 5.8f). These two tracers are very similar, they have the same general structure and identical molecular weights but they differ markedly in the way the 'iodo-tag' is linked to the drug analogue. In the Bolton–Hunter tracer the link is via an amide bond but in the other tracer an *N*-alkyl link has been formed. These different methods of linking result in very different stereochemistries and electron densities around the N atom which has a significant effect on their binding to the antisera as discussed below.

The data in Table 5.3 shows the titres and assay sensitivities resulting from three of the four possible combinations of sera and tracer. Sensitivity is quoted in terms of a limit of detection (LoD) which is the concentration of ICI 160181 that gave 10 per cent depression of binding. Antisera raised against the hemisuccinate conjugate in combination with the Bolton–Hunter tracer, both of which have an amide linkage, i.e. a homologous assay system, gave a reasonable titre of 1/1750 but the sensitivity was very poor. The Bolton–Hunter tracer in combination with antisera raised against the glutaraldehyde conjugate gave a much reduced titre, unfortunately the sensitivity of this heterologous system was never determined. Interestingly the titres with the *N*-alkyl linked tracer were reversed in order of magnitude in comparison to the Bolton–Hunter tracer, but both sera gave a very sensitive assay. The relatively high titre and low sensitivity seen with the hemisuccinate derived antisera and the Bolton–Hunter tracer is thought to be the result of bridge recognition as both the immunogen and the tracer (Figures 5.8c and 5.8e, respectively) had an extra and common antigenic determinant (the amide linkage) in contrast to the analyte ICI 160181 (Figure 5.8a). The combination of an antiserum raised against the glutaraldehyde conjugate and an *N*-alkyl linked tracer were used to give a sensitive and specific assay. A similar phenomenon has been reported in the literature in the development of immunoassays for testosterone (White *et al.*, 1985) and adrostenedione (Nordblom *et al.*, 1981). These examples reinforce the view expressed earlier

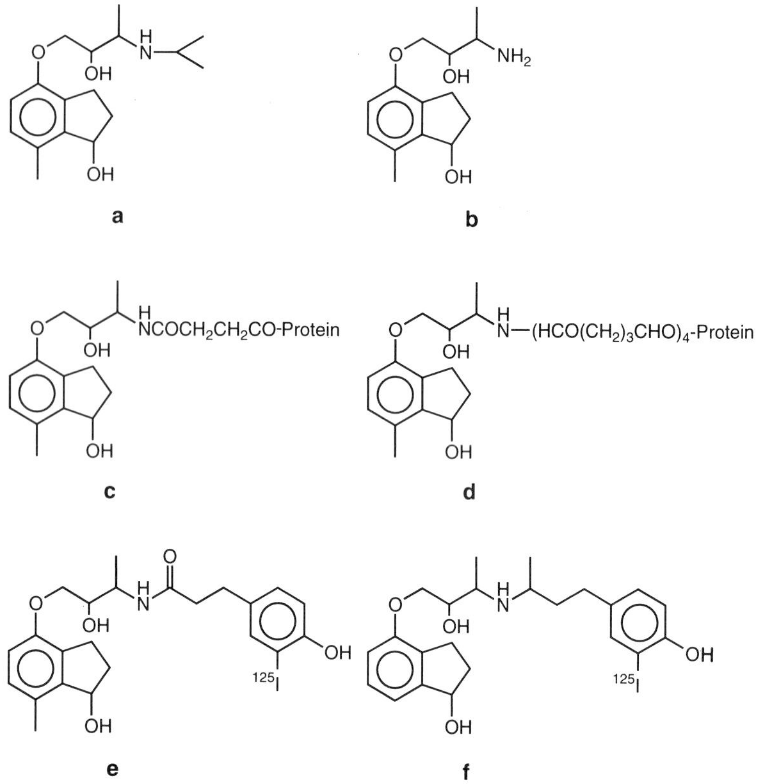

Figure 5.8 (a) the β_2-agonist ICI 160181; (b) the primary amine hapten ICI 193833; (c) an immunogen prepared from ICI 193833 and BSA using a hemisuccinate linkage; (d) an immunogen prepared from ICI 193833 and BSA using a glutaraldehyde linkage; (e) a radiotracer prepared from ICI 193833 by reaction with Bolton–Hunter reagent; (f) a radiotracer prepared from ICI 193833 by reaction with an *N*-alkylating agent and then subsequent iodination.

that for successful assay development it is necessary to prepare a number of different conjugates and tracers in order to guarantee success.

If a number of antisera have been produced but the requisite specificity cannot be obtained, then bridge recognition can be used in a positive manner. The following example shows how chemical modification of the tracer has been used in the past to 'tune' the specificity of an assay for the drug amphetamine (Mason *et al.*, 1983). In

Table 5.3 Antisera titres and assay sensitivities obtained with four different combinations of antisera and radiotracers

	Bolton–Hunter tracer		*N*-alkyl tracer	
Conjugate link	titre	LoD*	titre	LoD*
Glutaraldehyde	1/200	nd**	1/1490	0.25
Hemisuccinate	1/1750	10	1/350	0.4

* Assay limit of detection in ng/ml.
** Not determined.

Table 5.4 Cross-reactivity (percentage)* of amphetamine and analogues in three assays using different tracers but the same antiserum

Compound	Tracer 1	Tracer 2	Tracer 3
Amphetamine	100	100	100
N-Methylamphetamine	250	167	69
Ephedrine	36	8	4
Chlorphetamine	4.5	8	0.4
Phenylpropanolamine	4	3	2
Phenelzine	4	0.5	0

* Cross-reactivity was measured at 100 ng/ml amphetamine.

this work four tracers were prepared with increasing similarity to the compound used to form the immunogen. The first of these, the most dissimilar to the immunogen, showed no binding to the antiserum. The other three (described as 1 to 3, Table 5.4) however all showed good binding, with the titre of the antisera increasing as the similarity between the tracer and the immunogen increased. The aim of this work was to produce an assay that was specific for the controlled drugs amphetamine and *N*-methylamphetamine but which would not detect the commonly prescribed drugs such as ephedrine and phenylpropanolamine. The data in Table 5.4 show how the specificity of the assay could be effectively 'tuned' by chemically modifying the tracer and introducing bridge recognition. The marked similarity between the tracer 3 and the immunogen, meant that the tracer was bound with greater affinity and hence it could only be displaced by those compounds which also possessed the same structural features, amphetamine and *N*-methylamphetamine in this case.

Monitoring iodination reactions

Although the synthesis of iodinated tracers *per se* can be relatively quick and straightforward, establishing which of the reaction products is the desired tracer of interest, and purifying this tracer can in the first instance be difficult. This section therefore is devoted to techniques and tips for monitoring iodination reactions and separating the reaction products to obtain the desired tracer in pure form and at high specific activity.

High-performance liquid chromatography (HPLC)

HPLC with its high resolving power is a useful tool for reaction monitoring, although the chromatographic run time can be a limiting factor if reaction times are short. Another problem with this approach relates to injection reproducibility. Radioiodine has a habit of sticking to plastic-type materials and the seals and rotors of the commonly used HPLC injection valves are no exception. This can frequently lead to 'ghost' peaks or apparent loss of radioactivity as the valve becomes 'conditioned'. At best this can be annoying and at worst highly infuriating as one tries to rationalise why peaks keep appearing and disappearing. A further problem is that the compound of interest may not be eluted from the HPLC column under the conditions used, or it may elute with exceptionally long retention such that it is lost in the background radioactivity. For these reasons the use of HPLC is not recommended here for reaction monitoring.

Thin-layer chromatography (TLC)

The method of choice for iodination reaction monitoring is thin-layer chromatography (TLC). TLC systems are usually available for the compound of interest and these serve as a useful starting point for monitoring any iodination reaction. In the author's laboratory chromatography is usually carried out using adsorption (normal-phase) type systems with silica gel as the stationary phase. Merck TLC plates (5 × 10 cm) have proved particularly useful, offering good resolution in a relatively short run time (typically 10 to 15 min for most systems). In this way a number of reactions can be readily monitored and results obtained whilst the reaction is still underway. TLC also has the advantage that it does not suffer the problems of carry-over as a result of 'memory effects' often seen with HPLC. Furthermore all the material spotted onto the plate will be visible, i.e. there are no problems of non-elution.

Typically, small samples of the reaction mixture, e.g. 0.1 to 0.5 μl, are spotted directly onto the plate. This is conveniently carried out using a 1 or 0.5 μl syringe which are obtainable from companies such as SGE, Milton Keynes, UK. Although the syringe becomes indelibly contaminated, this poses no problem as unbound radioactivity can be washed out between samples using a suitable solvent, such that cross contamination is negligible. As small sample volumes are used in this procedure, the spotting of aqueous buffered reaction mixtures is also possible without detriment to the chromatography. Also spotting of the reaction mixture onto the plate effectively stops the reaction. Application of the starting material, e.g. sodium ^{125}I-iodide or Bolton–Hunter reagent, to the TLC plate facilitates the identification of the spots and location of the desired tracer and reaction by-products.

Location of the radioactive materials as spots on the TLC plate can be effected in a number of ways. Some laboratories will possess radio-scanners or linear analysers which, as well as giving precise quantitative radioactivity measurements, will also provide Rf data on all detected spots. These instruments are rather costly and not readily available in every laboratory.

A simpler and more versatile alternative is the use of a modified scintillation meter. All laboratories carrying out work with radioiodine should have a scintillation meter suitable for the detection of gamma radiation, e.g. a series 900 Minimonitor fitted with a type 42A X-ray probe from Mini-Instruments Ltd, Burnham-on-Crouch, Essex, UK. This type of instrument is essential for contamination monitoring, but by simple modification of the probe head this can be readily converted into a sensitive and specific TLC radiochemical scanner capable of giving rapid semi-quantitative information. The modification merely requires the placing of a piece of lead sheet approximately 2 to 3 mm thick over the photographic lens cap that acts as the probe cover. In the centre of this lead shield is cut a narrow slit, typically 7 × 2 mm, through which the radiation can pass. In use, the modified probe is head is passed along the underside of the TLC plate, following the track of the spot, from the origin to the solvent front. The probe head is orientated so that the widest part of the slit is at right angles to the chromatographic track.

By monitoring the detector signal, either from the meter or via the audible output, the spots can be detected and marked on the surface of the plate with a soft pencil. This system offers reasonable resolution and good sensitivity; spots of approximately 100 nCi can be easily detected. Greater sensitivity can be obtained by increasing the length of the slit from 7 × 2 to 7 × 5 mm, although this will result in a small loss in resolution. Location of all spots on the TLC plate is very rapid, and the technique also gives semi-quantitative data. As well as being used for monitoring reactions to determine yield etc., this approach is particularly useful for assessing the purity of radiochemical reagents prior to their use.

Figure 5.9 shows the results of monitoring a conjugation reaction between a derivative of an angiotensin converting enzyme (ACE) inhibitor and Bolton–Hunter reagent, using two different TLC systems. The first employs a non-polar mixture of hexane and ethyl acetate (1 : 1). In this system the Bolton–Hunter reagent runs with an Rf of 0.50. By making two applications of Bolton–Hunter reagent and over-spotting one with ammonia solution (approx. 1 µl of 25%) it is possible to produce the major by-product of the conjugation process, 3-^{125}I-iodo-4-hydroxy-phenylpropionic acid. In the ethyl acetate/hexane system this compound has poor mobility and runs with an Rf of 0.09. It is easily identified however and distinguished from the highly polar desired product which does not run and is detected at the origin.

The second system in Figure 5.9 was selected because it gave reasonable migration of the precursor (and the labelled compound). In this system the non-polar Bolton–Hunter reagent runs near the solvent front (Rf 0.92) closely followed by the

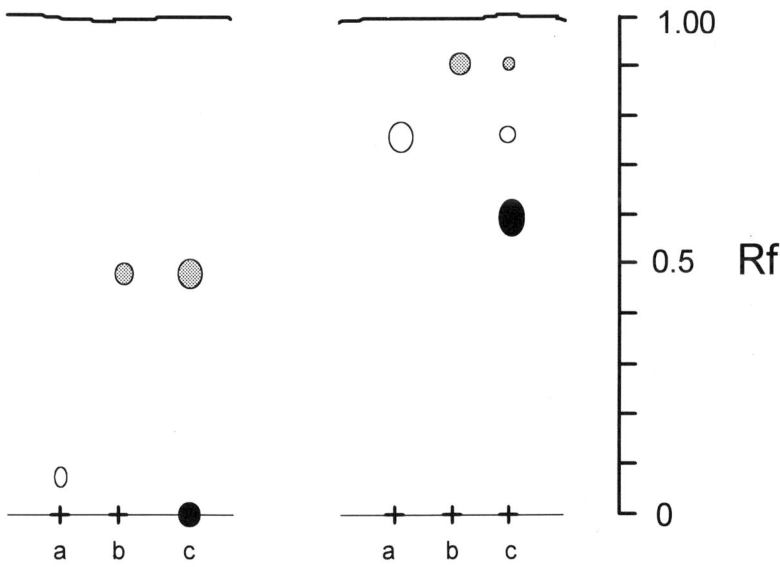

Figure 5.9 TLC chromatograms obtained following the reaction of an ACE inhibitor analogue with Bolton–Hunter reagent. The plates were Merck silica gel run in ethyl acetate/hexane (1/1) – (A) – and acetonitrile/water (60/40) – (B). The samples were (a) Bolton–Hunter reagent overspotted with ammonia solution to give 3-^{125}I-iodo-4-hydroxyphenylpropionic acid, (b) Bolton–Hunter reagent and (c) the reaction mixture sampled after 5 min. The radioactive spots were detected using a modified scintillation meter.

propionic acid by-product (Rf 0.77). The desired radiotracer is clearly visible at an Rf of 0.62 and well separated from the other materials.

Purification of tracers

Iodinated tracers

Once prepared it is usual practice to purify the crude radiolabelled material. This purification serves several different functions. First it removes reaction debris or by-products which may subsequently chemically degrade the tracer, e.g. metabisulphite. It also removes labelled but non-antigenic impurities, e.g. ^{125}I. Most importantly, however, it can be used to increase the specific activity of the tracer through the removal of antigenic material which may or may not be radiolabelled.

In certain instances where high sensitivity and as a consequence high specific activity are required, thorough purification is necessary. This may not always be that simple, as shown by the data in Table 5.2, which lists the antigenic and radioactive components present after conjugation of ^{125}I-iodohistamine to THC-11-oic acid using the mixed anhydride procedure (Law *et al.*, 1982). The unlabelled histamine and its derivatives were the result of carry over of histamine from the iodination reaction. The large number and wide range of materials present (seven in total) necessitated a selective purification procedure in order to obtain a tracer with maximal specific activity. Purification was effected in this instance by solvent extraction followed by paper chromatography, although HPLC would have been equally satisfactory.

Gel permeation chromatography has been used widely in the past, particularly for the purification of labelled peptides and proteins. This process serves to separate the low-molecular-weight iodide from the high-molecular-weight labelled tracer. In the labelling of small molecules this type of technique is of limited use and it will not be discussed further.

Solvent extraction

When a high specific activity tracer is not required it is possible to effect partial purification through simple solvent extraction. This procedure has been successfully applied in the radioiodination of morphine and 4-hydroxyphenobarbitone described above (Mason *et al.*, 1981; Mason and Law, 1982). By careful control of the aqueous pH prior to extraction the resulting extract only contained drug related material (labelled and unlabelled). Although this resulted in tracers with specific activity lower than theoretical because of the presence of unlabelled material, they were found to be perfectly adequate for the intended assay without extensive purification.

Thin-layer chromatography (TLC)

Although the small masses involved in radioiodinations allow the use of analytical TLC plates for preparative work, there are a number of problems associated with this approach which preclude its general use. The removal of the radioactive spot from the TLC plate necessitates scraping the silica. This is a potentially hazardous procedure, giving rise to radioactive particulate material. Given the relative buoyancy of silica in air, carrying out this type of procedure in a fume cupboard would merely serve to scatter the material everywhere.

A more practical alternative is the use of ITLC (instant thin-layer chromatography) materials from Gelman, Ann Arbor, Michigan, USA. The ITLC plates are made of glass fibre impregnated with silica, or silicic acid. They allow reasonable loadings, and very fast separations (hence the name) with adequate resolution. Their great advantage however is that they can be cut with scissors without producing radioactive silica gel dust or flakes. Thus once the spot has been located on the plate it can be simply cut from the sheet of ITLC material and eluted with an appropriate solvent.

Elution of the radioactive material is conveniently brought about by hanging the strip of ITLC material from the end of a bent hypodermic needle connected to a syringe (Figure 5.10), and passing a suitable solvent through it. Elution is normally accomplished in high yield, typically greater than 95 per cent, through the use of a highly eluotropic solvent. This can be either the mobile phase enriched with the polar component or an alcohol containing a small amount of acid or base. The more obvious procedure of soaking the piece of cut plate in a solvent with or without sonication is not recommended as this is much less efficient than the above method.

The only disadvantages associated with the use of the ITLC materials relate to the lower resolution than that seen with standard silica gel plates, and the lower

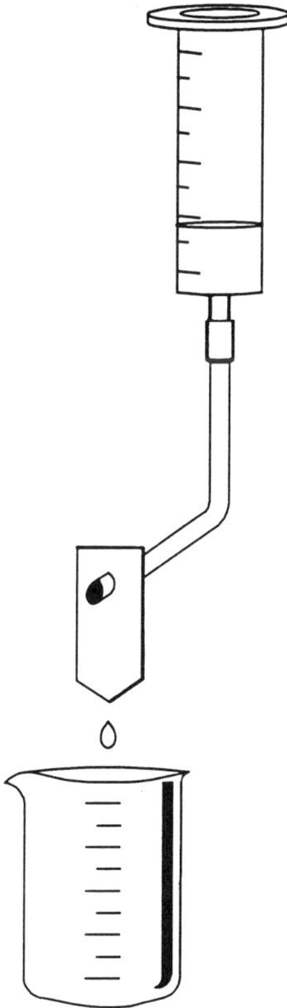

Figure 5.10 A method for the elution of radioactive material from a section of ITLC plate.

polarity of the stationary phase which necessitates the use of more weakly eluotropic solvents than would be used on standard silica phases. These disadvantages however are more than compensated for by the simplicity of use.

High-performance liquid chromatography (HPLC)

When the reaction mixture to be purified is complex, requiring high separating power, preparative HPLC is the obvious choice. Using reversed-phase HPLC, most aqueous reaction mixtures can be injected directly onto the column with the minimum of pretreatment. Memory effects, leading to cross contamination can be a particular problem especially if the same column and injection system are used for both analytical and preparative work, where the amounts of radiolabelled material injected can be up to 10^5-fold different.

Experience has shown that the major source of carry-over between injections results from binding of radioiodide and radiotracers to the seals and rotors in Rheodyne-type injection valves. In an attempt to overcome this problem we have investigated the use of on-column injection, a technique used in the early days of HPLC. Although successful in overcoming the problem of carry-over, technical problems associated with the injection technique itself meant that it was less than satisfactory for routine use. A more satisfactory solution, where analytical and preparative separations are required, is to use a separate injection valve and column system for each type of procedure and in so doing avoid the problem altogether.

Detection following an HPLC separation can be effected in a number of ways. Technically the simplest method is to collect the eluent as it elutes from the column using a standard fraction collector. The radioactivity in each fraction can then be determined using a hand-held scintillation monitor or if more precise data is required using a gamma counter. The data so generated can then be used to plot a radiochromatogram giving the retention volume and yield of the various components.

The use of a gamma counter for assessing the radioactivity in HPLC fractions has one major disadvantage however, especially if the fractions are counted directly. The relatively large amounts of activity used in radioiodinations can result in the maximum count rate of the gamma counter being exceeded. Should this happen the data may look rational, but the overall radiochemical yield will be artificially reduced, with that of the high yielding components being most affected. This problem can be easily overcome however by selecting for counting small aliquots of each fraction, although this adds an extra stage into the procedure. It is also still necessary to ensure that the count rate of the detector is not exceeded.

An alternative procedure exists when multi-head gamma counters are used. In this case the plastic cassette holding the samples is simply raised out of the counting wells and the counts for the sample giving the highest counts checked. If the counts do not fall on raising the samples then the count rate was saturated and the sample casset should be raised further and the procedure repeated. When the count in the most active sample is seen to fall the detector is no longer being saturated and meaningful counts will be obtained from all samples at that position.

Although the above methods can be satisfactory, the optimal method, both for analytical or preparative HPLC applications is the use of an online radiochemical monitor designed for gamma-emitting isotopes. There are a number of systems available, such as the Beckman 170 Radiochemical Monitor, or the Gamma-ram from Lablogic. Although these are relatively sophisticated microprocessor controlled systems, the detector itself is merely a modified scintillation probe which employs a sodium iodide scintillator and a photomultiplier tube. The flow cell, which in the Beckman instrument is simply the PTFE or stainless steel tubing forming the exit from the HPLC column, is brought into close contact with the detector head. The controller module gives an output in two forms (Figure 5.11). The first is a typical analogue chromatographic signal which is fed to a chart recorder to give a radiochromatogram. The second is a numerical output to a printer which lists the retention times and the percentage of radioactivity associated with each peak. The detectors can also be connected to a fraction collector which is then started at the point of injection. This can also be set to collect timed fractions or by peak (as in the example shown). Although relatively expensive (approximately £5000), the use of such instruments is highly recommended as it greatly simplifies the isolation of the desired product.

Any mode of HPLC can be used for tracer purification, although reversed-phase HPLC (RP-HPLC), the most widely used form of the technique, is particularly appropriate for the purification of iodinated radiotracers. Direct iodination of a molecule or conjugation to iodohistamine for example will generally increase the lipophilicity of the tracer in relation to the starting material. This increase in lipophilicity is accompanied by an increase in retention on a RP-HPLC column. If a RP-HPLC system is available for the starting material then this could be used for purification of the tracer in the knowledge that the tracer will elute later than the starting material. To ensure that all the radioactive material is eluted from the column the use of gradient elution is recommended, at least in the first instance while the method is under development. Using this approach the crude tracer is injected onto the column and eluted with around 10 column volumes of eluent low in organic modifer, i.e. around 10 per cent methanol, suitably buffered to give good chromatographic performance for the starting material or preferably the tracer, when this can be predicted. Using a standard 100 × 4.6 mm column, 10 column volumes would be 10 to 12 ml. The procedure is then repeated using 10 column volumes of, for example 30, 60 and finally around 90 per cent methanol. In this way all the radioactivity should be eluted from the column. Because the eluent is invisible to the radiochemical detector a flat chromatographic base line will be obtained.

Where it is considered necessary to monitor the cold starting materials as well as radioactive materials a UV detector can be connected in series with the radiochemical detector. Because of the large volume flow cells typically employed with radiochemical detectors the UV detector should always be the first in line connected directly to the HPLC column. In adopting such an approach it must be accepted that the flow cell and associated connection tubing of the UV detector may become contaminated with radioiodine and be difficult to decontaminate. As a result of this contamination problem it may be necessary to commit the detector full time to radioactive work.

Using the above recommended methods most tracers can be routinely prepared and purified to high specific activity in a few hours.

Tritiated tracers

Following custom synthesis, tritium labelled tracers can be supplied as a crude reaction mixture which requires some purification to give a usable tracer. The separa-

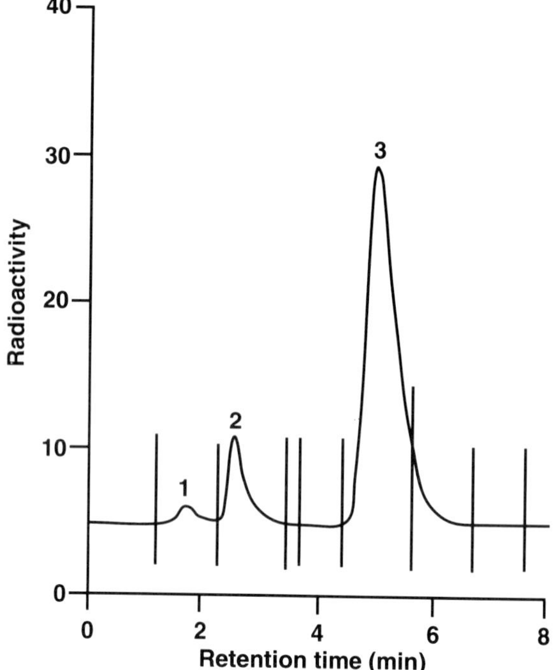

AUTO COUNT START

FLOW RATE	: 1.000 ML/MIN	CELL LENGTH	: 26.00 CM	TUBE I.D.	: 0.763 MM
VOLUME	: 118 UL	RESIDENCE TIME	: 0.1188 MIN	NORM FACT	: 1.0000E+ 0
SCALE	: 200.0 KCPM	OFF SET	: 0.100 KCPM	BACKGROUND	: 0.500 KCPM
EXIT LENGTH	: 66.00 CM	FRAC TIME	: 1.200 MIN	FRAC DELAY	: 0.301 MIN

PEAK NUMBER	FRACTION NUMBER	FRACTION CPM*NORM FACT	RETENTION TIME	PEAK CPM*NORM FACT
	1	**********		
	2	1549		
	3	-2.580E+1		
1	4	11197	1.73	11197
2	5	41794		
2	6	1149	2.56	42943
	7	3397		
3	8	255415		
3	9	28579	4.92	283994
	10	6781		
		RUN TOTAL 349837	RUN TIME 7.83	PEAK TOTAL 338135

PEAK NUMBER	PERCENT OF TOTAL
1	3.31
2	12.70
3	83.99

Figure 5.11 Typical output from a Beckman 170 radioactivity detector. The upper half shows the analogue output following separation of a crude reaction mixture. Three radiolabelled compounds are identified. The lower part of the figure shows the digital output which identifies the peaks and their relative proportions etc. The third peak, the desired radiotracer, is shown to be produced in more than 80 per cent yield.

tion and purification procedure used will depend very much on the nature of the compound and the complexity of the reaction mixture. In general any of the procedures discussed above with respect to radioiodine can be used here, although HPLC would usually be the method of choice. As the crude reaction mixture may contain many curies of tritiated material care must be exercised in the handling and purification of this material.

Tritiated tracers on storage, even under optimal conditions, will frequently undergo radiolysis to give impurities which may adversely affect the assay. As a result of tritium exchange reactions the major impurity may frequently be tritiated storage solvent, e.g. tritiated water or ethanol. Such volatile impurities can be removed by gentle evaporation in a stream of nitrogen, taking care to ensure that the radioactive vapours given off are well contained or preferably trapped for subsequent disposal. Where other impurities are present some form of chromatographic separation will be necessary.

Figure 5.12(A) shows an HPLC chromatogram of a sample of ^{3}H-xamoterol which on storage in ethanol underwent partial decomposition. The material shows two major impurities in addition to the ^{3}H-xamoterol, the first of which is ^{3}H-ethanol. When used in an immunoassay this impure tracer not only gave reduced binding, but more importantly it resulted in very high assay blanks since the low-molecular-weight ^{3}H-ethanol did not absorb to the charcoal used in the separation procedure. The presence of the non-volatile impurity (peak 2) necessitated the use of a chromatographic clean-up procedure to purify the tracer for immunoassay work.

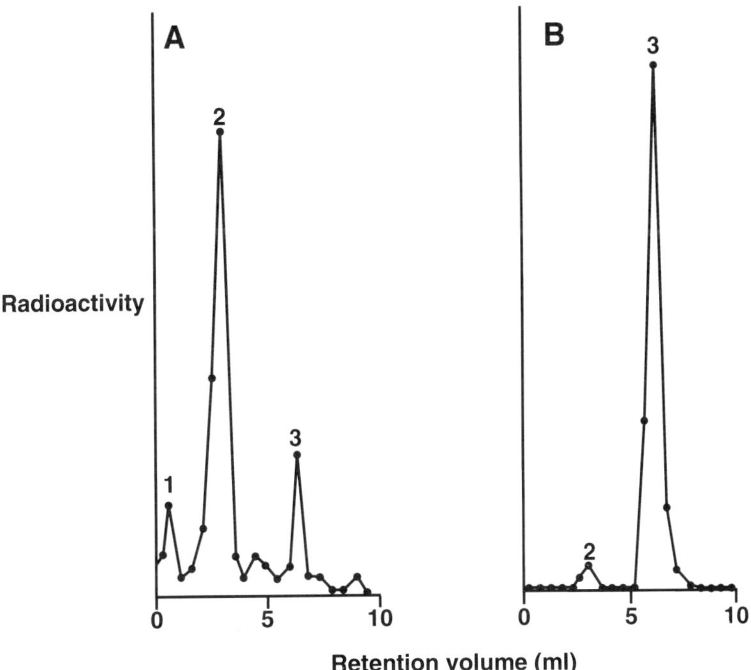

Figure 5.12 Radiochromatograms of ^{3}H-xamoterol after several years storage in ethanol (A) and after purification by HPLC and storage in ethanol for 3 months (B). Peak 1 = ^{3}H-ethanol, 2 = unknown impurity, peak 3 = ^{3}H-xamoterol.

To minimise the injection of large amounts of radioactivity onto the HPLC column the ^{3}H-ethanol was first removed with a stream of nitrogen in a fume cupboard. The residue was then redissolved in HPLC eluent, chromatographed and the eluent collected as 0.5 ml fractions. Small aliquots of each fraction (ca. 5 μl) were then taken for scintillation counting. On the basis of this data three fractions corresponding to the xamoterol peak were combined and diluted with ethanol to give a stock solution of ^{3}H-xamoterol. Repeat HPLC analysis of this material gave the chromatogram shown in Figure 5.12(B) which clearly shows the sample to be relatively pure.

Tracer assessment

Tracer assessment involves determination of the purity and specific activity of the tracer and ultimately determining that the tracer actually gives the desired assay characteristics.

Tracer purity

If the purification of the tracer is carried out by HPLC for example and peaks associated with both hot and cold materials can be identified, then it can be assumed that the tracer is totally pure with 100 per cent of theoretical specific activity. Where a less effective purification has been carried out, the purity can be checked using any of the chromatographic techniques mentioned above. If HPLC is employed care should be taken to ensure that the injection valve and column are free of radioactive contamination which could lead to underestimation of purity.

An alternative though somewhat cruder method of checking purity is to incubate the tracer with an excess of antiserum, typically a 1/10 or a 1/100 dilution. If the binding is high, i.e. greater than 90 per cent, it is probable although not certain that the tracer has reasonable radiochemical purity. If the binding is low then the radiochemical purity is probably also low and equal to the level of binding seen with an excess of antiserum. There are other reasons for low binding to an excess of antiserum, such as the tracer being non-antigenic resulting from some structural change taking place on iodination. Alternatively the tracer could contain a large excess of cold antigenic material, i.e. it has low specific activity. If the approaches outlined above have been followed then low binding should indicate low purity.

Tracer specific activity

The specific activity of ^{125}I tracers is somewhat difficult to determine, especially if the tracer is chemically different to the analyte, and as a result the binding affinities of the two are different. Under these conditions the only unequivocal way of determining specific activity is to prepare and compare both hot and cold tracer (i.e. the analyte labelled with ^{125}I and also the natural isotope of iodine; ^{127}I). The method of comparison can be any sensitive quantitative analytical technique, even the immunoassay in which the tracer is to be used (Morris, 1976). The problem of radioactive contamination, especially if expensive analytical instrumentation is used, seriously limits the analytical approaches that can be taken. The simplest procedure however, is to use a well characterised and powerful separation procedure at the purification stage and therefore make the not unreasonable assumption that specific activity is 100 per cent of theoretical!, i.e. 2200 Ci/mmol.

After determining that the tracer has good chemical and radiochemical purity it is still necessary to demonstrate that it gives the desired assay performance. Despite the tracer having high specific activity, if it has structural features which are common to the immunogen but not to the analyte, then reduced assay sensitivity or inappropriate specificity may ensue (see the examples discussed above under bridge recognition). It is essential therefore that the effect of the tracer on the assay characteristics is fully evaluated and understood before validation begins.

Stability of radiotracers

The optimum conditions for the storage of radiotracers to ensure maximal stability will vary, not only with the isotope, but also with the nature of the labelled compound. The rates of decomposition of tracers used for immunoassays as quoted by Amersham International plc are given in Table 5.5. To be able to reproduce these optimal data a number of precautions have to be taken.

As with most radiolabelled tracers the higher the specific activity, the poorer the radiochemical stability. The specific activity of the tracer should therefore be no greater than is necessary for the assay for which it is intended. The rates of all chemical reactions are reduced with decreasing temperature (approximately twofold for each 10°C), and in general reducing the temperature at which a radiotracer is stored can improve its stability through reducing the rate of primary external or secondary chemical effects. However, exceptions do exist and each tracer should be investigated to determine the optimal conditions for storage. An interesting example is presented below where the lowest storage temperature was not that which conferred greatest stability on the tracer.

The effect of temperature

The optimum conditions for the storage of an antibiotic metabolite labelled with Bolton–Hunter reagent was studied (Ballard *et al.*, 1996). The data in Figure 5.13 show the stability of the tracer over a 2 month storage period, determined in this instance by antiserum binding which should be around 50 per cent for freshly prepared tracer. It can be seen that although reduced temperature has some effect on

Table 5.5 Typical rates of decomposition of radiotracers used in immunoassays stored under optimal conditions

Nuclide	Rate of decomposition
^{14}C	1–3% per year
^{3}H	1–3% per month
^{125}I	5% per month

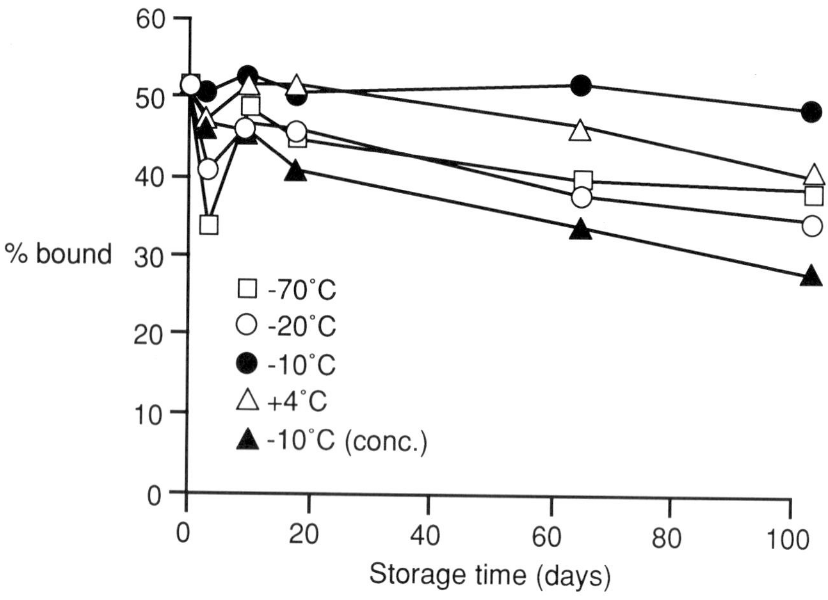

Figure 5.13 Stability data for an iodinated antibiotic derivative stored in acetonitrile/phosphate buffer at different temperatures. All samples were 10 μCi/ml except (conc.) which was 300 μCi/ml. Stability is indicated by the level of binding to antisera.

stability, optimal storage was achieved at −10°C, and not at −20°C or −70°C as would have been predicted. This is explained in this case by the fact that at temperatures below −10°C the storage solvent (acetonitrile/phosphate buffer) froze, and it was this change of state that actually promoted decomposition. Although temperature played some part (compare −10°C with 4°C and −20°C with −70°C), in this instance the optimal storage temperature was the lowest that could be achieved without inducing freezing of the solvent, i.e. −10°C. Similar effects have been reported in the past for ^{3}H-labelled thymidine (Evans and Stanford, 1963). The data in Figure 5.13 also show clearly the effect of concentration on stability. As well as temperature being important, maximal stability was only achieved when the radioactive concentration was 100 μCi/ml or less. It is worth noting in this example that the tracer was actually stable and usable for in excess of 100 days. In the author's experience this is typical for small molecules labelled with ^{125}I.

The effect of storage solvent

The storage solvent can also have a profound effect on the stability of the tracer. Figure 5.14 shows stability data for a ^{125}I-labelled ACE inhibitor, assessed in this instance by binding to excess antisera. The interesting point about this compound is that the poor stability was exhibited in assay buffer which would generally be considered advantageous, in contrast to methanol (data not shown) where the compound showed excellent stability for at least 4 months. The decomposition process in this case was first order with 50 per cent of the antigenic activity being lost in around 20 days.

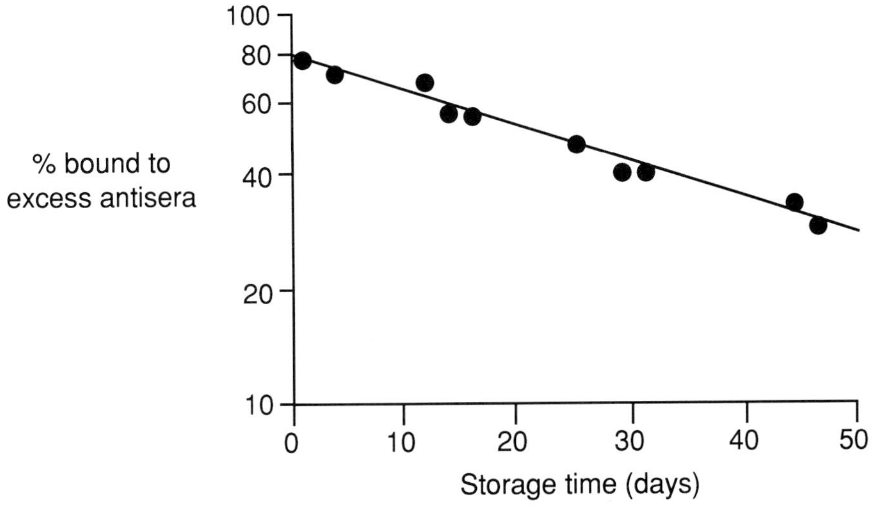

Figure 5.14 Stability data for an iodinated ACE inhibitor stored in assay buffer: phosphate 0.1 M, pH 7.4, containing BGG (0.2%). Stability is indicated by the level of binding to an excess of antisera.

Effect of storage container

The storage vessel can also play an important role in tracer stability. In a number of examples in our laboratory the use of plastic containers as opposed to glass has been found to lead to greater tracer stability. In particular polyethylene liquid scintillation vials have been found to be especially effective in conferring improved stability on a variety of radiotracers. The deleterious effects of glass containers may be attributable to the catalytic effect of the hydroxyls on the glass surface.

As the process of self-radiolysis occurs through reactive intermediates, such as hydroxyl radicals etc., the avoidance of aqueous solutions is recommended where possible. If aqueous media must be used then the inclusion of radical scavengers such as ethanol, or *N,N′*-dimethylthiourea is recommended. The latter has been recently shown by NEN (Kirshenbaum *et al.*, 1989) to be highly effective in stabilising tritiated compounds, although it has not been evaluated with ^{125}I-labelled compounds.

As part of any assay development programme it is necessary to define clearly the optimum conditions for storage of the radiotracer. It is necessary to investigate the influence of solvent, temperature, container type (e.g. plastic or glass) and concentration. Where problems occur the use of radical scavengers may need to be studied. This work should be initiated as soon as relatively stable assay conditions have been defined. It must be borne in mind however during the initial stages of the assay development, that the tracer may not be stored under optimal conditions. Therefore, day to day changes in assay parameters such as binding at zero dose and non-specific binding may not be because of the assay variable being investigated, e.g. antibody dilution or separation method, but they may actually be artefacts resulting from tracer decomposition. In general when there is no evidence to the contrary, keep the radioactive concentration and temperature low, use simple alcohols as solvents and store in plastic containers.

Conclusions

The preceding discussions have focused very much on ^{125}I which has a lot to offer as a tracer for immunoassay. If a ^{3}H tracer is available, having been synthesised for other purposes, perhaps then this could be investigated initially. In terms of specific activity it will not give the same assay sensitivity afforded by a ^{125}I tracer, but it may be suitable for some assays.

Where high sensitivity is required then ^{125}I is the tracer of choice and the following scheme, which is a summary of the foregoing discussion, represents a good overall approach to tracer synthesis and purification.

The favoured approach to iodination involves the use of Bolton–Hunter reagent, therefore arrangements should be made to have a suitable primary or secondary amine in the molecule to be labelled. If the same amine is to be used for immunogen synthesis, then to avoid any potential problems associated with bridge recognition the protein linking chemistry must be carefully selected. The use of conjugation reactions which lead to an amide linkage in the immunogen should be avoided and a method such as the glutaraldehyde procedure used.

Initially the iodination should be carried out on a small scale to determine the optimum reaction conditions, i.e. solvent, pH, reaction time etc. This can be conveniently done by sub-aliquoting the Bolton–Hunter reagent into small septum-sealed vials (32 × 6 mm I.D.) such as an HPLC microinjection vial (e.g. 03-CVG from Chromacol, London, UK). Using this approach 10 small scale reactions using 50 μCi in 10 μl of solvent can be carried out from a 0.5 mCi sample of the iodination reagent. TLC is the method of choice for monitoring the reaction and in many instances this can be modified to give a preparative procedure. To produce a high specific activity tracer the use of HPLC is strongly recommended.

The tracer should be characterised in terms of purity, binding characteristics and its ability to generate the necessary assay specificity. The stability of the tracer should not be assumed but carefully defined with respect to storage solvent, temperature, concentration and container.

References

Ballard, P., Stafford, L. E. & Law, B. (1996) *J. Pharm. Biomed. Anal.*, **14**, 409.

Bolton, A. E. & Hunter, W.M. (1973) *Biochem. J.*, **133**, 529.

Corrie, J. E. T., Hunter, W. M. & MacPherson, J. S. (1981) *Clin. Chem.*, **27**, 594.

Evans, E. A. & Stanford, F. G. (1963) *Nature*, **209**, 762.

Foster, N. I., Dannals, R., Bruns, H. D. & Heindel, N. D. (1981) *J. Radioanal. Chem.*, **65**, 95.

Fraker, P. J. & Speck, J. C. (1978) *Biochem. Biophys. Res. Commun.*, **80**, 849.

Gilby, E. D., Jeffecoate, S. L. & Edwards, R. (1973) *J. Endocrinol.*, **58**, 20.

Goddard, C. P., Law, B., Mason, P. A. & Stead, A. H. (1986) *J. Label. Compds.*, **23**, 383.

Grassi, J., Maclouf, J. & Pradelles, P. (1987) In: Patrano, C. & Peskar, B. A. (eds) *Radioimmunoassay in Basic and Clinical Pharmacology.* Springer-Verlag, Berlin.

Hunter, W. M. & Greenwood, F. C. (1962) *Nature*, **194**, 495.

Kirshenbaum, K., Blanchette, M. & Rigdon, M. (1989) *DuPont Biotech Update*, **4**, 8.

LANGONE, J. J. (1980) *Methods in Enzymology*, **70**, 221.
LAW, B., MASON, P. A., MOFFAT, A. C. & KING, L. J. (1982) *J. Label. Compds.*, **19**, 915.
MASON, P. A. & LAW, B. (1982) *J. Label. Compds.*, **19**, 357.
MASON, P. A., LAW, B. & ARDREY, R. E. (1981) *J. Label. Compds.*, **18**, 1497.
MASON, P. A., LAW, B. & MOFFAT, A. C. (1983) *J. Immunoassay*, **4**, 83.
MASON, P. A., ROWAN, K. M., LAW, B. & MOFFAT, A. C. (1984) *Analyst*, **109**, 1213.
MORRIS, B. J. (1976) *Clin. Chim. Acta*, **73**, 213.
NARS, P. W. & HUNTER, W. M. (1973) *J. Endocrinol.*, **57**, 47.
NORDBLOM, G. D., WEBB, R., COUNSELL, R. E. & ENGLAND, B. G. (1981) *Steroids*, **38**, 2.
PILLAI, M. R. A., GUPTE, J. H., JYOTSNA, T. & MANI, R. S. (1987) *J. Radioanal. Nucl. Chem.*, **116**, 193.
SEEVERS, R. H. & COUNSELL, R. E. (1982) *Chem. Rev.*, **82**, 575.
TANTCHOU, J. K. & SLAUNWHITE, W. R. (1979) *Prep. Biochem.*, **9**, 379.
(1980) *J. Immunoassay*, **1**, 129.
WHITE, A., SMITH, G. N., CROSBY, S. R. & RATCLIFFE, W. A. (1985) *J. Steroid Biochem.*, **23**, 981.
WOLTANSKI, K. P., BESCH, W., KEILACKER, H., ZIEGLER, M. & KOHNERT, K. D. (1990) *Exp. Clin. Endocrinol.*, **95**, 39.
WOOD, F. T., WU, M. M. & GERHART, J. C. (1975) *Anal. Biochem.*, **69**, 339.
YALOW, R. S. & BERSON, S. A. (1960) *J. Clin. Invest.*, **39**, 1157.

6

Radioimmunoassay development and optimisation

B. LAW

Zeneca Pharmaceuticals, Macclesfield

R. A. BIDDLECOMBE

GlaxoWellcome Research and Development, Beckenham

Introduction

This chapter will concentrate on the steps needed to develop and optimise a competitive radioimmunoassay, making the assumption that a high quality tracer is available. The general principles that will be outlined are also applicable to other immunoassays, such as fluoro- and chemiluminescent immunoassays. The development and optimisation of enzyme-linked immunosorbent assays (ELISA), which are different in a number of respects to competitive radioimmunoassays, will be dealt with separately (Chapter 7).

The initial discussion will focus primarily on the development of a liquid-phase RIA since this is the simplest and hence the quickest and easiest to establish. The final selection of assay format, which relates principally to the separation stage, i.e. solid or liquid phase, is influenced by the required sensitivity and precision as well as the expected sample throughput, available equipment, financial constraints and personal preferences. Consideration will be given to solid-phase formats in the section on optimisation.

Before beginning the assay development work it is important to have a clear idea of the exact use to which the assay is to be put as this will have some influence on development goals such as precision and sensitivity.

The first experiment in the development of a new assay using a collection of untested reagents is probably the most difficult of all to design and execute successfully. The outcome of this first experiment and hence the success of the development work will not only be affected by the quality of antibody and tracer but a wide range of other factors such as buffer type and molarity, protein additives, incubation volume and temperature as well as incubation time, separation system and sample matrix; to mention but a few. Inappropriate selection of any one of these could lead to erroneous conclusions being drawn and perfectly good antibody reagents being discarded under the mistaken assumption that they are useless. It is essential therefore that the starting conditions are carefully selected to give the maximum chance of obtaining the desired outcome. This can only be done through experience and the expertise on which this chapter is firmly based. It is worth pointing out that the conditions selected and the assumptions made at this early stage can have an enormous influence on the final assay. Through inappropriate choice of starting conditions it is possible to obtain a working assay but this may not be the most optimal assay. It is worth remembering then that in immunoassay development, where you start from ultimately controls where you end up!

The development and optimisation of an assay can be divided into five distinct phases:

1 Selection of basic operating conditions, e.g. tracer concentration, buffer, incubation temperature etc.
2 Selection of separating system(s)
3 Assessment and selection of antisera
4 Introduction of matrix
5 Optimisation of assay conditions to give the desired assay characteristics

Sample matrix is not introduced until a working assay has been established in buffer. This decision is based on the fact that analysis of analyte in a matrix other than assay buffer can be a difficult procedure and hence to avoid complicating the early stages of assay development this stage is considered separately.

It is strongly recommended that before performing any experimental work a written plan of the proposed experiment is prepared which should be firmly adhered to. All dilutions, volumes and incubation times should be recorded; it is also important to take note of batches of reagents etc. It is all too easy to generate meaningless results because small changes have not been recorded. Although this may seem obvious, it is a major reason for wasted time and muddled development work.

Equipment for RIA

One of the big advantages of RIA is that apart from a counter, the equipment required is readily available in most laboratories. Some care however needs to be taken in the selection of certain items and guidance is given below.

Assay tubes

For most assays, polystyrene or polypropylene disposable test tubes will prove satisfactory although care needs to be exercised with certain analytes, particularly those which are highly lipophilic. These types of compounds can non-specifically adsorb to plastics resulting in high non-specific binding (nsb). This adsorption phenomenon is related to the surface energy of the plastic and in this respect polypropylene is probably superior to polystyrene in that it has a lower surface energy (van Krevelen, 1990) and in the authors' experience is less adsorbing. If high tube binding is observed it is worth investigating tubes from different manufacturers or even different batches from the same manufacturer as batch-to-batch variability can be a problem. Glass tubes have been widely used in the past although in most laboratories these have been replaced by a range of plastic tubes, which are easier to dispose of. When used for radioiodine counting, glass tubes also have the disadvantage of giving around 25 per cent less counts than plastic tubes, depending on the thickness of the tube wall.

In terms of size, tubes of 75 mm in length with a diameter of 10 or 12 mm are widely used. The wider diameter is preferred as this allows better access to the bottom of the tube with a pipette tip. Tubes with conical bottoms are also preferred as these give a more compact pellet at the separation stage, however some counters have difficulties with these types of tubes and some form of adapter may be necessary. Ultimately the choice is dictated by that available from the manufacturers: companies such as Sarstedt (Leicester, UK) and LIP (Shipley, UK) offer a reasonable selection.

A selection of racks capable of holding up to around 200 assay tubes, as well as standard solutions and antibody dilutions will also be required, these can be obtained from companies such as Denley (Billingshurst, Sussex, UK).

Pipettes

For most work a set of air displacement pipettes capable of delivering volumes from 10 μl to 5000 μl is required. If the samples to be dispensed are highly viscous or pipetting of mobile organic liquids is required, then positive displacement pipettes covering a similar range are recommended.

For repetitive dispensing a repeat dispenser such as the Eppendorf multipette is highly recommended. From a single filling it can dispense 50 aliquots of 50 μl, 100 μl or 250 μl for example, with excellent precision and accuracy.

Vortex mixers

For small scale development work a standard laboratory vortex mixer will prove adequate. When working with large batches of tubes however, a multivortex mixer such as the Multi-tube Vortexer from Alpha Laboratories (Eastleigh, Hants, UK) is particularly useful. It is important however to test the mixing efficiency of such an instrument since this is controlled somewhat by the tubes and the design of the racks which must hold them reasonably tightly.

Centrifuges

Most laboratory centrifuges capable of achieving gravitational accelerations of at least $2500 \times g$ and taking at least 80 tubes are acceptable, many laboratory centrifuges are capable of handling around 220 tubes in one batch. To ensure good batch-to-batch reproducibility some form of temperature control is essential. This is particularly important if the centrifuge capacity is small and large assays have to be spun in several batches, resulting in increasing centrifugation temperatures for each successive batch.

Aspirator

One of the advantages of using ^{125}I tracers is that following separation of bound and free it is a relatively simple matter to count precipitates. The supernatant is

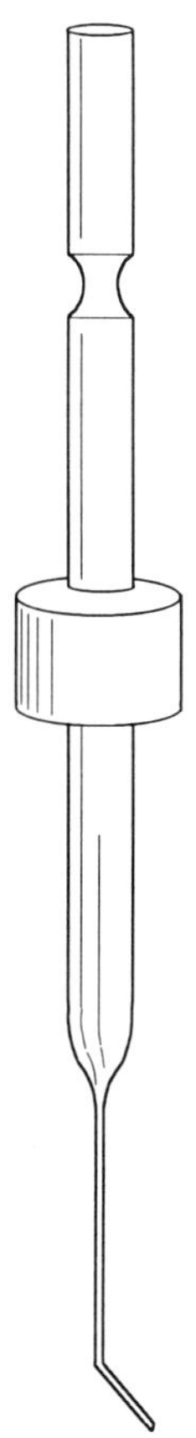

Figure 6.1 A simple aspirator made from a modified glass Pasteur pipette for removing supernatants from assay tubes.

conveniently removed using an aspirator connected to a vacuum source. The aspirator can be a glass or metal tube (approximately 100 mm long) with a narrow end, and a movable stop to control the depth the tip reaches into the assay tube. The example shown in Figure 6.1 is constructed from a glass Pasteur pipette. The capillary tube has been shortened and the end rounded in a flame. A movable piece of rubber tubing has been added to act as a stop. The kink at the end of the tube is important to allow the removal of all the supernatant with minimal disturbance to the precipitate.

If disposal of radioactive waste via the drains is permissible then the vacuum source can be a simple water-jet driven device where the radioactive waste goes directly down the drain, being diluted with large amounts of water in the process. If direct disposal via the drain is not permitted then any vacuum source can be used, either a vacuum pump or a water jet with the waste being collected in a trap.

Counters

If tritium is used as the tracer then any one of a number of commercially available counters will suffice, there being little to choose between them. However, the more recently introduced multi-head beta scintillation counters offer a significant advantage, especially when counting times are long. The range of gamma counters available is probably narrower than that of beta counters, but because of the simpler technology involved they all tend to be multi-head counters with generally 12 to 16 counting wells. Counters such as the NE 1600 (NE Technology Ltd, Reading, Berks, UK) have the added simplicity of having no moving parts. Although the samples have to be loaded by hand, the fact that counting times are relatively short, usually less than one minute, and the fact that sixteen samples can be counted simultaneously means that results are generally produced faster than samples can be loaded. As this instrument also produces results on an integral strip printer (as well as via an RS232 interface) results can be obtained very quickly. Because access to the instrument is very simple it is particularly useful for counting one-off samples or small batches associated with assay development work.

To summarise, a basic set of equipment for RIA is given below:

- A set of pipettes capable of accurately and precisely dispensing volumes from 10 μl to 5000 μl and an Eppendorf multipette for repetitive dispensing
- Polypropylene or polystyrene assay tubes, 75 × 12 mm
- Racks to hold approximately 200 tubes
- A vortex mixer or a multivortex mixer
- A refrigerated centrifuge capable of $>2500 \times g$ with suitable carriers to hold the assay tubes
- A manual loading gamma counter for radioiodine detection, such as an NE 1600

Tracer mass

A simple approach when using an iodine tracer is to employ a concentration of labelled analyte which gives a useful number of counts, such as 25 000 cpm per assay tube. Alternatively choose a mass of labelled analyte equal to the mass of analyte in the assay tube at the midpoint (ED_{50}) of the preferred calibration range. This second approach is only valid when the assay is incubated to equilibrium. Furthermore, the assumption is made that the antibody has equal affinity for the tracer and the analyte. This is rarely the case with heterologous tracers employing enzyme, fluoro- and most iodine labelled analytes. If the latter approach is adopted the resultant counts should not be too low since counting error is proportional to one over the square root of the number of counts. For example the coefficient of variation (CV% or RSD) on 10 000 counts is only 1%, however this rises to 3.2% on 1000 counts and on 100 counts it is 10%.

The same rationale applies to tritium tracers, in this instance however the affinity for the tracer and analyte will be the same, therefore selecting a tracer concentration equal to the midpoint on the calibration range is a rational approach. However it is important to have a clear idea of how the assay is going to be used. If speed and throughput are important then go for an adequate number of counts that can be obtained in five minutes. If sensitivity is a key development goal then keep the mass of tracer low and accept long counting times. To avoid the need to reoptimise the tracer concentration at a later stage some workers would employ two concentrations of tracer approximately fivefold apart.

Buffers and buffer additives

In the process of setting up an assay, selection of the buffer system is often taken for granted. The analyst will often select a buffer that worked well the last time or a buffer that is already available in the laboratory, possibly being used for another procedure. Different buffers can give markedly different results with the same set of reagents. The data in Figure 6.2, which presents four different antibody dilution curves, show how both the buffer type and the protein additive (particularly the latter) can have an effect on the evaluation of antisera. The four curves were all generated using the same antisera and tracer, but with different combinations of buffer and protein additives. The combination, phosphate buffer/bovine serum albumin (BSA) gave the highest levels of binding, closely followed by Tris buffer/BSA. Using gelatine in combination with either buffer type, however, gave much reduced binding such that the antiserum appeared worthless.

Whilst it is impossible to avoid such problems many workers are unaware of the effect different buffers can have on the assay performance, as shown by the limited reports in the literature. A recommended approach is to use initially a limited number of well-characterised buffers; if binding seems unusually low or matrix problems are in evidence (see below) then other buffers should be tried. Table 6.1 lists a number of common assay buffers used in immunoassay work.

A wide range of buffers for use in biological systems can also be found in *Geigy Scientific Tables* (Lenter, 1984). It is worth noting also that buffers based on Tris have relatively high temperature coefficients (approximately 0.04 pH units/°C) which could be a problem if the incubation temperature is varied widely. We generally use NaN_3 (0.1%) as a preservative, some workers prefer thiomersal (0.1%). To avoid

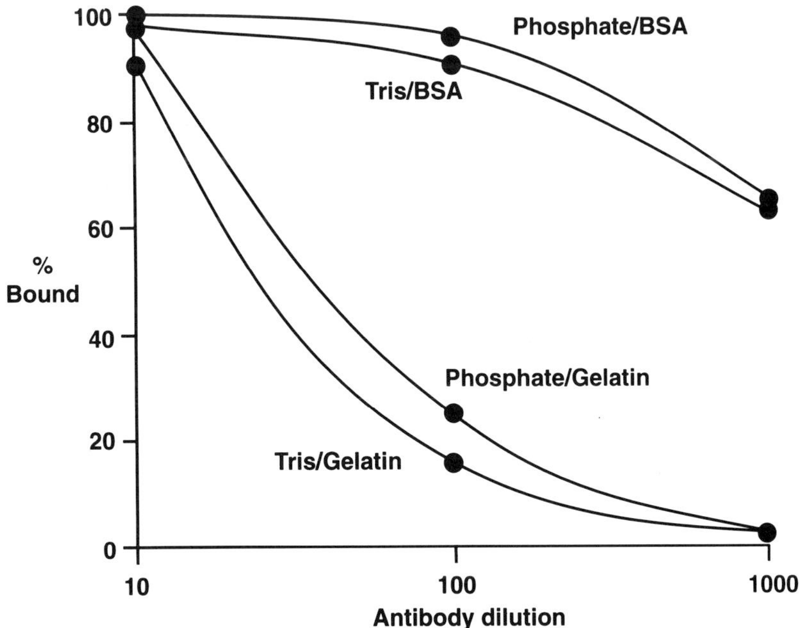

Figure 6.2 Four antibody dilution curves, generated using the same antisera and tracer but with different combinations of buffer (phosphate or Tris) and protein (BSA or gelatin) additive.

Table 6.1 Buffers commonly used for radioimmunoassay

Buffer type	pH	Molarity#	Prepared from
Phosphate	5.0	0.1	KH_2PO_4 (13.5 g), Na_2HPO_4 (0.114 g) and H_2O (1 l)
Phosphate	6.0	0.1	KH_2PO_4 (12.1 g), Na_2HPO_4 (1.576 g) and H_2O (1 l)
Phosphate	7.0	0.1	KH_2PO_4 (5.62 g), Na_2HPO_4 (8.34 g) and H_2O (1 l)
Phosphate	7.4	0.1	KH_2PO_4 (2.68 g), Na_2HPO_4 (11.40 g) and H_2O (1 l)
Phosphate	8.0	0.1	KH_2PO_4 (0.504 g), Na_2HPO_4 (13.7 g) and H_2O) (1 l)
Phosphate buffered saline	7.4	0.15	KH_2PO_4 (0.2 g), $Na_2HPO_4 \cdot 12H_2O$ (2.9 g), NaCl (8.0 g), KCl (0.2 g) and H_2O (1 l)
Borate	8.6	0.1	H_3BO_4 (6.18 g), sodium hydroxide solution (1 M, 29 ml) and H_2O (971 ml)
Tris*	7.2**	0.05	Trizma HCl (7.02 g), Trizma base (0.67 g) and water (1 l)
Tris*	8.0**	0.05	Trizma HCl (4.44 g), Trizma base (2.65 g) and water (1 l)
Tris*	8.5**	0.05	Trizma HCl (2.21 g), Trizma base (4.36 g) and water (1 l)
Tris*	9.0**	0.05	Trizma HCl (0.76 g), Trizma base (5.47 g) and water (1 l)

The molarity of the buffer can be varied by adjusting the relative proportions of the active ingredients, although this can have a small effect on the actual pH.

* Trizma is the Sigma brand name for Tris (tris(hydroxymethyl)aminoethane).

** The pH quoted is that for 25°C.

problems associated with variability in the ionic strength from sample to sample, we have usually employed a buffer of high ionic strength (e.g. 0.1 M).

It is common practice in immunoassays to add additional reagents such as proteins, detergents and non-specific binding competitors to the basic buffer. These additives serve one of several purposes. A non-specific gamma globulin or albumin is often added to 'stabilise' antisera, where because of high titres the sera may be diluted several millionfold with the concomitant risk of loss of antibody through adsorption to container walls etc.

Where the analyte in question is lipophilic and has poor water solubility the addition of a carrier protein such as bovine serum albumin (BSA) or a detergent such as Tween 80 or Triton (e.g. Teale *et al.*, 1975; Albro *et al.*, 1979) may be added to solubilise the analyte and tracer.

In our experience BSA (and by inference other albumins) have proved highly variable and an assay which works with one batch of BSA may not work well with the next batch, even though it is the same material prepared nominally by the same procedure from the same manufacturer. Table 6.2 lists a range of typical buffer additives and their intended function in the assay. Table 6.2 also includes some reagents which are used to minimise matrix effects, these will be discussed in more detail below.

In practice we would recommend the simple approach: unless there is good reason to the contrary the use of buffer additives should be kept to a minimum. In the first instance we would only add bovine gamma globulin (BGG) at a concentration of 0.2%. This serves to 'protect' the antisera and to bulk up the precipitate

Table 6.2 Materials commonly used in radioimmunoassay buffers along with their function in the assay

Material	Function
BGG	'Carrier' protein for antiserum and bulking agent for precipitiation separation methods.
BSA	'Carrier' protein for antiserum, can also help to solubilise analyte and tracer thereby reducing nsb.
Gelatin	'Carrier' protein for antiserum.
Detergent e.g. Triton, Tween CHAPSO, etc.	Solubilises tracer and analyte and reduces nsb, also reduces surface tension thus aiding decanting.
8-Analino-1-naphthalene sulphonic acid (ANS)	Competes with tracer and analyte for non-specific binding and specific binding sites, e.g. those on cortisol carrier protein.
Analogue of analyte	Reduces nsb by competing with tracer and analyte for binding sites on assay tube, also can compete with the analyte and tracer for binding sites on non-specific proteins.
Ethylenediamine acetic acid (EDTA)	Chelates metals (e.g. Ca) which may interfere with antibody binding.
Sodium azide	Antibacterial and preservative.

Table 6.3 The relative merits of commonly used RIA separation procedures (the more plus signs the better)

Separation method	Cost	Versatility	Robustness	nsb level	Speed	Practicality/ automatability
PEG	+++	++++	++++	+++	++++	+++
Ammonium sulphate	++++	++++	++++	++	+++	+++
Charcoal	++++	++++	+++	+++	++	++
Second antibody	++	+++	+++	+++	++*	++++
Solid-phase second antibody	+	++	++++	++++	+++	+++
Solid-phase primary antibody	++	NA	++++	++++	++++	+++

* Can be improved using PEG-assisted separation or by simultaneous addition of first and second antibody.

Table 6.4 B_0 and non-specific binding (nsb) values obtained with different separation procedures in a RIA for propranolol

Separation method	B_0 (%)	nsb (%)	net binding (%)
Charcoal	26	9	17
Solid-phase second antibody	23	15	8
PEG	34	8	26
Ammonium sulphate	76	65	11

when fractional precipitation methods are used to separate bound and free (see 'Separating systems' below).

Separating systems

Although a wide range of separation procedures have been used and reported in the literature, few have found widespread use either for assay development work or in a routine assay. The commonly used separating methods can be divided into three categories: adsorption methods, e.g. charcoal; fractional precipitation methods, e.g. polyethylene glycol (PEG) and ammonium sulphate; and second antibody methods, which can either be liquid-phase or solid-phase.

Separating systems are assessed in terms of their efficiency and practicality. The efficiency of separation is the accuracy with which the bound and free are classified. The practicality of the separation procedure is measured in terms of the speed, simplicity, applicability, reproducibility and cost; inevitably this will be somewhat subjective. Table 6.3 gives a list of the commonly used separation procedures and their relative merits. The procedures based on second antibodies or solid-phase first antibodies are unsuited to antibody evaluation.

The criteria used to select a separating procedure for development work can be different to those which would dictate the ultimate selection of a separation method for a routinely used assay. During assessment of antibody and the initial stages of development it is essential to choose a method which will work with any antibody concentration, i.e. PEG, charcoal, or ammonium sulphate. It is also desirable to choose a method which requires the minimum of optimisation and hence will work with most analytes and buffers etc. In this latter respect the PEG procedure comes out best, although to cover all eventualities it is sensible to try more than one approach since there are occasions where these procedures can give very different data or where one works but the others do not. This fact is clearly seen in the data for a propranolol assay (Table 6.4) where the zero dose binding (B_0) and non-specific binding (nsb) levels using four different separation methods vary widely.

The following discussion will consider the major separation procedures in more detail. It is worth bearing in mind that no separation system is 100 per cent efficient. In every assay, steps must be taken to measure this efficiency and the degree to which bound is misclassified as free and vice versa.

Fractional precipitation methods

All fractional precipitation methods follow a simple principle: when the primary reaction is complete, the separation agent is added at a concentration which causes 'salting out' and precipitation of the antibody fraction, whether or not it has antigen bound to it. The free fraction remains in solution and the precipitate can be spun down, compacted and the radioactivity determined in the pellet (bound fraction) or supernatant (free fraction). Practically, it is very easy to aspirate the supernatant to waste and leave a radioactive pellet. In the case of ^{125}I-labelled tracers this pellet can be counted directly.

Fractional precipitation methods act by reducing 'free water' in the system, i.e. the water able to form a solvation shell around a dissolved molecule and keep it in solution. A protein molecule's ability to attract water molecules depends very much on its overall electrostatic charge, which is determined by the isoelectric point of the molecule and the pH of the medium. Antibody molecules carry little charge at neutral pH and hence they are easily precipitated by low concentrations of separating reagent, such as half-saturated ammonium sulphate or around 18% PEG 6000.

Fractional precipitation techniques score high in terms of practicality, they are applicable to a wide range of analyte types and importantly they can be used with any dilution of antisera. It is important with these techniques to measure the degree of non-specific binding which can result from one of two main causes. First, tracer can bind non-specifically to proteins derived from the sample or the buffer. When precipitated, this radioactivity is misclassified as bound. Unduly high non-specific binding can be reduced by washing the precipitate with the precipitating agent. This approach is not always effective, however, and it can make the assay unnecessarily tedious, so avoidance of the problem through changes to the assay conditions or separation procedure would be recommended. The second form of non-specific binding is not actually binding, but is the result of tracer being physically trapped in the protein complex as it is compacted into a pellet. In this case washing of the precipitate with the separating agent is highly effective at removing this entrapped material.

The non-specific binding would normally be determined by setting up B_0 tubes, but instead of adding antisera, adding a similar dilution of control sera, or if the antisera are used at a dilution in excess of 1/2000, assay buffer can be used. The bound and free would be separated in the standard manner (see PROCEDURES 1 and 2 for details), and any material bound must be bound non-specifically because of the absence of antisera.

Ammonium sulphate

Ammonium sulphate is widely used to fractionate and separate proteins by precipitation (Harlow and Lane, 1988) and the use of ammonium sulphate in RIA is a logical extension of this process. Addition of an equal volume of ammonium sulphate to an antibody solution at neutral pH will result, after a short incubation, in precipitation of the gamma globulins. The precipitate is compacted by centrifugation. It can still be fragile however, needing care when aspirating. With some analytes, especially lipophilic molecules, high non-specific binding can be a problem. Like the PEG separation procedure discussed below inclusion of 0.2% BGG in the buffer is necessary to bulk up the mass of precipitate. The use of antisera at high dilution without added BGG to the incubation medium can result in no precipitation! When working with ^{125}I tracers the bound would be counted in the precipitate but with ^{3}H tracers the supernatant containing the free would be counted.

PROCEDURE 1 Separation of bound and free using ammonium sulphate

Reagents

- Saturated aqueous ammonium sulphate prepared by mixing ammonium sulphate (≥200 g) with distilled water (250 ml)

NB. The assay buffer must contain BGG at a concentration of around 0.2% w/v.

Method

To each assay tube (excluding total counts), add an equal volume of ammonium sulphate solution. Briefly vortex each tube until the contents are milky white and homogeneous. Incubate at room temperature for 10 to 15 min and then centrifuge all tubes for 15 min (2500 × g) at room temperature. If a ^{125}I tracer is being used, aspirate the contents of each tube to waste (with the exception of the total tubes) and count the precipitates. Count all tubes for an appropriate length of time to give sufficient counts for good precision.

If a ^{3}H tracer is being used it is necessary to add ammonium sulphate to the total tubes which are vortexed but *not* centrifuged. After the other tubes have been centrifuged, a fixed aliquot is removed from each tube (typically 650 or 700 µl from 750 µl) and transferred to a counting tube, scintillation cocktail added and the samples counted.

Polyethylene glycol 6000 (PEG)

PEG was first introduced by Desbuquois and Aurbach (1971). It works with a wide range of analytes from small-molecular-weight compounds such as amphetamine, to relatively large peptides such as parathyroid hormone, molecular mass 9425 Daltons. It also works well with different structural types such as highly polar antibiotic metabolites (Ballard *et al.*, 1996) and lipophilic compounds, for example tetrahydrocannabinol (Law *et al.*, 1984). Although assay parameters such as buffer, pH and ionic strength do have some effect on the efficiency of PEG separation (Desbuquois and Aurbach, 1971; Sourgens *et al.*, 1979) in our experience PEG can be used with the minimum of optimisation providing the following guidelines are followed. The final PEG concentration in the separation mixture should be at least 17.5% w/v, and to ensure complete precipitation it is essential that a gamma globulin is included in the assay buffer. We recommend BGG at a concentration of 0.2% in the buffer giving a concentration of around 0.16% in the incubation medium. A recommended method for the use of PEG is given is PROCEDURE 2. This separation procedure works at any temperature, it is fast (samples can be spun immediately after mixing), and it works for any dilution of antisera. It is also possible to obtain relatively low non-specific binding even with very lipophilic compounds.

PROCEDURE 2 Separation of bound and free using PEG

Reagents

- Polyethylene glycol, molecular weight 6000 (PEG 6000) (27.5% w/v) in distilled water containing NaN_3 (0.1%) as preservative

NB. The assay buffer must contain BGG at a concentration of around 0.2% w/v.

Method

To each assay tube (excluding the total counts) add two volumes of PEG (i.e. add 0.5 ml PEG to 0.25 ml incubation mixture). Briefly vortex each tube until the contents are milky white and homogeneous. Centrifuge all tubes for 15 min (2500 × g) at room temperature. If a ^{125}I tracer is being used aspirate the contents of each tube to waste (with the exception of the total tubes). This should be done in two stages. The bulk of the liquid is first removed with the aspirator, moving quickly from one tube to the next. Because of the viscous nature of the solution some residual liquid will run down the side of the tube, collecting in the bottom, above the precipitate. Return to the first tube and removing each tube in turn from the centrifuge rack, use the aspirator (with the stop set so that the bottom of the tube can be reached) to remove the last drop of liquid. At this stage the tube can be transferred to the original rack. Count all tubes for an appropriate length of time to give sufficient counts for good precision.

If a ^3H tracer is being used it is necessary to add PEG to the total tubes which are vortexed but *not* centrifuged. After the other tubes have been centrifuged, a fixed aliquot is removed from each tube (typically 650 or 700 µl from 750 µl) and transferred to a counting tube, scintillation cocktail added and the samples counted.

Charcoal

The use of charcoal was first described by Herbert *et al.* (1965). It has been widely used for the separation of low-molecular-weight compounds and for many years was the mainstay of most steroid RIAs. It relies on the principle that only the tracer and not antibody or antibody-bound tracer are adsorbed onto the charcoal surface.

Although it is still used in many laboratories charcoal has a number of disadvantages compared with the precipitation methods. The contact time (the length of the incubation time with the charcoal) needs to be precisely controlled for reproducible separation. This is especially so with low affinity sera where prolonged contact times can lead to the charcoal stripping the bound antigen from the antibody, particularly when incubated at room temperature. Incubation temperature and time as well as the amount of charcoal required and the presence or absence of proteins (in the sample and buffer) all need optimising and controlling for reproducible results.

Charcoal is usually used in the form of 'dextran coated charcoal' with the addition of dextran to the charcoal suspension. The concentration of charcoal in the suspension is normally around 0.5% with dextran being added at 1/10 of this concentration. The dextran was originally thought to give a sieving effect, preventing the adsorption of the large-molecule-weight antibodies (Herbert *et al.*, 1965). This has now been refuted (Binoux and Odell, 1973; Boxen and Tevaarwerk, 1982) and dextran is now included as it is thought to make the charcoal stickier permitting easier centrifugation into a pellet and giving improved precision. When employing charcoal it is essential to determine the efficiency of the adsorption. As well as giving an indication of the misclassification error this parameter is also useful diagnostically, especially in relation to problems of tracer purity. The efficiency of adsorption is sometimes referred to as an assay blank and frequently, though incorrectly, as non-specific binding. It is determined by setting up a B_0 tube, but instead of adding antisera adding a similar dilution of control sera, or if the antisera are used at a dilution in excess of 1/2000, assay buffer. The bound and free would be separated in the standard manner (see PROCEDURE 3 for details). The difference between the total counts and the assay blank tube represents the efficiency of the separation procedure.

As discussed above the effective use of charcoal is dependent on a number of factors, many of which can only be determined and optimised once the assay has been developed. Based on the collective experience of the authors the conditions outlined in PROCEDURE 3 will prove generally useful and will serve to demonstrate that antisera have been produced and that a working assay is possible.

PROCEDURE 3 Separation of bound and free using charcoal

Reagents

- Suspending buffer, typically this would be the same as that used for the assay (without addition of additives) although in practice any buffer can be used. Once selected this buffer should be held constant
- A suspension of charcoal (Norit A) (0.5% w/v) in buffer containing dextran T70 (0.05% w/v) at 4°C

Method

If working at room temperature is preferred then at the end of the primary incubation add to each assay tube (excluding total counts) two volumes of dextran-coated charcoal suspension (i.e. add 0.5 ml charcoal to 0.25 ml incubation mixture). To the total count tubes add the equivalent volume of buffer. Briefly vortex each tube and incubate for around 10 min at ambient temperature.

Alternatively, first bring the temperature of the assay tubes to around 4°C by incubating them in an ice-water bath for around 30 min. Then add the charcoal and after vortex mixing incubate the samples at 4°C for 20 to 30 min. After incubation the tubes are centrifuged for 15 min (2500 × g) at the incubation temperature, i.e. 4°C.

If a ^{3}H tracer is being used remove a fixed aliquot from each tube (typically 650 or 700 µl from 750 µl), transfer to a counting tube and add scintillation cocktail. Care should be taken during this process since the charcoal pellet is relatively buoyant and it is easily disturbed with a careless pipetting technique. If a ^{125}I tracer is being used the supernatant in each tube is aspirated to waste (with the exception of the total tubes), once again with care. Count all tubes for an appropriate length of time to give sufficient counts for good precision. In contrast to the precipitation methods, counting the supernatant gives bound and counting the charcoal pellet gives free.

If charcoal is to be used for much of the development work then some form of optimisation should be carried out. Using the exact assay conditions to be employed in further work, the optimal incubation time and mass of charcoal which gives effective adsorption of free tracer whilst having minimum effect on antibody-bound tracer should be determined. This is simply carried out using a series of B_0 and assay blank tubes. Typically charcoal incubation times between 5 and 120 min would be used with the concentration of the charcoal suspension being varied between 0.1 and 5.0% w/v. It is important that the temperature and the protein concentration are fixed and controlled, although if necessary these can also be varied as part of the optimisation work. Once the assay conditions and the amount of charcoal have been selected they must be kept constant, if conditions are changed then the charcoal concentration must be reselected. It is also worth setting aside a large batch of charcoal since batch-to-batch variability will necessitate re-optimisation if the batch of charcoal is changed.

Second antibody methods

Second antibody methods, whether liquid or solid phase, but particularly the former, require some optimisation. Since at the early stages of assay development the quality of the antisera is very much unknown these procedures are inappropriate, for example most solid-phase second antibodies can only be used with primary antisera dilutions of greater than 1/2000. Once the assay has been developed however, these techniques come into their own since they can give precise assays with very low non-specific binding. Second antibody methods will be discussed further under 'Assay optimisation' below.

Assay conditions

In the initial stages of method development it is recommended that small total incubation volumes are used, typically 0.25 ml. This is conveniently made up from solutions of tracer (0.1 ml) and antiserum (0.1 ml) with sample or standard (0.05 ml). This has the advantage of giving fast kinetics, enabling short incubation times to be used (less than an hour) so that experiments can be carried out rapidly. Small incubation volumes can predispose the assay to matrix effect problems if the sample volume is relatively large. Ultimately the assay incubation volume may be around twice that recommended here. However, providing the inclusion of the matrix is delayed in the assay development process the use of small incubation volumes is convenient and advantageous.

Unless there are good reasons to do otherwise, i.e. the analyte shows temperature-dependent instability, it is recommended that all incubations are carried out at room temperature. Although some variation in normal laboratory temperature will occur this should not lead to any serious problems at this stage. It is claimed that the antibody–antigen interaction is largely entropy as opposed to enthalpy driven (Vining *et al.*, 1981) hence there is little change in antibody affinity and hence assay sensitivity when using elevated temperatures. This could be disputed by some workers and if desired a range of temperatures can be investigated. However, incubation at room temperature, as opposed to 4°C for example, leads to faster attainment of equilibrium, hence quicker assays and faster assay development. Furthermore working at room temperature is technically simpler and requires less equipment than incubating at 4°C or 37°C.

Assessment of antibodies

The first practical step in the assay development programme involves assessing the specificity, titre and potential sensitivity (affinity) of a number of candidate antisera. Specificity is assessed by determining the cross-reactivity of related compounds, metabolites and endogenous compounds. Most workers employ the method of Abraham (1969). The procedure for determination of the cross-reactivity is fully described in the chapter on assay validation (Chapter 9).

The titre is simply the dilution of antisera that will bind a defined fraction (typically 50 per cent) of a given mass of tracer. Some workers refer to the dilution of the antisera in the assay tube, i.e. the final dilution; however, most reports refer to the dilution of the antisera in the antiserum reagent, i.e. the working dilution. Whilst the former is more correct, the latter convention will be adopted here.

The sensitivity of an assay, which is ultimately related to the affinity of the antisera, is dependent on the assay conditions and any work at this stage will only give an indication of what is ultimately attainable.

The affinity of the antisera can be determined by incubating increasing amounts of tracer with a fixed amount of antibody and then analysing the data using a Scatchard plot (Scatchard, 1949). This form of analysis gives the antibody binding constant which is a measure of the strength of the antibody–antigen interaction, which for most antibodies is in the range 10^6 l/mol to 10^{12} l/mol. The Scatchard analysis also gives the concentration of the antibody binding sites and indicates whether the sera is mono- or polyclonal.

Unfortunately, measuring antibody affinity is of little value since it is dependent on assay conditions, such as incubation time and possibly temperature as well as pH and ionic strength of the incubation medium. Furthermore if a heterologous tracer is being used then the affinity is that for the tracer and not the analyte. Selection of an antiserum with a high affinity for the tracer may ultimately result in an insensitive assay (Rowell *et al.*, 1979). Conversely selection of a serum having low affinity for the tracer may result in the generation of a non-robust assay. The determination of affinity constant has little meaning, except when tritiated tracers are being used. Even then it is only one of several parameters that need to be considered.

Most workers approach antibody assessment by first selecting sera based on titre, following the old adage that 'biggest is best'. As a measure of antisera quality this is certainly not true. In our laboratory we have developed and successfully used an assay which employed an antiserum with titre of only 1/200! (Ballard *et al.*, 1996). Using this traditional approach the 'best' antisera would be used to generate calibration series which would then be optimised in terms of sensitivity, and cross-reactivity tested. This is very much a sequential approach involving a great deal of iteration, especially if the initially selected serum does not give the necessary assay characteristics. Using an approach employed in a number of laboratories, including our own, it is possible to generate data on all three parameters: titre, cross-reactivity and sensitivity, in a single experiment with the minimum amount of experimental work. This approach also leads to early but well-reasoned selection of the best all-round antisera.

The recommended approach which is outlined in detail in PROCEDURE 4 involves generating an antibody dilution curve for each antiserum, along with a series of displacement curves. A displacement curve is an antibody dilution curve to which has been added a test compound, either the analyte or a related compound for which lack of cross-reactivity in the assay is critical. If a concentration of analyte equivalent to the required limit of detection is added to the displacement curve, the serum which gives the best sensitivity and the dilution at which this is obtained is readily identified. This serum would be the one where the displacement between the antibody dilution curve and the displacement curve with added analyte is greatest.

PROCEDURE 4 Evaluation of antisera

This procedure assumes a single antiserum is being evaluated using six serial dilutions from 1/10 to $1/10^6$. The method involves generating four curves: (A) an antibody dilution curve, (B) a displacement curve with analyte, (C) a displacement curve with a potential cross-reactant and (D) an assessment of non-specific binding across the antiserum dilution range.

Equipment

The standard equipment as described above is required. In terms of assay tubes, two are required for the total activity and four sets of 12 tubes (6 duplicate pairs) are required for each of the curves

Reagents

- Assay buffer selected to be compatible with the separation procedure
- Assay buffer minus additives such as protein for the preparation of standard solutions
- Radiotracer diluted in assay buffer to give around 25 kcpm per 100 μl
- Control non-immune serum (from a non-immunised animal) serially diluted in assay buffer from 1/10 to $1/10^6$
- Antiserum diluted serially in assay buffer from 1/10 to $1/10^6$
- Analyte of interest diluted in assay buffer (minus additives) to a concentration at or around the desired assay limit of detection
- Potential cross-reactant diluted in assay buffer (minus additives) at a concentration around 100-fold above that of the analyte of interest

Method

The following method assumes PEG or ammonium sulphate is being used for the separation of bound and free. If charcoal is used then the procedure will need modifying in accordance with PROCEDURE 3 above.

Add analyte diluent (50 μl) to the tubes to be used for the dilution curve (A) and the nsb determination (D). Add the analyte solution (50 μl) to all the tubes for the displacement curve (B) and the cross-reactant solution (50 μl) to the cross-reactivity displacement tubes (C).

Add radiotracer solution (100 μl) to all tubes. Add the solution of non-immune serum (100 μl) to the tubes for the measurement of nsb (D) and antiserum solution (100 μl) to the remaining tubes (A to C) with the exception of the total tubes. Vortex mix and incubate at room temperature for at least 1 h.

Carry out the separation of bound and free as described in PROCEDURE 1 or 2 above. Aspirate the supernatant to waste and count the precipitates for around 60 s. Plot percentage of radioactivity bound versus the logarithm of serum dilution.

Some typical results from such an experiment are shown in Figure 6.3 and a number of features are readily apparent. First the conditions used give relatively low non-specific binding (nsb less than 5 per cent) providing the dilution of the sera is greater than 1/100. The immune serum shows a good level of binding at antibody dilutions of less than 1/1000, which suggests that the tracer is pure as well as indicating a good antibody response and high titre. Comparison of the antibody dilution curve (A) and the analyte displacement curve (B) suggests that the maximum displacement occurs at an antiserum dilution of 1/7500 to 1/10 000. The curve with the added potential cross-reactant shows virtually no displacement, indicating that this compound is unlikely to cause interference in the assay under the present conditions.

Although very useful, the above approach has been criticised by Ekins (1981) who rightly claims that displacement alone is not a good measure of sensitivity, as the precision of the response should also be taken into account. However, to generate precision data at this stage would not only involve considerable extra work but

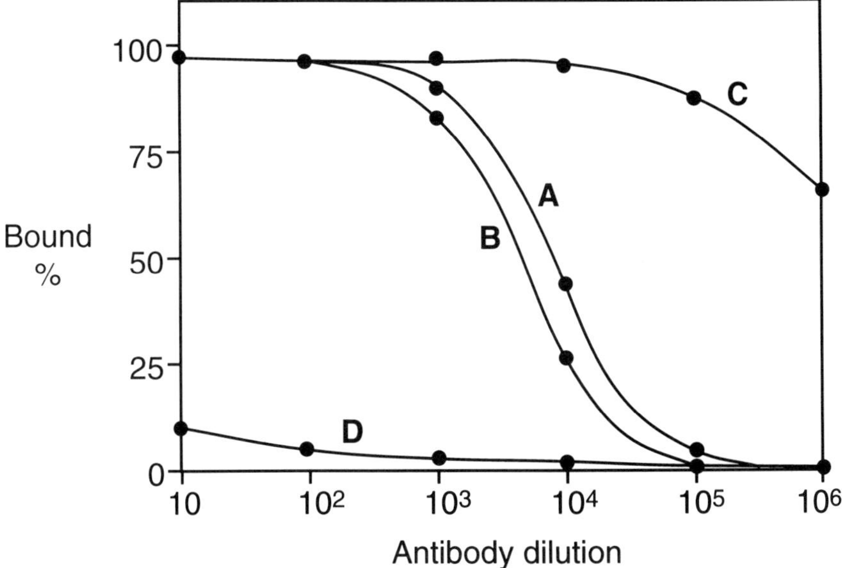

Figure 6.3 The results of antiserum assessment as carried out in PROCEDURE 4, showing an antibody dilution curve (A), a displacement curve using analyte (B), a displacement curve including a potential cross-reactant (C) and a curve showing non-specific binding (nsb) (D).

the data would probably be meaningless since subsequent optimisation of the assay would probably lead to marked changes in precision.

In contrast to the data presented in Figure 6.3 the results of the evaluation may be equivocal: binding may be low or non-existent, non-specific binding high or specificity or sensitivity poor. If the immunogen has been well characterised, the hapten known to be immunogenic and the tracer structure commensurate with good binding, then it is likely that the assay conditions are at fault. The recommendation at this stage would be to carry out simple antibody dilution curves under a variety of conditions. Try a different separation procedure, also different buffer types or a buffer pH $\pm$ 2 units around that employed initially. The ionic strength of the buffer could be changed as could the added protein if one has been used. If non-specific binding is high then it may be useful to determine if this is binding to the assay tubes or proteins in the serum or buffer. If necessary these can be changed or competitors added (see Table 6.2 above and the section on introduction of matrix).

If the first experiment has been successful, in that one or two suitable sera have been identified, then further work should focus on these sera with the aim of defining the assay limitations.

As mentioned earlier the specificity of a serum and the level of binding are dependent on the incubation time. At this stage it is probably worth carrying out some limited optimisation of the incubation time, if only to allow standardisation for future experiments. This is conveniently done by repeating the initial experiment with the serum or sera of choice (probably using a maximum of three). Extra antisera dilutions can be introduced around the point of maximum displacement to allow more precise definition of the required titre. Furthermore, additional related compounds can also be tested for cross-reactivity. This experiment should be set up in duplicate and one set of tubes incubated for around 2 h and the other for at least

16 h, i.e. overnight. The results of this and the previous experiment will give an indication of the reaction kinetics. Providing specificity is not a serious problem then a suitably short incubation time can be selected for future experiments. It may also be possible from this experiment to reduce the number of sera for further study.

Once the sera of choice and the dilution which gives the required sensitivity have been defined, then the next stage is to set up a calibration series. This is normally done using a logarithmic distribution of standards. For example, if the required limit of detection is 1 ng/ml then a series of standards having the concentrations 0, 0.5, 1, 2, 4, 8, 16, 32, 64 and 128 ng/ml would be prepared in assay buffer. These would then be used to generate a calibration series using the previously defined conditions and incubation time.

Introduction of matrix

The development, up until this stage, has been carried out using relatively simple conditions since the introduction into the assay of plasma or extracts of tissue, soil or cereal can seriously disrupt the binding and lead to a situation where the assay is apparently unworkable. Such an example involved the assay for ICI 215001, a β_3-agonist (Ballard *et al.*, 1994). Figure 6.4 shows two calibration graphs, the first for standards prepared in assay buffer gave a good level of binding and sensitivity. The second, which employed standards prepared in human plasma, gave binding which was much reduced such that the assay was effectively unworkable in the state shown. By taking the development a step at a time and delaying the addition of sample matrix, it was immediately apparent where the problem lay and reference conditions, i.e. those without matrix, were available for comparison.

The problem demonstrated in Figure 6.4 was found to be the result of plasma proteins effectively competing with the antibodies and actually reducing the binding of tracer to the antibodies (Ballard *et al.*, 1994). This problem was overcome by altering the pH of the incubation medium and adding in a competitor which displaced tracer from the plasma proteins without competing for antibody binding sites.

The competition between plasma proteins and specific antibodies for the analyte is a well documented phenomenon in the area of steroid immunoassay (Pratt *et al.*, 1975; Brock *et al.*, 1978). The addition of 8-anilino-1-naphthalenesulphonic acid (ANS) to the incubation buffer at a concentration of around 200 μg/ml can reduce this non-specific binding. At the extreme however ANS has a detrimental effect on the antigen–antibody interaction (Brock *et al.*, 1978). An alternative method involving an analogue of the analyte as a specific displacement agent has been used in a number of steroid immunoassays (Pratt *et al.*, 1975, 1978). This strategy must be used with care since there is potential for cross-reactivity.

Modification of the assay buffer type, pH, molarity etc., can also have a positive effect on matrix problems. Where the effect of the matrix is mediated through the separation procedure then changing conditions may also help eliminate matrix problems.

As a general rule the maximum incorporation of sample into the assay incubation volume is 10 per cent, although in the authors' experience this can often be doubled without serious problems (Mason *et al.*, 1982; Law *et al.*, 1984). Reducing the proportion of the sample included in the assay is one way of minimising matrix

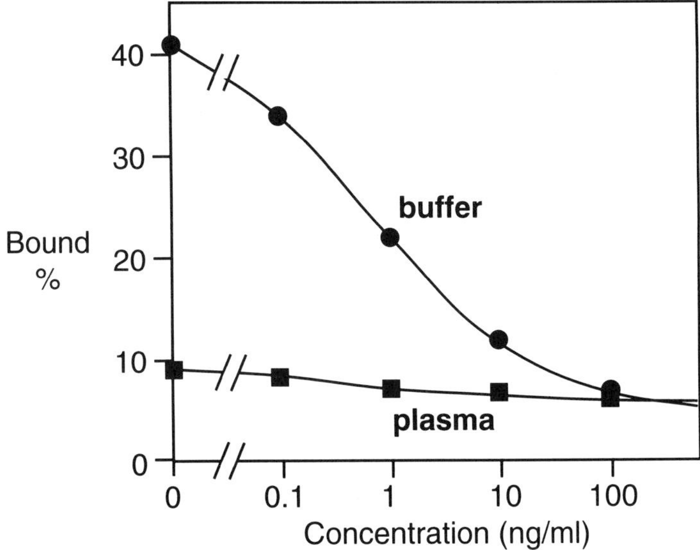

Figure 6.4 Calibration graphs for ICI 215001 using standards prepared in phosphate buffer (0.1 M, pH 7.4) and human plasma. The same volume (50 μl) of each standard was employed in a total assay volume of 250 μl.

effects, although this approach is limited for a number of reasons. First there is a minimum volume which can be reliably pipetted, around 10 μl. Although sample volumes can be effectively reduced by dilution, prior to addition to the assay this may adversely affect sample throughput etc. Such changes must also be considered in terms of their effect on assay sensitivity. Rather than reducing sample volumes, the incubation volume can be increased. However, doubling the incubation volume effectively reduces the reagent concentrations by a factor of two resulting in a doubling of the incubation time.

A quick way of assessing the effect of matrix in an assay is to overspike buffer standards with matrix. This can be conveniently achieved without affecting the overall assay incubation make-up by employing the following method. Add standards in buffer as normal but prepare either the antiserum or tracer at double the normal concentration and add half the amount. The deficiency in volume can then be made up by addition of an appropriate volume of matrix. Using this procedure it is possible using standard assay conditions to evaluate the effect of several different matrices without the need to prepare standards in each of these different samples.

Once matrix has been introduced into the assay it is worth rechecking sensitivity and specificity since these may change. At this stage it is also sensible to assess the overall assay precision across the calibration range, which can be conveniently done by generating a precision profile as advocated by Ekins and co-workers (1983).

Most computerised data-capture and processing systems include the necessary software to generate a precision profile. To obtain meaningful data it is essential that there is a good spread of analyte concentrations across the calibration range. One way of ensuring this is to assay 10 calibration series in a single assay. This can usually be achieved in under 180 assay tubes. If the software is not available to generate a precision profile as defined by Ekins then the following simple approach can be applied. Either count the 10 sets of curves and generate a mean calibration set and then read each curve, in turn, off the mean curve. Alternatively count one set as the calibration series and then read the other 9 sets of standards plus the original set off the calibration curve, thus generating 10 concentration values at each standard point. Each of these ten values is then meaned, the CV calculated and plotted against concentration to give the precision profile. The use of precision profiles will be discussed further in the section on optimisation below.

Defining incubation time

It is necessary at some stage to qualify the data already generated and accurately determine the required incubation time. This information will also give an indication of the likely throughput of the assay since for most methods much of the analysis time is taken up by the incubation.

The incubation time which had been previously defined would be used as a general guide and study would be made around this time period. Assuming a provisional incubation time of 3 h a typical protocol for determining the incubation period is given in PROCEDURE 5.

PROCEDURE 5 Determination of the minimum incubation time

Materials and equipment

These are as previously described

Method

Set up a series of duplicate assay tubes for 9 zero standards, 9 high standards and 9 nsb tubes. Add the appropriate standard to each tube followed by tracer. Add antiserum or buffer as appropriate to one batch of tubes (zeros, high standards and nsbs) at time t = 0, then at times 2, 4, 5, 6, 6.5, 7, 7.5 and 8 h. Immediately after the addition of the antiserum to the 8 h tube add the separation agent to all tubes and carry out the separation.

Using the above procedure gives incubation times of 0, 0.5, 1, 2, 3, 4, 6 and 8 h. The binding for the three types of tube are plotted against incubation time to give typical curves as shown in Figure 6.5.

Although the data in Figure 6.5 suggests that binding was reaching a plateau after 3 h, an incubation time of 75 min (minimum) was selected for convenience. This choice was substantiated by additional work which showed that the results from real samples was independent of incubation time over the range 70 min to 3 h.

The above approach, which is widely used, has been criticised by Vining *et al.* (1981), since it is based on a measure of the analyte (tracer)/antibody association rate and does not take into account the dissociation rates. Failure to consider the latter parameter can lead to an increase in cross-reactivity. Where assay specificity is of major importance the experiment described in PROCEDURE 5 should be carried out with the addition of an extra set of tubes containing an amount of cross-reactant that reduces the binding at zero concentration by around 50 per cent. Under these circumstances the binding will be seen to rise more slowly and an incubation time can be selected that minimises cross-reaction.

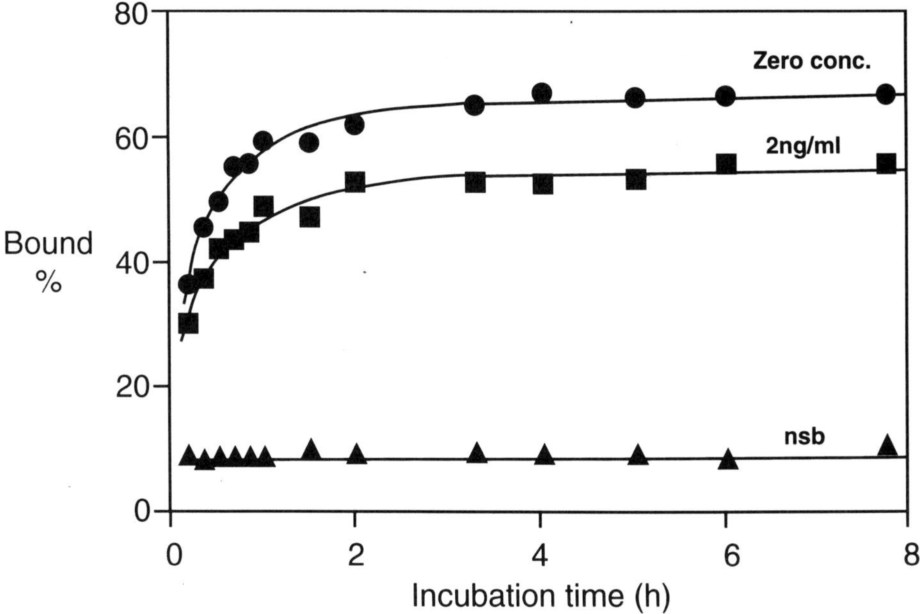

Figure 6.5 The effect of increasing incubation time on the level of binding in an assay for delta-9-tetrahydrocannabinol metabolites. Two dose levels were studied along with non-specific binding.

Assay optimisation

After the basic assay has been established and the matrix introduced, it is generally necessary to carry out some form of optimisation. This optimisation is an iterative process whereby the assay is fine tuned to give the required sensitivity, specificity, speed etc. It should be borne in mind that very few immunoassay variables can be changed independently. For example increasing the incubation temperature to effectively speed up the assay can alter the specificity and change precision. In general most variables will have some effect, either positive or negative, on precision, and reassessment after every major change using the precision profile as mentioned above is necessary.

Optimising for practicality

Separation methods

The initially developed assay may not be ideal for routine application where several hundred samples per day may have to be assayed. One aspect which has a profound effect on sample throughput and general practicality is the separation procedure. In our hands PEG has proved particularly useful in giving good precision and relatively low nsb with a wide range of small-molecular-weight analytes. Ammonium sulphate is similarly efficient and it has been successfully used in a number of commercial RIA kits (e.g. Roche Diagnostics Abuscreen for barbiturates and opiates). However there will undoubtedly be occasions where these methods give unsatisfactory performance and alternative separation methods have to be found. There is also a drive to use solid-phase techniques with their greater adaptability to automation, which can be difficult with PEG because of the viscosity of the reagent. For a general discussion and a critical evaluation of separation methods the interested reader is referred to Ratcliffe *et al.* (1974), Cameron *et al.* (1975), Brown *et al.* (1980), Walgraeve *et al.* (1986) and El-Gamal and Landon (1988). The following discussion will focus on some of the alternative separation procedures not hitherto discussed.

Solid-phase first antibody

In this approach the first antibody is attached to a solid phase, either the surface of an assay tube or a small particle such as a cellulose bead. Inclusion of magnetisable ferric oxide in the particle permits separation using a magnet rather than a centrifuge. This approach has been used in our laboratory and although giving very good precision it offers no real advantage over some of the other more simple techniques.

The use of solid-phase first antibody necessitates a good supply of high titre sera, which needs to be purified prior to linking. As the reagent is totally analyte specific it would only be applied to a well developed assay assured of continuous use.

Second antibody methods

A common and widely used separation procedure involves the use of an antibody raised against the primary antibody. This so-called second antibody reacts with primary antibody-bound antigen to produce an insoluble macromolecular complex which can be precipitated and counted. Liquid-phase second antibody systems offer great efficiency, i.e. they minimise misclassification errors, have broad applicability and good reproducibility. The main disadvantages are cost (the second antibody is generally used at a titre of around 1/20 to 1/40), and speed (long second incubations are normally required). It is possible in certain assays to speed up liquid-phase second antibody separations by one of two methods. First, the primary and second antibodies can be added simultaneously and in certain instances in a combined pre-precipitated form (Hales and Randle, 1963; Brown *et al.*, 1980). A second and widely used approach is addition of PEG to the second antibody separation mixture to give a final concentration of about 5 per cent (Hartman *et al.*, 1982). This so called PEG-assisted second antibody method is not only faster, incubation times are reduced from 24 to 2 h, but the amounts of second antibody reagents are also reduced.

Second antibody methods do require careful optimisation with respect to the concentration of the second antibody, carrier serum and the incubation time. A typical optimisation is given in PROCEDURE 6.

PROCEDURE 6 Optimisation of a second antibody separation procedure

Reagents

- Anti-species IgG diluted in assay buffer 1/12, 1/24 and 1/48
- Normal serum of the same species as the primary antibody, diluted in assay buffer 1/50, 1/100, 1/200 and 1/400
- Standard RIA reagents

Method

For each incubation time to be studied, a series of 12 B_0 and 12 nsb tubes are set up in duplicate. For convenience these should be arranged in a 4 by 3 matrix as shown below. These tubes are incubated to equilibrium and then a fixed aliquot (0.1 ml) of the normal serum dilutions is added to a series of tubes and this is combined with the same volume of the second antibody dilutions using the matrix design below.

		Working dilution of normal serum			
		1/50	1/100	1/200	1/400
Working	1/12				
dilution of	1/24				
2nd antibody	1/48				

The tubes are mixed and incubated for various times (typically 1 to 24 h for a new assay). Following centrifugation at 2000 × g for 30 min the supernatant is aspirated to waste and the precipitate counted if ^{125}I is being used or the supernatant sampled if a ^{3}H tracer is being employed.

The highest dilution of second antibody which gives the greatest specific binding and the lowest nsb in the shortest time period would be selected for use in the assay.

As seen above the second antibody is used at relatively low dilution which necessitates frequent reoptimisation as new batches are introduced.

Solid-phase second antibody methods

The coupling of second antibody to a particulate material such as cellulose gives all the advantages of liquid-phase second antibody separations plus the speed and simplicity to compare with precipitation methods. Incorporation of magnetic particles may obviate the need for centrifugation. Although these reagents can be produced in the laboratory a number of them are available commercially, and optimisation is very straightforward.

Scintillation proximity assays (SPA)

SPA is an assay format which has been recently introduced by Amersham International. It is in essence a second antibody method but without the need for a separation step! This novel approach is thus able to convert a standard heterogeneous RIA into a homogeneous method with all the attendant advantages this brings.

The SPA reagent consists of a small bead containing a scintillant molecule. Chemically attached to the surface of these microspheres is the second antibody (either anti-rabbit, anti-mouse, anti-sheep or protein A). Only tracer molecules which become bound to the surface-linked second antibody and hence are in close proximity to the bead will induce the scintillant to emit light. Thus only antibody-bound drug is counted; the free drug being too distant from the beads to induce scintillation, is not detected.

This procedure will work with weak β-emitters such as ^{3}H, ^{14}C, as well as ^{125}I through the Auger electrons produced by this last isotope. The SPA reagent can be added after the completion of the primary incubation or simultaneously with the first antibody and tracer. In the latter approach it is not usually necessary to increase the incubation time significantly thus the speed of the assay is maintained. The second generation microbeads are relatively buoyant, so continuous agitation of the assay tubes is unnecessary.

After the final incubation the tube is counted and only bound material registers. As well as avoiding the need for a separation of bound and free this approach also does away with the need for scintillant if ^{3}H or ^{14}C tracers are used. By carrying out the assay in a microtitre plate complete automation of the assay is possible following the introduction of multi-head β-counters by Canberra Packard (Pangbourne, Berks, UK) and Wallac (UK) Ltd (Milton Keynes, UK) capable of taking microtitre plates. Because no separation takes place the antibody–antigen reaction is still proceeding whilst the samples are being counted. It is essential therefore, especially when counting times are long, to ensure that the assay is incubated to equilibrium to prevent assay drift.

Some optimisation of the mass of microbeads will be needed when converting an existing assay to the SPA format, also because of the lower counting efficiencies with SPA (typically 20 to 25 per cent for ^{3}H) longer counting times or some other adjustment to the assay may be necessary. One serious, though not insurmountable problem that has been encountered, particularly with the microtitre plate format, is a significant increase in nsb. The inclusion of surfactants such as Tween or Triton however, seems to overcome this problem.

Optimising for sensitivity

Having an assay with too much sensitivity is rarely a serious problem, the converse is normally the rule. Should this arise, however, there are a number of relatively straightforward approaches that can be used to effectively desensitise the assay.

The first and most obvious suggestion is to reduce the sample size (this will also have the added benefit of minimising matrix problems). This approach is limited only by the minimum volume of sample that can be precisely pipetted. We would not recommend using anything less than 10 μl, even with automated pipetting devices. Samples can always be diluted but this adds an extra stage (and extra error) into the assay procedure, which may be unacceptable.

The other approach is to use increased concentrations of antisera and/or tracer. Either of these approaches will lead to desensitised assays with the calibration curves shifted to the right. If the approach outlined under antibody selection was used then some data on the effect of antibody concentration on sensitivity should be available. If necessary, further antibody dilution and displacement curves can be generated with different concentrations of tracer. If increased concentrations of tracer are used the situation may arise where unacceptably high counts are being added to each assay tube (greater than 50 000 cpm). Under these circumstances it may be necessary to dilute the tracer with cold material, effectively reducing the specific activity of the tracer. It is essential however that the antibody affinity for the tracer and the 'cold' diluent are identical. One disadvantage of using concentrated reagents is that antisera and tracer will be consumed at a much faster rate, which may impact on long-term assay viability.

As already mentioned, insufficient sensitivity is the usual problem as analysts are required to determine lower and lower analyte concentrations. When sensitivity is limited, increasing sample size is generally the first line of attack, although it may be difficult to increase the volume of sample to much greater than 10 to 15 per cent of the incubation volume without incurring matrix interference problems.

Assuming that the optimal antibody concentration has been selected from the initial experiment then optimisation will centre around the tracer. Additional displacement curves should be run with reduced concentrations of tracer; the reduced counts will then have to be offset with increased counting times to ensure precision is maintained. Alternatively it may be possible to increase the specific activity of the tracer through more sophisticated purification techniques or higher incorporation of the tracer atom, i.e. the use of di-iodo Bolton–Hunter reagent.

Much of this work can be carried out using simple experimental protocols. For example the binding need only be determined at two concentrations of analyte: zero and the desired sensitivity. The displacement in binding along with the precision of the binding parameters will give a good measure of the likely sensitivity.

Where assay sensitivity still remains limited even after optimisation as outlined, then more radical solutions should be sought. Reducing the affinity of the antisera for the tracer, by chemical modification of the tracer or the bridge, may improve sensitivity (Rowell *et al.*, 1979). This approach however can result in an increase in imprecision.

Where the poor sensitivity is the result of bridge recognition effects leading to higher affinity for the tracer than analyte then purification of the sera may offer a solution. Albro *et al.* (1979) and Knight *et al.* (1985) describe methods for the removal of bridge recognising antibodies. In the former, the method is based on affinity chromatography, in the latter the method is solution based. Knight *et al.* (1985) showed a threefold improvement in the sensitivity of an assay for cotinine following serum purification.

The use of non-equilibrium methods has also proved useful in certain instances for increasing assay sensitivity (Samols and Bilkus 1963; Mason *et al.*, 1984). This approach involves mixing the antiserum and sample and then after a predetermined delay, the tracer. With non-equilibrium assays the time delay before adding tracer and then carrying out the separation are critical. This approach is assay dependent and its usefulness would have to be determined for each analyte. Once again there is a downside, which in this case is reduced specificity.

Pretreatment of the sample by extraction and/or concentration is an obvious way of improving the sensitivity of any assay. However this approach tends to be used as a last resort with immunoassays, since it detracts from one of the major benefits of immunoassay methods which is high sample throughput and it leads to more complex assay procedures. Extraction of the sample sometimes leads to aggravated matrix problems as a result of concentrating of interferents or solvent impurities which may affect the assay. The success of such an assay can be very dependent on the batch of extraction solvent used. Extraction however does confer one advantage in that it can improve specificity by selective removal of specific interferents, this is discussed in more detail below.

Optimising for specificity

Specificity is ultimately a function of the antiserum which is controlled by the structure of the hapten and immunogen that were used to generate it. If the structure of the hapten and the resultant immunogen was such that the antiserum recognises a related compound then it may not be possible to obtain the desired specificity. If the problematic cross-reactivity was a chance occurrence because of some quirk of the animal's immune system, then full evaluation of all available sera may offer an alternative with the desired or near acceptable specificity characteristics. This is one good reason for using as many animals as possible when raising antisera.

It has been clearly shown that short incubation times can lead to significantly increased cross-reactivity (Vining *et al.*, 1981), typically three- to fourfold but occasionally up to tenfold where very short incubation times have been employed. For maximum specificity therefore it is important that the assay is incubated to equilibrium and that the effect of incubation time is investigated. Vining and co-workers also reported an increase in cross-reaction with increasing incubation temperature, therefore if specificity is a problem this should also be investigated.

Various assay parameters such as added protein, ionic strength of buffer etc. can have some bearing on assay specificity through specific and non-specific effects. It is difficult to predict when such variables will be of importance or whether their investigation will prove fruitful. In general it would be expected that analytes or cross-reactants which were highly protein bound would be expected to show some change in binding characteristics as the make-up of the incubation medium was changed.

One parameter that can have a marked and predictable effect is the pH of the assay medium. Many analytes are charged at physiological pH and since electrostatic interactions are the strongest of the intermolecular forces it is probable that the antibody binding site bears a complementary charge to that on an analyte molecule. Thus by varying the pH of the incubation medium about the pK_a of an ionisable functional group on the analyte or cross-reacting molecule, the degree to which these molecules bind to the antibody can be altered and the assay specificity modified.

Although the quality of the antiserum is the major factor controlling specificity, the structure of the tracer also has some influence as was discussed in Chapter 6. Greatest specificity should be achieved with the tracer for which the antiserum has the highest affinity (Rowell *et al.*, 1979).

Instances can occur where, despite taking all the necessary precautions when raising the sera and trying the approaches discussed above, it is still not possible to obtain the necessary specificity. Where the problem is the result of a known interferent, such as a metabolite, then a number of approaches still exist to be tried which may be far from ideal but which may actually solve the problem. The first of these is extraction.

Where the interfering compound has physico-chemical properties different to the analyte then it may be possible to extract one or other of these from the sample. For example if the interferent is a polar metabolite, then it should be possible to extract the parent compound from the sample using a non-polar solvent leaving the polar interfering compound behind. The extract can be concentrated, the solvent removed and the residue dissolved in buffer for introduction into the assay. Such an approach has been successfully applied to the analysis of ondansetron in the presence of cross-reacting metabolites (Wring *et al.*, 1994). Through the use of sophisticated extraction procedures based on solid-phase methods it should also be possible to extract polar interferents and leave the parent compound intact in a near original sample. The particular approach adopted will be compound dependent and discussion of this type of analysis is outside the scope of this chapter.

Where extraction procedures are inappropriate because of similarity in the properties of the analyte and interferent then it may be necessary to resort to HPLC purification. This has been used on a number of occasions in the authors' laboratories and there are also many reports in the literature covering a wide range of analytes (e.g. Law *et al.*, 1984; Pellegatti *et al.*, 1992). A further advantage of this approach is that the retention properties of the analyte can give some form of identification, which can be a valuable asset to the method in the forensic context.

On occasions, i.e. in drug screening, it may be desirable to have a non-specific assay with broad ranging cross-reactivity. Under such circumstances the opposite strategy to that outlined above would be adopted. It may also be possible by reducing the antiserum affinity for the tracer through chemical modification of the latter to broaden the specificity of an assay.

Optimising for precision

Depending on the intended use of the assay a high level of precision may or may not be required. For example if the assay is used to screen fungal cultures for active metabolites then it is unlikely that precision would be an issue. However, if the method is used to generate pharmacokinetic data or plasma drug levels in criminal cases then a high level of precision is required.

The precision profile as discussed above is the best way to evaluate precision both within and between assays or days.

The data in Figure 6.6 show two precision profiles generated with different separation methods for the peptide urogastrone. The profiles show the level of preci-

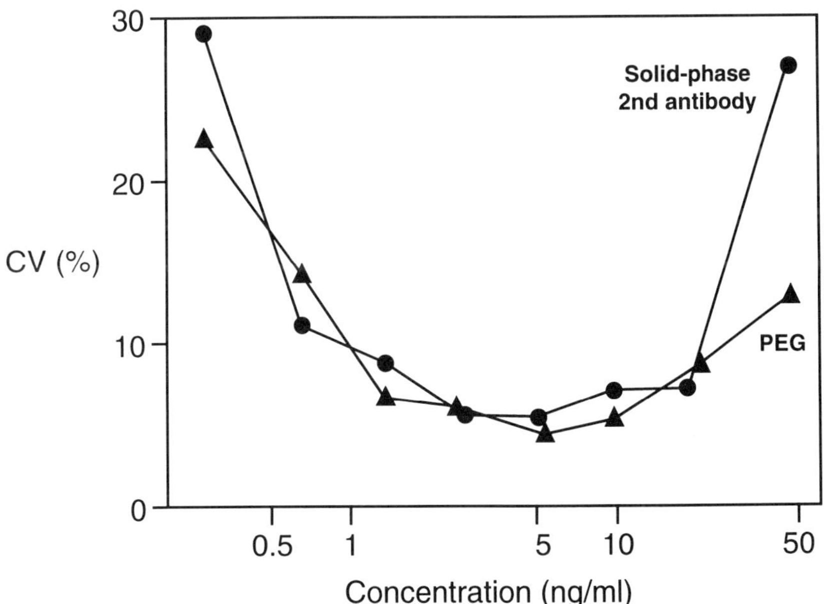

Figure 6.6 RIA precision profiles generated with an assay for the peptide urogastrone. The profile obtained using a PEG separation method was found to be superior to separation using solid-phase second antibody.

Table 6.5 Precision data obtained following the analysis of 10 calibration series in a single run. The assay tubes were processed in three separate batches resulting in assay drift

Calibration series	Centrifugation batch	Concentration (ng/ml)			
1	1	7.3	14	31	88
2	1	7.1	15	31	81
3	1	7.5	15	30	80
4	2	7.8	16	30	101
5	2	7.6	16	32	92
6	2	8.0	15	34	111
7	2	7.9	17	33	104
8	3	8.4	17	32	115
9	3	8.3	16	36	111
10	3	8.2	16	35	87
	Mean	7.8	16	32	97
	S.D.	0.43	0.95	2.1	13
	CV (%)	5.5	6.0	6.4	13.5

sion achieved using PEG (which was employed for the assay development work) to be superior, at least at the extremes of the calibration range, to that generated using a solid-phase second antibody procedure. Employed in this way, the precision profile is a useful tool for monitoring variation in performance resulting from changes to assay parameters, such as pipetting technique, new batches of separating agent, incubation temperature or even different operators.

Precision profiles can also be useful in diagnosing problems such as drift, i.e. variation in the concentration of a fixed standard across an assay. A number of assay methods, particularly those with time-dependent separation methods, such as charcoal, can suffer from drift. The data in Table 6.5 taken from an assay for an ACE inhibitor, show the calculated concentrations for four of the standard concentrations measured in 10 calibration series. The overall level of precision is reasonable (CV approximately 5 to 14 per cent), but closer inspection of the data shows that it is aggravated by drift. This is clearly shown by the data for the nominal 32 ng/ml standard which increases from 31 to 35 ng/ml over the 10 calibration series. Similar changes are evident for the other standards. The problem in this case was traced to the fact that an unrefrigerated microcentrifuge was used to spin the samples after the addition of PEG. Because of the limited capacity (40 tubes) it was necessary to carry out the centrifugation in three batches. The significant warming of the centrifuge over the three batches caused a drop in binding for each subsequent batch which resulted in a drift in concentration from batch 1 to batch 3. This manifested itself, when viewed across the whole assay, as poor precision.

Optimising for accuracy

Inaccuracy can occur through one of two factors which reveal themselves in different ways. Wherever possible an immunoassay method should be compared with a selective physico-chemical method, e.g. HPLC, using both real samples and spiked samples (see Chapter 9). If the immunoassay is found to give higher results than HPLC for real samples but not for spiked samples then the suggestion is that the assay is not specific and there are cross-reacting materials (e.g. metabolities) present in the sample which are absent from the spiked standards. It is possible that the ratio of concentrations obtained by the two techniques may be constant for all samples. In drug bioanalysis however, it is more likely that this ratio will change with time since drug/metabolite ratios inevitably increase with time after dosing.

If high results are obtained from both real samples and spiked samples then the evidence suggests the presence of an endogenous cross-reacting interferent in the matrix. If either high or low results are obtained compared with the reference technique then some form of matrix problem exits. If it is the former then the reader is referred to the section above on 'Optimising for specificity'. The matrix problem can be clearly demonstrated by spiking a series of individual samples with compound and analysing them. If these samples give results significantly different to that expected or show a high degree of variability then a matrix effect has been confirmed. Should this occur the reader is referred to the section on 'Introduction of matrix'. If the effect cannot be overcome the bias can be averaged by preparing the calibration standards in an 'average matrix' using pooled samples.

Conclusions

An immunoassay is a complex interaction of many factors which must be carefully and systematically evaluated for successful optimisation. A logical well-documented approach is essential to develop precise, accurate, sensitive, specific and robust assays in a timely manner. Although this chapter has dealt specifically with development and optimisation of a competitive radioimmunoassay the basic principles are universally applicable.

References

Abraham, G. E. (1969) *J. Clin. Endocrinol. Metab.*, **29**, 866.

Albro, P. W., Luster, M. I., Chae, K., Chaudhary, S. K., Clark, G., Lawson, L. D., Corbett, J. T. & McKinney, J. D. (1979) *Toxicol. Appl. Pharmacol.*, **50**, 137.

Ballard, P., Malone, M. D. & Law, B. (1994) *J. Pharm. Biomed. Anal.*, **12**, 47.

Ballard, P., Stafford, L .E. & Law, B. (1996) *J. Pharm. Biomed. Anal.*, **14**, 409.

Binoux, M. A. & Odell, S. E. (1973) *J. Clin. Endocrinol. Metab.*, **36**, 303.

Boxen, I. & Tevaarwerk, G. J. M. (1982) *J. Immunoassay*, **3**, 53.

Brock, P., Eldred, E. W., Woiszwillo, J. E., Doran, M. & Schoemaker, H. J. (1978) *Clin. Chem.*, **24**, 1595.

Brown, T. R., Bagchi, N., Ho, T. T. S. & Mack, R. E. (1980) *Clin. Chem.*, **26**, 503.

Cameron, E. H. D., Hillier, S. G. & Griffiths, K. (eds) (1975) *Steroid Immunoassay.* Proceedings of the 5th Tenovus Workshop, Cardiff, April 1974, Alpha Omega Publishing, Cardiff, UK.

Desbuquois, B. & Aurbach, G. D. (1971) *J. Clin. Endocrinol.*, **33**, 732.

Ekins, R. (1981) *Ligand Quarterly*, **4**, 33.

Ekins, R. P. (1983) The precision profile: its use in assay design, assessment and quality control. In: Hunter, W. M. (ed.) *Immunoassays for Clinical Chemistry.* Churchill Livingstone, Edinburgh, pp. 76–105.

EL-GAMAL, B. A. & LANDON, J. (1988) *Clin. Chim. Acta*, **173**, 201.

HALES, C. N. & RANDLE, P. J. (1963) *Biochem. J.*, **88**, 137.

HARLOW, E. & LANE, D. (1988) *Antibodies: a Laboratory Manual.* Cold Spring Harbor Laboratory, New York, USA, p. 298.

HARTMAN, D. J., COTISSON, A., GUILLOUX, L. & VILLE, G. (1982) *Radioimmunoassay and Related Procedures in Medicine*, Proceedings of an International Symposium, IAEA, Vienna, Austria, pp. 123.

HERBERT, V., LAU, K. S., GOTTLIEB, C. W. & BLEICHER, S. J. (1965) *J. Clin. Endocrinol. Metab.*, **25**, 1375.

KNIGHT, G. J., WYLIE, P., HOLMAN, M. S. & HADDOW, J. E. (1985) *Clin. Chem.*, **31**, 118.

VAN KREVELEN, D. W. (1990) *Properties of Polymers.* Elsevier, Amsterdam, p. 233.

LAW, B., MASON, P. A., MOFFAT, A. C. & KING, L. J. (1984) *J. Anal. Toxicol.*, **8**, 14.

LENTER, C. (ed.) (1984) *Geigy Scientific Tables*, Vol. 3. Ciba Geigy Ltd, Basle, Switzerland, pp. 58.

MASON, P. A., LAW, B., POCOCK, K. & MOFFAT, A. C. (1982) *Analyst*, **107**, 629.

MASON, P. A., ROWAN, K. M., LAW, B., MOFFAT, A. C., KILNER, E. A. & KING, L. A. (1984) *Analyst*, **109**, 1213.

PELLEGATTI, M., BRAGGIO, S., SARTORI, S., FRANCESCHETTI, F. & BOLELLI, G. F. (1992) *J. Chromatogr.*, **573**, 105.

PRATT, J. J., WIEGMAN, T., LAPPOHN, R. E. & WOLDRING, M. G. (1975) *Clin. Chim. Acta*, **59**, 337.

PRATT, J. J., BOONMAN, R., WOLDRING, M. G. & DONKER, A. J. M. (1978) *Clin. Chim. Acta*, **84**, 329.

RATCLIFFE, W. A., CHALLAND, G. S. & RATCLIFFE, J. G. (1974) *Ann. Clin. Biochem.*, **11**, 224.

ROWELL, F. J., PAXTON, J. W., AITKEN, S. M. & RATCLIFFE, J. G. (1979) *J. Immunol. Methods*, **27**, 363.

SAMOLS, E. C. & BILKUS, D. (1963) *Proc. Soc. Exp. Biol. Med.*, **115**, 89.

SCATCHARD, G. (1949) *Ann. N.Y. Acad. Sci.*, **51**, 660.

SOURGENS, H., WINTERHOFF, H., KEMPER, F. H. & AENSTOOTS, F. (1979) *Clin. Chim. Acta*, **97**, 179.

TEALE, J. D., FORMAN, E. J., KING, L. J., PIALL, E. M. & MARKS, V. (1975) *J. Pharm. Pharmacol.*, **27**, 465.

VINING, R. F., COMPTON, P. & MCGINLEY, R. (1981) *Clin. Chem.*, **27**, 910.

WALGRAEVE, H., VAN BEEK, E., CRIEL, G., VAN BRUSSEL, K. & DE LEENHEER, A. (1986) *Insect Biochem.*, **16**, 41.

WRING, S. A., ROONEY, R. M., GODDARD, C. P., WATERHOUSE, I. & JENNER, W. N. (1994) *J. Pharm. Biomed. Anal.*, **12**, 361.

7

Enzyme-linked immunosorbent assay (ELISA) development and optimisation

B. LAW and M. D. MALONE

Zeneca Pharmaceuticals, Macclesfield

R. A. BIDDLECOMBE

GlaxoWellcome Research and Development, Beckenham

Introduction

The term ELISA (enzyme-linked immunosorbent assay) was introduced by Engvall and Perlmann (1971) to describe a subset of the widely used immunoassay technique. ELISAs are distinguished from other immunoassays such as RIA by the use of an enzyme label linked either to the antigen or the antibody. This label in conjunction with a suitable substrate produces the assay signal. ELISAs are distinguished from other enzyme immunoassay (EIA) methods by the fact that one of the reagents is bound to a solid phase. In practice this solid phase usually takes the form of a 96-well microtitre plate. This gives the ability to handle many samples at one time and it facilitates automation of the assay. For a full discussion on all aspects of EIA the reader is referred to a number of books on the subject (Tijssen, 1985; Kemeny and Challacombe, 1988; Kemeny, 1991).

Many different enzymes have been used as tracers in ELISAs (Gosling, 1990; Porstmann and Kiessig, 1992), including urease, alkaline phosphatase, horseradish peroxidase (HRP) and β-galactosidase. Each of these can be employed with a number of substrates to generate an assay signal which usually takes the form of a coloured dye. Substrates which yield fluorescent or chemiluminescent products have also been used (Gosling, 1990).

The ELISA technique has principally been applied to the determination of proteins and other large-molecular-weight species. However, two formats have also been developed for the analysis of low-molecular-weight analytes of less than 1000 Dalton (Tijssen, 1985). These consist of one with the antigen as the immobilised component and the other with the antibody immobilised.

In the immobilised antigen ELISA, the analyte (or a suitable hapten) is linked to the solid phase indirectly. This linking is effected by preparing a hapten–protein conjugate which can be physically adsorbed onto the surface of the solid phase. The design and synthesis of this hapten–protein conjugate is crucial to the successful development of the ELISA.

There are many more steps in an antigen-immobilised ELISA than in a comparable RIA and these are shown in Figure 7.1. The first stage of the assay involves adsorbing the hapten–protein conjugate (plate conjugate) to the solid phase, which is known as sensitisation. The plate is then washed and vacant binding sites on the plate are often blocked by a suitable inert protein which is included in the buffer. The plate is then washed again and analyte-specific antiserum is then incubated in the wells together with standards or samples containing the analyte. This is the primary antiserum incubation. The antiserum used in this incubation is diluted such that the amount of antibody is limited compared with the amount of immobilised antigen bound to the plate. Added analyte then competes with the immobilised antigen for the antibody binding sites. The amount of antibody bound to the immobilised antigen at equilibrium is inversely related to the concentration of added analyte. Following a further washing stage (which is effectively the separation of bound and free) the enzyme-labelled antibody is added to detect the primary antibody bound to the immobilised antigen. This is known as the second antibody incubation. The plates are further washed and a response developed using a suitable substrate. A calibration curve is obtained similar to that of a competitive RIA with decreasing colour for increasing analyte concentrations.

The assay format with the analyte immobilised has a number of advantages over the alternative which are worthy of discussion. In the immobilised antibody approach an analyte–enzyme conjugate has to be prepared for every newly developed assay. When employing the immobilised antigen approach recommended here however, the enzyme-labelled second antibody can be obtained commercially. Furthermore, if the specific or first antibody is always raised in the same species, then the same enzyme-labelled second antibody can be used with every assay. In effect it is a 'universal tracer', lending significant advantages of cost and convenience. With the immobilised antibody approach it may be necessary to purify the antiserum before this can be linked to the solid phase, especially when only a small population of the specific antibodies are present in the sera. When the antibody is immobilised

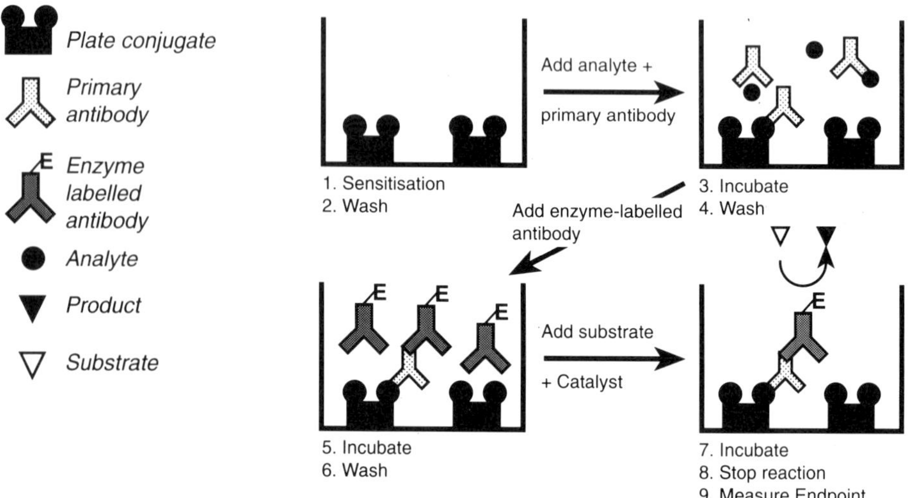

Figure 7.1 Schematic diagram for an immobilised antigen ELISA.

on the plate, there is often a significant reduction in affinity (Arends, 1971) coupled with a dramatic reduction in binding capacity (Butler *et al.*, 1992). The denaturation of the antibody which leads to the loss of binding can obviously occur with other proteins (Pesce and Michael, 1992), however with multivalent plate conjugates this should be less of a problem. Finally with the immobilised antigen method, the matrix is washed away before the enzyme–antibody complex is added. In the antibody immobilised format the enzyme-labelled antigen and the matrix are present simultaneously (Figure 7.2). Thus should the sample contain any noxious agents or irreversible enzyme inhibitors then the resultant signal could be affected and a spurious result obtained.

The immobilised antigen approach has been used extensively and successfully in the authors' laboratories and the development of ELISAs employing this approach will form the basis of this chapter. Initially the reagents and equipment particular to ELISA will be described, followed by a discussion of the major stages of assay development. Five major stages will be considered, these are:

1 The selection of a suitable carrier protein and production of the plate conjugate
2 Selection of the initial assay conditions
3 Assessment of the antisera
4 Introduction of matrix
5 Optimisation of assay conditions with matrix present

This chapter will concentrate in the main on stages 1, 2 and 5 in the list above, since these aspects of assay development are specific to the ELISA format. The conditions for the preparation and purification of the plate conjugate are essentially the same as those for the preparation of immunogens (Chapter 3) although some important differences will be outlined.

The assessment of the antiserum and the subsequent development and in part the optimisation (steps 3 to 5 above) are similar to those described in Chapter 6 for RIA.

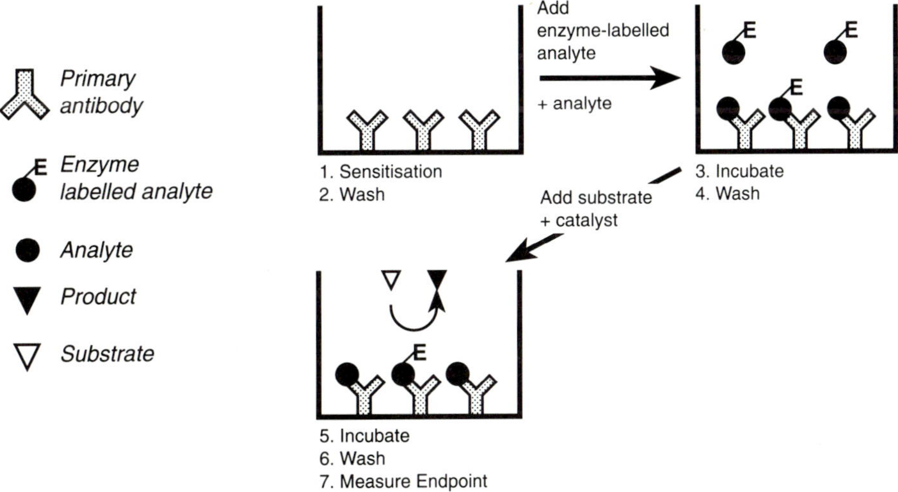

Figure 7.2 Schematic diagram for an immobilised antibody ELISA.

Reagents and buffers for ELISA

Enzyme-labelled antibodies

Although it can be relatively simple to prepare antibody–enzyme conjugates (see Tijssen, 1985; Kemeny, 1991 for methods), for those delving into ELISA for the first time the use of pre-prepared reagents is recommended. A wide range of enzyme-labelled anti-IgG reagents are commercially available for use as indicator reagents in immobilised antigen ELISAs. The most common of these contain HRP, alkaline phosphatase or β-galactosidase. These are available linked to IgG (often from donkey) and directed against IgG from the major species used for reagent antibody production, i.e. sheep, rabbit and goat.

Each of these enzymes can be utilised with a variety of substrates. Most of the commonly used substrates give rise to soluble coloured products which can be readily detected by spectrophotometric means. Table 7.1 lists the three most commonly used enzymes along with their possible substrates. HRP is probably the most popular, and its use is recommended here and by other workers (Porstmann and Kiessig, 1992) principally because of its low cost and the fact that it gives a stable coloured end product.

Some workers have used substrates which give rise to fluorescent or chemiluminescent products (e.g. Shalev *et al.*, 1980). For example, 4-methylumberliferyl derivatives can give reaction products with alkaline phosphatase that can be detected at 100-fold lower concentrations than the conventionally used nitrophenyl phosphate. The increased sensitivity of detection for these materials however is rarely converted into a comparable increase in assay sensitivity (Porstmann and Kiessig, 1992) and hence their use is not recommended at this stage.

Table 7.1 Commonly used enzymes in ELISA and their substrates

Enzyme	Substrate	Comment
Alkaline phosphatase (EC 3.1.3.1)	*p*-Nitrophenyl phosphatase	Enzyme present at low levels in serum
Horseradish peroxidase (HRP) (EC 1.11.1.7)	*m*-Phenylenediamine/H_2O_2	Carcinogen
	o-Phenylenediamine (OPD)/H_2O_2	Mutagen
	2,2′-Azino-bis(3-ethyl-benzthiazoline-6-sulphonic acid) disodium salt (ABTS)/H_2O_2	Mutagen
	3,3′,5,5′-Tetramethylbenzidine (TMB)/H_2O_2	Non-carcinogenic* Non-mutagenic*
	o-Toluidine/H_2O_2	Carcinogen?
	o-Dianisidine/H_2O_2	Carcinogen
	p-Hydroxycinnamic acid/luminol/H_2O_2	Chemiluminescent
β-Galactosidase (EC 3.2.1.28)	*p*-Nitrophenyl galactose	Enzyme not normally present in mammalian fluids
	4-Methylumbelliferyl-β-D-galactose (MUG)	Fluorescent

* Bos *et al.* (1981).

Most manufacturers of indicator antisera suggest dilutions to be used with their reagents. However, whilst the recommended dilution may give an acceptable rate of colour development, this may be at the expense of a high degree of non-specific colour. It is recommended that the most appropriate dilution for a particular assay/reagent combination is investigated and optimised.

In our experience manufacturers often make 'improvements' to their products, such as changing the enzyme:antibody ratio or providing the reagent in a purer form. These changes may alter the non-specific binding characteristics of the product and also the rate of colour development. In such circumstances we have usually found it necessary to re-optimise the incubation conditions for the enzyme-labelled reagent. It is strongly recommended therefore that all new preparations are checked, and if necessary the appropriate assay conditions re-optimised to regain the required assay characteristics.

Assay buffers

A wide variety of buffers are used in ELISAs, including those for sensitisation, primary and secondary incubations as well as for blocking, washing and developing the colour. Although there appears to be a great degree of latitude in the type of buffers that can be used, on occasions even for the sensitisation buffer (Geerligs *et al.*, 1988; Porstmann and Kiessig, 1992), the use of the appropriate buffer at certain stages can be important for successful assay development. For example, the colour development buffers often have their own specific characteristics, especially with respect to the pH optima (Porstmann and Kiessig, 1992). Because sodium azide can be an inhibitor of HRP it is not generally used as a preservative in the substrate development buffer, and for convenience many workers prefer to avoid this preservative completely when working with this enzyme. Where a preservative is required, thiomersal at a concentration of around 0.1 per cent can be used. In practice however we do not use a preservative but prepare buffers on a weekly or 2 weekly basis.

Detergents are included in all buffers (with the exception of the sensitisation buffer) where they act to reduce non-specific binding of proteins to the plastic surface (Engvall and Perlmann, 1972). Their action is thought to be the result of a reduction of the surface tension of the incubation media, thus inhibiting hydrophobic interactions between proteins from the reagents, sample or buffers with the uncoated plastic surface. If a detergent is used effectively then it may be possible to omit the use of a blocking buffer (Bullock and Walls, 1977). However the detergent concentration should be kept as low as possible since too high a concentration may interfere with the antibody–antigen binding.

A variety of detergents have been used in ELISAs including the Tweens: 20, 40 and 80 as well as Brij 35 and Triton X-100. By far the most widely used detergent is Tween 20 which is effective at concentrations of less than 0.05 per cent.

Sensitisation buffers

For sensitisation of the plate most workers employ a carbonate buffer (pH 9.8, 0.1 M). Some workers claim adsorption to be relatively independent of pH, ionic strength or buffer type (Geerligs *et al.*, 1988; Porstmann and Kiessig, 1992) whilst others hold the opposite view (Tsang *et al.*, 1980). We have found phosphate buffer (pH 7, 0.1 M) with or without the addition of sodium chloride to be useful in a number of assays and this will be used here.

Incubation buffers

The nature of the incubation buffer used can have a marked effect on both specific and non-specific binding. Generally, neutral or near-neutral buffers are used, the most popular being phosphate, phosphate/citrate and tris(hydroxymethyl)amino-methane (Tris). We recommend a standard phosphate buffered saline (PBS), and to help minimise matrix interference the overall concentration is kept high with the phosphate at least 0.05 M, and the sodium chloride up to 0.3 M.

Blocking buffers

A variety of agents have been successfully employed as blocker in ELISA including gelatin, casein, BSA and even powdered milk, usually in the concentration range 0.1 to 1.0 per cent. The buffer is normally phosphate or Tris based. When required we have found phosphate buffered saline containing sodium caseinate (0.1 per cent) to be very effective.

Although blocking buffers can be used in a separate blocking step, when required it is generally convenient to include the blocking protein in the incubation buffers.

Washing buffers

For plate washing, the same phosphate buffer as used for incubation is recommended without the sodium chloride but with the addition of the detergent Tween 20 (0.05 per cent).

Substrate development buffers

Most enzyme/substrate combinations have their own special buffer requirements particularly with respect to pH and the need for cofactors. It is important that these are determined before trying an enzyme for the first time. For the development of the substrate 2,2′-azino-bis(3-ethylbenzthiazoline-6-sulphonic acid) disodium salt (ABTS) employed in the examples quoted here, an acetate buffer (pH 4.2, 0.1 M) is used along with hydrogen peroxide as the cofactor. When working with the enzyme HRP, a non-ionic detergent (e.g. Tween 20 or Triton X-100) is usually included in the substrate development buffer as this allows development at a temperature above the normal optimum of 15°C (Tijssen, 1985).

Stop solution

In the assays described here using HRP, sodium azide at a concentration of 10 mM is used as the stop solution to end the enzyme reaction. A number of alternatives have been employed such as sulphuric acid (4 M), although the use of sodium cyanide is not recommended.

Commercially available reagents

A number of companies, in particular Sigma (Poole, Dorset, UK) and Pierce Warriner (Chester, Cheshire, UK) supply a wide range of reagents, many specifically designed for ELISA work. These include not only enzymes, antibody–enzyme conjugates, activated proteins and purified detergents but even pre-prepared blocking buffers. Although the cost of some of these materials may be higher than those prepared in-house, their use does help minimise the risk of failure for anyone intending setting up an ELISA for the first time.

Equipment for ELISA

Microtitre plates

ELISAs can be carried out in a variety of ways with the solid phase in the form of a tube, dip-stick, bead or membrane. However the convenience and low cost associated with the use of the microtitre plate is responsible in part for the rapid development and growth of ELISA. Microtitre plates are self-contained units usually consisting of 96 wells, arranged in 8 rows (horizontally) by 12 columns (vertically). Each well has a maximum capacity of approximately 300 µl of which up to 200 to 250 µl is effectively usable.

Microtitre plates are widely available in one of two plastics, namely polystyrene and polyvinylchloride (PVC). Flexible PVC microtitre plates have been reported to have the greatest capacity to bind protein (Kemeny, 1991). They also have the advantage that they can be cut up with scissors if the radioactive content of wells is required to be counted, for example when checking protein binding capacity. However, for most work we have successfully used rigid polystyrene plates and our choice is also reflected in a survey of the recent literature which shows polystyrene to be preferred over PVC. A number of manufacturers now produce individual wells which can be inserted into a suitable holder. These can be useful where there is a need to set up small numbers of tests and a full plate is not required.

Batch-to-batch differences between plates is much less common than it used to be. Nevertheless, it is a good idea to buy plates in bulk and test new batches in parallel with old ones. This should be carried out using a robust established, but discriminating, assay. Some manufacturers supply certificated microtitre plates where the adsorption of IgG across the 96 wells has a coefficient of variation of less than 5 per cent and all results within 10 per cent of the mean. The use of these certificated plates is recommended.

Another common problem with microtitre plates is the occurrence of edge effects which are manifested in increased signal in the outer wells. These effects are thought to be caused by temperature differentials across the plates and are evident when chilled reagents are used. Because of the insulating properties of the polystyrene, the outer wells reach ambient temperature faster than those in the middle of the plate. This problem can usually be eliminated by ensuring all reagents are at room temperature prior to adding to the wells. However, if the problem persists then the use of the outer wells of the plate should be avoided such that the plate is effectively reduced to 60 wells, i.e. 6 × 10. It is also recommended that plates are not stacked as this can effectively insulate the inner wells, further increasing the temperature differential. The use of long incubation times or continuous agitation should help ensure that thermal equilibrium is attained across the plate.

In our laboratories we use MaxiSorp F96 certificated polystyrene plates from Nunc (obtained in the UK through Life Technologies Ltd, Paisley, UK).

To prevent evaporation and possible contamination during the long incubations the plates should be covered. Many workers use purpose-made adhesive films such as Seal Plate Films (Anachem Ltd, Beds, UK). However where these are highly adhesive there may be problems actually removing them and for this reason a number of workers simply use domestic 'cling film'.

Pipettes

For most work it is suitable to use air displacement pipettes capable of delivering from 10 µl up to 100 µl. To minimise pipetting operations the use of multi-channel pipettes is recommended. These are similar to the standard single pipettes but with either 12 or 8 channels to allow multiple dispensing or pipetting, either across or down a microtitre plate. It needs to be borne in mind however that calibration of the multipipettes can be a tedious task.

Washing apparatus

ELISAs involve numerous wash steps which can be conveniently and simply carried out by flooding the plate using a squeezy bottle. After a defined period the waste solution is merely flicked out of the wells into a waste container.

Where more precise control or a less messy procedure is desired then one of the proprietary wash systems can be used. Such a device is the Immunowash-12 (Nunc), which has 24 nozzles arranged in pairs which fit across the 12 rows of the plate. One set of nozzles are connected to a reservoir and are used to dispense buffer into the wells using a simple siphon system. The other set of nozzles are connected to waste via a water-jet-driven vacuum pump and are used to aspirate the wash solution to waste.

Detectors

The quantification of the assay end point merely involves reading the absorbance of the coloured solution in the plate well. A range of plate readers are available which incorporate a suitable spectrophotometer to allow precise measurement of this coloured solution. These readers are fully automatic such that the whole plate can be read and 96 optical density measurements returned within 2 to 3 min. To allow detection of the full range of coloured reaction products most plate readers incorporate a series of filters with different wavelength cut-offs. A plate reader with filters set at 405, 450 and 490 nm will be suitable for the vast majority of the enzyme/substrate combinations which are used. Some automated systems such as the Biomek 1000 (see below) also have in-built detection systems.

As an alternative to stopping the reaction prior to reading, a kinetic plate reader can be used. With this type of system the rate of the enzyme reaction is determined rather than the colour at the end point. This approach should give greater precision since the tight control of the time course of the enzyme reaction is no longer required. Where the stopped reaction approach is to be employed, access to a kinetic plate reader during assay development can also be useful since this can allow the substrate incubation process to be studied and the stop time to be optimised.

Plate shakers

One limitation of solid-phase assays is the slow attainment of equilibrium compared with a solution-based system: this often leads to long incubation times (Franz and Stegemann, 1991). To a degree this can be overcome by gently agitating the plates during the incubation phases. The use of some sort of shaker or mixer is considered essential at the colour development stage to ensure that the colour is distributed evenly in the well and precise absorbance measurements are made. A quick mix is also recommended prior to the start of each incubation. A number of suitable mixers/shakers are available commercially and some of the automated systems (see below) and modern plate readers have a variable shaking facility built in.

Automated systems

Where high sample throughput is required then the use of some form of automation is strongly recommended. Because the separation of bound and free in an ELISA merely involves washing the plate, total automation of the process is possible in contrast to conventional RIA methods.

Most automated ELISA instruments are essentially liquid handling devices which are capable of carrying out all the pipetting operations of an ELISA. One widely used instrument which offers full automation is the Biomek 1000 Automated Laboratory Workstation (Beckman Instruments (UK) Ltd, Berks, UK). This instrument can dispense volumes in the range 20 to 200 μl with excellent accuracy and precision with the facilities to vary the rate of aspiration and dispensing which can be useful when handling viscous samples. In addition, this particular system will wash the plates and measure the optical density response at the end of the assay. The use of such equipment not only gives better assay precision compared with manual analysis but the monotony associated with carrying out the assay is virtually eliminated.

Plate conjugates

Small-molecular-weight species, particularly polar molecules, do not readily bind to plastics. Where they do, their small size precludes the ready access of an antibody, such that direct attachment of an antigen to a solid phase to give an antigen-bound ELISA is not possible. Most proteins however show considerable hydrophobic character which results in strong non-covalent binding to plastic surfaces. Thus, providing the analyte can be chemically linked to a protein, the resultant conjugate can be bound to the surface of a plastic microtitre plate. A variety of proteins have been used as carriers for the antigen and the methods of conjugation are similar to those employed in immunogen formation.

Table 7.2 Molecular masses and iso-electric points (pI) of various proteins used in the preparation of plate conjugates

Protein	Molecular mass (Dalton)	Iso-electric point
Bovine thyroglobulin	670 000	4.6
Immuno gamma globulin	150 000	4–5
Casein	375 000	4–5
Human serum albumin	68 000	4.7
Ovalbumin	43 000	4.7
Poly-D-lysine	1 000–300 000	NA
Haemocyanin	1 000 000	5–6.4
Bovine serum albumin	68 000	4.6–4.9

NA = not applicable.

Carrier proteins

Table 7.2 shows the variety of proteins which have been used as carriers in immobilised antigen ELISAs, together with their molecular masses and iso-electric points (pI). Of the proteins tabulated, the most commonly used are bovine serum albumin (BSA), bovine thyroglobulin, keyhole limpet haemocyanin (KLH) and poly-D-lysine. Assays based on these different proteins vary considerably in their characteristics, especially the non-specific binding and detection limits.

Since any antisera raised against a hapten–protein conjugate will contain antibodies to the protein as well as the hapten, it is essential that the protein used in the production of the immunogen is completely different to that used in the plate conjugate. Failure to do so will lead to increased non-specific binding and seriously compromised sensitivity, since antibodies will also bind to the carrier protein (Briand *et al.*, 1985).

Incorporation ratio

The conjugation or incorporation ratio of the plate conjugate has been reported to be an important factor controlling the assay sensitivity. The degree of incorporation determines the physical distance between the adjacent hapten or analyte molecules which are chemically linked to the surface of the protein. If the distance between adjacent hapten molecules is similar to the distance between the two binding sites of the antibody then bivalent binding of the antibody to the plate conjugate can occur. Bivalent binding interactions have been reported to have affinity constants which are 100 to 1000 times greater than the corresponding monovalent binding (Karush and Hornick, 1973). Thus if the incorporation ratio is very high, a poor sensitivity will result since the analyte will be unable to compete effectively with the hapten–protein conjugate for the antibody. It is recommended therefore that incorporation ratios are kept low, certainly less than those used in the production of immunogens.

In our laboratory, plate conjugates involving poly-D-lysine (molecular mass 50 000 Dalton) having an incorporation ratio of 6 : 1 and bovine thyroglobulin (molecular mass 670 000 Dalton) with a ratio of 22 : 1 have produced assays with similar sensitivity to that of RIA. Thus incorporation ratios of this order are recommended.

Preparation of plate conjugates

Methods for producing plate conjugates are essentially the same as those for immunogen preparation described in Chapter 3 and any of the methods described there can be used. In order to keep the incorporation ratio to a minimum it is recommended that the hapten to protein reactant ratio is reduced by at least a factor of two compared with that used to produce immunogens. Alternatively, the reaction time can be reduced.

It is strongly recommended that the incorporation ratio is measured using one of the available techniques (Chapter 3) so that the influence of the incorporation ratio on sensitivity can be determined.

Bridge recognition

To minimise bridge recognition (see Chapter 6) it is important that the chemical bridge linking the hapten to the protein in the immunogen and the plate conjugate are different. This is even more important than in RIA since in ELISA both the immunogen and the plate conjugate have the same chemical nature. It is particularly important in ELISA therefore to have a range of linking procedures available and if possible a range of haptens bearing different reactive groups. However, it appears to be accepted that bridge recognition can be reduced or minimised when the length of the bridge in either conjugate is less than four atoms.

Other literature indicates that the degree of bridge recognition can vary across a series of polyclonal antisera from different animals immunised with the same immunogen and that the effect is generally less of a problem for antisera taken later in an immunisation schedule. Thus careful screening and selection of the 'right' antiserum is an extremely important factor in determining the assay quality.

Irrespective of which conjugate is nominally the immunogen and which the plate conjugate, it is recommended that both are employed as immunogens and injected into animals. Any sera obtained against one conjugate can be evaluated using the other as the plate conjugate and *vice versa.* It is important to bear in mind in evaluating sera produced in this way that meaningful results will only be obtained if both the chemical linking group, i.e. the bridge, and the protein are different in the immunogen and the plate conjugate (Briand *et al.*, 1985).

Assay development

Defining the starting conditions

Like the development of an RIA, the first experiment in setting up an ELISA can also be critical, with inappropriate selection of these starting conditions possibly leading to perfectly good reagents being rejected. In contrast to RIA, ELISA has many more variables which need to be fixed before beginning the assay development. Foremost amongst these is the plate conjugate concentration, which along with the incorporation ratio effectively controls the mass of hapten in the assay system. Varying the plate conjugate concentration is therefore equivalent to varying the mass of tracer in a RIA.

The optimum conjugate concentration for a particular assay is dependant on a number of factors and certain assumptions have to be made at this stage. In terms of assay sensitivity the optimum concentration should be as low as can be precisely detected using an enzyme-labelled antibody. However, a very low concentration of conjugate will leave the plate surface uncoated, which may lead to high non-specific binding if appropriate measures are not adopted. Conversely, a high concentration of conjugate not only results in reduced assay sensitivity but it can also lead to poor precision since some of the conjugate will only be loosely held by protein–protein interactions once the plate surface is saturated. These protein–protein interactions are weaker than those between the plastic and the protein and desorption of the plate conjugate can occur. It should be noted that the optimum concentration of protein to saturate the surface is dependent on the nature of the protein (Cantarero *et al.*, 1980).

In practice we would use an initial plate conjugate concentration of 5 μg/ml. This is within the concentration range of 1 to 10 μg/ml recommended by Voller *et al.* (1979) and is similar to that recommended by other workers (Tsang, *et al.*, 1980; Herrmann, 1981). This approach has worked well with a range of plate conjugates derived from small synthetic polymers such as poly-D-lysine (60 000 Dalton) to large natural proteins such as bovine thyroglobulin (670 000 Dalton).

In order to minimise non-specific binding to the plate a detergent is incorporated into all buffers subsequent to the sensitisation stage. No blocking protein is used at this initial stage although its use may be indicted later (see below). The concentration of the indicator reagent (second antibody–enzyme conjugate) is fixed using the manufacturer's recommended dilution. Incubation times are kept constant, and to facilitate rapid evaluation during this early stage in the development process, these are kept as short as is practicable.

Antiserum assessment

The first stage in the assay development is to assess the antisera for titre, specificity and sensitivity, very much as described for RIA in the previous chapter. This involves carrying out a series of antibody dilution curves, along with displacement curves for the analyte of interest and any compounds for which cross-reactivity is considered critical. A suggested method for antiserum assessment is given in PROCEDURE 1 below. The method describes the evaluation of two different sera using a single microtitre plate. The antibody dilution curves give the titre, and by running displacement curves with solutions of the analyte at the desired limit of detection an indication of the likely sensitivity is obtained. The process is carried out in a similar manner to that for RIA with all tests being performed in duplicate.

PROCEDURE 1 Initial assessment of the primary antiserum for titre and sensitivity

Reagents

- Sensitisation buffer is phosphate (0.05 M, pH 7.0) prepared from Na_2HPO_4 (4.17 g), KH_2PO_4 (2.81 g) and water (1000 ml)
- Incubation buffers for both primary and secondary incubations are phosphate (pH 7.0, 0.1 M) containing sodium chloride (0.15 M) and Tween 20 (0.05 per cent). These are pre-

pared from Na_2HPO_4 (8.34 g), KH_2PO_4 (5.62 g), sodium chloride (8.77 g), Tween 20 (0.5 ml) and water (1000 ml)

- Wash buffer is the same as that used for the incubation
- Substrate development buffer is acetate (pH 4.2, 0.1 M) containing Tween 20 (0.1 per cent v/v) prepared from sodium acetate trihydrate (0.325 g), acetic acid (0.436 ml), Tween 20 (0.1 ml) and water (100 ml)
- Plate conjugate dissolved in the sensitisation buffer at a concentration of 5 μg/ml
- Specific antiserum serially diluted in the incubation buffer 1/10 to $1/10^8$
- A control, non-immune serum diluted in a similar manner to the antiserum
- Analyte dissolved in the incubation buffer at a concentration near the preferred assay limit of detection
- Horseradish peroxidase–second antibody conjugate (Sigma, Dorset, UK) diluted in PBS containing Tween-20 (0.05 per cent) according to the manufacturer's instructions
- Hydrogen peroxide solution (30 per cent)
- Substrate solution: 2,2′-azino-bis(3-ethylbenzthiazoline-6-sulphonic acid) disodium salt (ABTS) (Sigma, Dorset, UK) dissolved in substrate development buffer (1.1 mg/ml)
- Stop solution prepared by dissolving sodium azide (0.65 g) in water (100 ml)

Equipment

- Polystyrene 96-well microtitre plates (certificated)
- Cellophane microtitre plate sealers
- Multi-head pipettes (8 or 12 channel) with capability to dispense up to 250 μl
- Washing apparatus
- Plate shaker
- Microtitre plate reader with 405 nm filter

Method

Add the plate conjugate solution (220 μl, 5 μg/ml) to all the wells of the plate, cover and incubate overnight at 4°C. The following day, aspirate the sensitisation solution to waste and wash the plate three times with wash buffer (300 μl). It is recommended that the wash solution is left in the well for a fixed time, typically 15 to 30 s, prior to aspirating to waste. Down the first two columns of the plate add the non-immune serum (200 μl), starting with the 1/10 dilution in the first row, the 1/100 dilution in the next row and so on with the $1/10^8$ in the last, the eighth row. Repeat the procedure for each of the antisera to be evaluated, filling four columns of the plate (two for the dilution curve and two for the displacement curve) with each serum. In this example the last two columns of the plate are not used. To the first two columns of the plate and all antibody dilution curve wells, that is the first two columns of each antiserum, add the simple buffer solution (20 μl) and to the displacement curve wells (the second two columns of each antiserum) add the analyte solution (20 μl). Cover the plate, mix gently and incubate at room temperature overnight. Aspirate to waste and wash three times with wash buffer.

Add to each well the second antibody–enzyme conjugate solution (220 μl) and incubate at room temperature for 3 h. Aspirate to waste and wash the plate three times with wash buffer. Mix a volume of hydrogen peroxide with the ABTS solution (18 μl to 10 ml) and then add this prepared substrate solution (220 μl) to each well and incubate at room temperature for a predefined interval (approximately 15 min) until a suitable colour intensity develops. Stop the reaction by the addition of the stop solution (20 μl) to each well and shake gently to ensure the colour is uniformly distributed in the wells and read the colour intensity at 405 nm.

Plot the optical density in each well against the log of the antiserum dilution to get an antibody dilution curve or a displacement curve, as shown previously in the assessment of antisera by RIA.

The layout of the plate can be readily altered from that described above. For example, to accommodate a narrower range of antisera dilutions (1/10 to $1/10^6$) these can be set up across the rows (rather than down the columns) with duplicates in adjacent wells in the same row. In this way it would be possible to test three sera per plate.

Unlike the RIA dilution curves shown in Chapter 6, there is often reduced binding at low antibody dilution in ELISA which appears as a 'hook' in the antibody dilution curve. The hook effect has been the subject of much study although the exact reason for this phenomenon is still unclear. In practice it is of little consequence however since most assays work with antiserum dilutions of greater than 1/1000. In contrast to RIA there is no 'total' signal which can be used to reference the sample and standard binding against. In ELISA the response for a given dilution of serum is compared with the maximum binding that is observed. Although the non-specific binding may be high at low serum dilution it rapidly falls off as the serum is diluted.

The data generated from these experiments is provisional and highly dependent on the experimental conditions used. However, a good indication should be obtained of which antisera contain useful antibodies. Furthermore, from the difference in optical density between the dilution curve and the displacement curve the antisera capable of giving the most sensitive assay can be selected. If displacement curves using potential cross-reactants are also carried out, then data on antiserum specificity will also be obtained.

When the initial experiment has gone well and one or two antisera are indicated as offering the requisite sensitivity and specificity, then calibration curves should be generated using these chosen sera at the indicated dilution. The assay conditions should be the same as those used in PROCEDURE 1. The first column of the plate can be set up with zero standards and non-specific binding wells (each in quadruplicate). Eight standards can then be set up down the next and subsequent columns depending on how many replicates are required. At this stage a more complete evaluation of sera specificity should also be carried out by evaluating the cross-reactivity of related materials and/or metabolites.

Although the assay may still be in prototype, once a calibration range has been defined the precision over this range should be determined by assaying multiple calibration series and generating a precision profile (see Chapters 6 and 9).

In a number of instances the experiment described in PROCEDURE 1 may not deliver the required result: binding may be low, sensitivity or precision may be poor, or non-specific binding so high as to mask the specific binding. In certain instances the cause may be readily apparent, for example a high level of absorbance in every well may indicate the use of too high a concentration of second antibody–enzyme conjugate. Where the reason is not immediately apparent then it will be necessary to carry out some investigation or optimisation of the experimental conditions. The most problematical stage in any ELISA is usually the sensitisation step (Kemeny, 1991). This should generally be investigated first since if non-optimal, it can affect all the above-mentioned parameters.

Optimisation of the sensitisation stage

Where the sensitisation stage is considered suspect then the experiment outlined in PROCEDURE 1 should be repeated using a range of plate conjugate concentrations with or without modifications to the sensitisation buffer (see below).

Reducing the concentration of the plate conjugate should improve sensitivity, whilst increasing the concentration will increase the limit of detection. There is an optimum with regard to the concentration of plate conjugate however. The stability of the adsorbed protein is greatest when adsorption takes the form of a monomolecular layer. When the protein concentration exceeds that required for monolayer formation a multilayered structure is produced. The resulting protein–protein interactions are weaker and can lead to poor precision as the protein desorbs during the assay procedure.

If the duplicates showed poor precision then this may be related to general handling procedures and pipetting etc. However it may also indicate the presence of protein–protein interactions (i.e. a too high a concentration of plate conjugate has been used) or that the interaction between the protein and plastic is poor.

Proteins are thought to adsorb to the plastic surfaces mainly by hydrophobic interactions, although charge is also thought to play a role (Shirahama and Suzawa, 1985; Kemeny and Challacombe, 1988). Therefore any change in the conditions which increases the hydrophobicity of the protein can be employed at the sensitisation stage. For example components which cause partial denaturation of proteins, e.g. 6 M guanidine hydrochloride (Lewis *et al.*, 1992), leading to exposure of hydrophobic regions may be suitable for inclusion in sensitisation buffers. Alternatively the ionic strength of the sensitisation medium can be increased. It is commonly believed that ionic components enhance the stability of the protein–plastic interactions by shielding repulsive charge-based interactions between neighbouring protein molecules, and several authors use high ionic concentrations as a consequence. However, the opposite has also been observed (Tsang *et al.*, 1980; Shirahama and Suzawa, 1985). If necessary the ionic strength of the sensitisation medium can be varied using sodium chloride or some other simple salt.

In the example in PROCEDURE 1 a sensitisation buffer of pH 7 phosphate was used, whereas most reports in the literature make use of carbonate (pH 9.8, 0.1 M). The reason for this is unclear but it probably relates to the fact that the first reported immunoassay using IgG-coated plastic was carried out using a carbonate buffer (Catt and Tregar, 1967). A range of proteins have been successfully immobilised using sensitisation buffers based on phosphate (Geerligs *et al.*, 1988), citrate (Geerligs *et al.*, 1988) and tris(hydroxymethyl)aminomethane (Tris) (Tsang *et al.*, 1980) under pH conditions often close to neutrality. If the sensitisation stage is considered to be problematic then it may be worth carrying out some basic optimisation experiments using a range of buffer types with and without added salts. A suitable carbonate buffer can be conveniently prepared by mixing a solution of

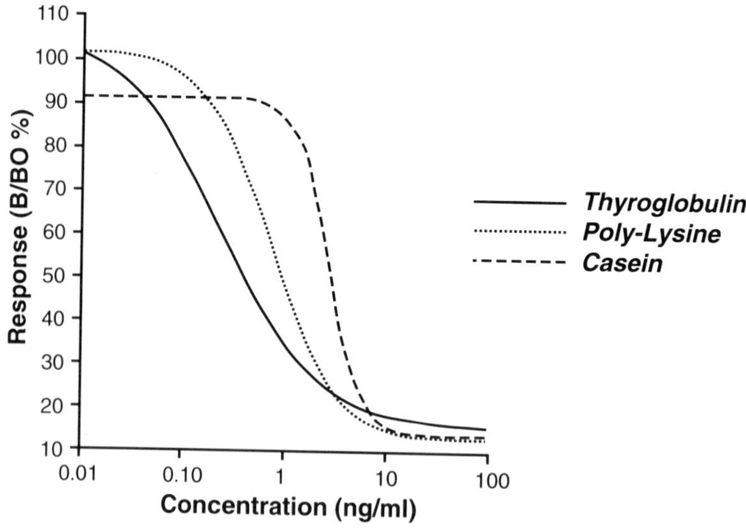

Figure 7.3 Calibration curves for an immobilised antigen ELISA using different proteins for the plate conjugate.

sodium carbonate (40 ml, 1.06 g/100 ml) with a solution of sodium bicarbonate (60 ml, 0.84 g/100 ml).

It is important to remember also that the nature of the protein itself can have a marked albeit unpredictable effect on the assay parameters, including the sensitivity. This is clearly shown by the data in Figure 7.3 which presents three ELISA calibration curves generated using identical conditions except for the nature of the conjugate protein. Although these results may change if different incubation buffers and pHs are used, they do demonstrate how the carrier protein can have a marked effect on assay sensitivity and dynamic range.

Optimisation of non-specific binding

If the non-specific binding is high, i.e. greater than 10 per cent of the maximum specific binding signal, then it is likely that the detergent is not being totally effective and some optimisation of the assay conditions is required. Although the concentration of detergent can be increased above that recommended (0.05 per cent) doing so may affect the antibody binding adversely at either the first or second stage.

In the PROCEDURE above we recommended three washes with a relatively short wash contact time. It may be possible to reduce non-specific binding by increasing the number of washes to five for example. Employing a greater number than this is unlikely to lead to any further reduction in non-specific binding and it may actually reduce specific binding and adversely affect precision and sensitivity. Increasing the length of the contact time, bearing in mind that some workers recommend contact times of up to 3 min (Bullock and Walls, 1977) or 5 min (Tijssen, 1985), and agitating the plate during washing can have a useful effect. However, some workers (Beumer *et al.*, 1992) have shown that if the washing conditions are carefully optimised it may be possible to reduce both the contact time and the number of washes.

When the simple approaches fail then the use of a blocking protein is probably required. Blocking proteins act by binding to uncoated plastic and thus preventing non-specific adsorption of the indicator antiserum. A separate blocking stage can be carried out after the sensitisation, but alternatively and more commonly, the blocking protein can be included in the first and second incubation buffers.

Buffers containing BSA at a concentrations of 0.05 to 0.5 per cent are commonly used as a blocking agents. However, it should be realised that many adults have IgG antibodies to BSA in their blood (Dise and Brunnell, 1987) which can result in high background readings when human samples are assayed. Another factor limiting the usefulness of BSA as a blocking protein is that many antisera are produced using BSA–analyte conjugates. Thus any resulting sera will also contain anti-BSA antibodies, once again leading to high background readings.

Other proteins suitable for blocking are gelatin and casein, at concentrations of around 0.1 to 1 per cent. In our experience gelatin often results in high background colours, possibly because of the presence of natural antibodies in sera which recognise collagen fragments. However, it should be noted that gelatins do vary markedly in their effectiveness depending on their source. The use of fish-skin gelatin has been recommended by Vogt *et al.* (1987). The use of casein for blocking is also popular and in our experience gives assays with the lowest background colour. Casein is thought to owe its effectiveness to its heterogeneous composition involving proteins of differing size, amino acid sequence and ionic charge.

The data in Table 7.3 (unpublished results) shows the effectiveness of various proteins in reducing non-specific binding to poly-D-lysine coated polystyrene. Whilst several of the proteins tested clearly reduce non-specific binding, others make the situation worse, namely bovine gamma globulin (BGG). This effect however is probably concentration dependent and this factor should be investigated for any protein used. In our experience, assays with poly-D-lysine as carrier give the lowest background colours using phosphate buffer containing sodium caseinate (0.1 per cent), and this is a combination we recommend.

Table 7.3 The effect of various buffer proteins on the binding of enzyme-labelled anti-sheep IgG to poly-D-lysine adsorbed onto polystyrene

	Binding*	
Buffer protein	Protein absent	Protein present†
Haemocyanin	0.44	0.22
Gelatin	0.41	0.23
Bovine gamma globulin	0.43	1.37
Polyglutamic acid	0.48	0.22
Sodium caseinate	0.46	0.19

* Binding is measured by the optical density response at 405 nm using the substrate *p*-nitrophenyl phosphate.

† The concentration of protein in the buffer was 2 per cent with the exception of sodium caseinate which was used as a saturated solution (approx. 0.1 per cent).

Optimisation of the primary antibody incubation

The time taken for a solid-phase immunoreaction to reach equilibrium is usually longer than that for the corresponding solution-phase reaction, since it is limited by the rate of diffusion of the antibody to and from the solid phase (Stenberg and Nygren, 1988; Franz and Stegemann, 1991). Consequently, long incubation periods, often overnight, are employed for the primary antiserum incubation stage of an ELISA. Indeed, it has been reported in the literature that in the absence of vigorous agitation an incubation time of 18 to 30 h is required compared with 20 to 30 min for an equivalent solution-phase assay (Franz and Stegemann, 1991). However, with agitation of the microtitre plate, reaction rates are increased and equilibration times can be significantly reduced (Boraker *et al.*, 1992; Franz and Stegemann, 1991; Pesce and Michael, 1992).

The reaction kinetics should be investigated and optimised for each assay. For this experiment a series of wells should be coated to allow for non-specific binding, zero standards and a concentration around the mid-point on the calibration curve to be measured at each time point in duplicate. At pre-defined times the contents of six wells would be emptied, washed and the necessary reagents added to give a non-specific binding, zero standard and mid-point standard test. The times would typically be 0, 3, 6, 9 and 23 h, i.e. the experiment would be spread across two days. One hour after the last batch of wells has been set up the contents of all wells are aspirated to waste and the assay completed as normal. Carried out in this way, the experiment will give primary incubation times of 1, 15, 18, 21 and 24 h. If the assay is found to have come to equilibrium by 15 h then the experiment should be repeated using a shorter overall time, i.e. 8 to 12 h. A similar approach would be adopted if elevated temperature or agitation is employed.

ELISA procedures are often carried out at 4°C although there appears to be no good reason for this. Incubations may be carried out at higher temperatures (e.g. 20°C to 40°C) for shorter periods of time without loss in assay sensitivity, and in the authors' laboratories, room temperature incubation is commonly employed.

Introduction of matrix

As discussed in Chapter 6 on RIA development the early introduction of matrix to the assay can lead to confounding effects which makes the development of the assay more difficult. The most straightforward approach in the authors' opinion is first to establish the basic assay conditions using standards prepared in buffer. It should then be apparent whether the assay target in terms of sensitivity, specificity and precision are at least achievable. The matrix can then be introduced and, providing there are no gross changes in the major assay parameters, limited further optimisation can then be carried out. Once the best sera have been selected a comparison should be made between standards prepared in buffer and matrix.

It is often found that matrix interference in ELISA is more pronounced than in RIA. This is because the total incubation volume in ELISA is generally smaller and there are many more factors that can be affected. As well as interfering with the antibody–antigen interaction the matrix components may alter the activity of the enzyme or potentiate non-specific binding effects. It is important therefore to prepare calibration standards in the same matrix as the samples. Furthermore, since matrix effects may vary from sample-to-sample, a pooled matrix should be used where possible. This will average or minimise the assay bias although sample to sample bias may still be evident.

Where the samples are highly proteinaceous, have high ionic strength or are generally 'dirty' then it is recommended that the proportion of matrix is kept below about 10 per cent of the total assay volume to minimise undesirable effects. Because of the limited usable volume of the microtitre plate wells (200 to 250 μl), only relatively small sample volumes, typically up to 20 or 25 μl, can therefore be assayed. This is in contrast to RIA, which is generally carried out in tubes where the total incubation volume can be increased to over 1 ml, and the volume of sample increased accordingly. Where the samples are relatively clean however, e.g. river water, the volume of sample added to the ELISA can be increased and the volume of first antibody decreased accordingly.

One report (Gissendorf, 1990) suggests that the incorporation of certain ions such as magnesium and calcium into ELISA buffers may help minimise matrix effects.

In the immobilised antigen ELISA the enzyme never comes into direct contact with the matrix so the potential for a matrix-induced change in the end point is reduced. HRP, the most commonly used enzyme marker, is relatively insensitive to small changes in pH, with activity varying very little over a pH range 2 units either side of the optimum. The peroxidase enzymes are, however, particularly sensitive to contaminating bacteria as well as sodium azide which is widely used as a preservative in buffers and sera.

Where the samples contain large-molecular-weight species such as proteins, then these may bind to exposed sites on the plastic. These same species can also bind to the plate conjugate itself, possibly occluding the hapten. Should they occur, these interactions can lead to changes in non-specific binding, sensitivity and precision. Following the introduction of matrix therefore, it is important to check for any variation in assay parameters such as those mentioned above. If variation is seen then re-optimisation may be necessary. As a minimum it is recommended that sensitivity and precision are re-checked following inclusion of the matrix.

Further assay optimisation

Once the basic assay has been established fine tuning of the assay parameters may be necessary to give the desired performance characteristics. Much of this work is comparable to that for RIA as discussed in the previous chapter.

Optimisation of the second antibody incubation

The enzyme-labelled second antibody incubation should ideally be optimised such that it is close to equilibrium and a maximal response obtained from the specific binding wells, together with low non-specific binding. Under these conditions the lowest limits of detection and quantification will be obtained. In PROCEDURE 1 an incubation time of 3 h along with the reagent dilution as suggested by the manufacturer (typically 1/1000 to 1/5000) was recommended. Although appearing to give a satisfactory and a workable assay these parameters should be fully investigated and optimised.

Typically second antibody incubation times from 30 min to 6 h would be investigated using a series of antiserum dilutions spanning those suggested by the manufacturer. A convenient and simple experiment would involve setting up a series of zero standard and non-specific binding wells for each time point/reagent dilution combination. These would then be given a long first incubation to ensure the system was at equilibrium. At a number of set intervals over a 5 h period (e.g. 0, 2, 4, 5 and 5.5 h) the appropriate wells would be emptied, washed and enzyme-labelled second antibody solutions added. Thirty minutes after the final addition (i.e. 6 h after the start) the contents of all wells would be aspirated to waste and the entire assay completed. Each enzyme-labelled antibody solution will then have been given an incubation time of 30 min, 1, 2, 4, and 6 h.

Specificity

In certain instances, buffer type and pH, as well as the characteristics of the assay proteins can have a possible though unpredictable effect on specificity. Where the required specificity is not apparent then these parameters should be investigated initially. If the requisite specificity cannot be achieved through assay modification then the use of an extraction procedure or an HPLC clean-up can be investigated. These approaches also have the advantage that they can help overcome matrix interference problems. Ultimately however, it may be necessary to try different antisera, re-immunise or even prepare new immunogens.

Sensitivity

Of the factors which control assay sensitivity the roles of the following have already been discussed:

- the plate conjugate protein
- the hapten–protein ratio in the plate conjugate
- the concentration of plate conjugate used for sensitisation

Like all immunoassays the sensitivity is ultimately linked to the affinity of the antibody. However, where this is high (i.e. greater than 10^{12} l/mole) and not considered limiting, then sensitivity can be affected by the quality of the second antibody–enzyme reagent. In such circumstances evaluation of reagents from other sources should be carried out or reagents can be synthesised in-house.

The obvious method of improving assay sensitivity through the use of a larger sample volume, will be limited by potential non-specific interference by the matrix. However if this secondary problem of matrix interference can by eliminated or reduced through changes in the assay conditions (e.g. buffer pH, plate conjugate protein) then significant improvements in sensitivity may be possible.

Precision

Poor pipetting precision or a sloppy or rough handling technique at any of the large number of pipetting or wash steps can have a serious negative impact on assay precision. A careful and methodical approach is therefore essential if good precision and low limits of quantification are to be achieved. The use of automated equipment can be particularly useful in ensuring that pipetting operations are reproducible and critical time periods are adhered to.

Microtitre plates which allow the covalent attachment of proteins may offer improvements in assay precision, since desorption of the plate conjugate during washing steps is eliminated. One such plate, Covalink (Nunc Ltd) has the polystyrene surface modified with secondary amine groups, which is reported to be ideal for binding molecules having carboxylic acid moieties. Conjugates can be linked to these derivatised plates using a suitable coupling procedure such as carbodiimide reaction (Sondergard-Andersen *et al.*, 1990).

Convenience

Although the number of stages and washes etc. may make ELISA seem unattractive compared with the relative simplicity of RIA, further work can often simplify the assay significantly. For example, where the assay shows low non-specific binding, it may be possible to reduce the number of washes used or the wash contact time. Either of these factors is relatively easy to study and optimise.

Through the use of a detector which is capable of kinetic measurements, the need for a stop solution can be dispensed with thus simplifying the assay procedure and possibly leading to improved precision. Where the end product is unstable or the stop reagent is not fully effective then the use of kinetic measurements could also lead to improved precision.

If assay speed is a major consideration then the assay can be run at a higher temperature; around 37°C. As well as resulting in faster attainment of equilibrium at the first and second antibody incubation stages, working at 37°C can result in sensitisation times being reduced significantly (Mushens and Scott, 1990) and even down to 1 h (Tsang *et al.*, 1980). Similarly agitation of the plate during the incubations will also result in faster attainment of equilibrium and a shorter overall assay time (Mushens and Scott, 1990). Reducing the incubation volume will also bring the assay to equilibrium faster with the possible disadvantage that matrix effects could be increased. In practice total assay volumes should not be less than 50 μl because of potential problems of evaporation which can be significant with such low volumes and uneven coating as a result of surface tension effects.

Before implementing any assay modification it is important to test its effect fully on the main assay parameters, such as precision and sensitivity. The precision profile as discussed in Chapters 6 and 9 is a powerful tool for the assessment of the effect on assay precision and limit of quantification.

Practical aspects of ELISA

Storage of coated microtitre plates

There is limited data on the storage of microtitre plates containing bound proteins. In the author's (BB) laboratory coated plates have been successfully stored at 4°C in a suitable buffer for up to 1 month. It has also been pointed out by Voller *et al.*

(1979) that dried protein-coated plates can be stored for a year or more with apparently no degradation if kept in air-tight waterproof packs. In practice we normally coat plates fresh the day before use, at least in the early stages of development. For convenience however, once the assay has been established evaluation of plate storage conditions should be carried out. One important factor controlling stability is the storage buffer which should contain some protein, typically as used in a blocking buffer.

Conclusions

Although ELISAs involve more stages than a comparable RIA they can be just as easy to perform and unlike most conventional RIAs they can be fully automated. The fact that the immunochemical reaction takes place at a solid phase often means that incubation times are longer, certainly longer than would be found with a liquid-phase assay. However, if plates are coated and stored then a well-optimised assay should be able to be completed in a typical 8 h working day.

The use of a solid-phase reagent means that the separation of bound and free can be effected by simply washing the plate. This allows simple and full automation of the whole assay procedure, from adding the samples to the wells to the generation of the calibration plot and assay results. Providing the primary sera for all assays are raised in a single species then one commercially available enzyme–antibody reagent can be successfully used with any analyte.

The ease of full automation plus the universal nature of the indicator reagent combine with the elimination of radioactivity to make ELISA a most valuable and versatile analytical tool.

It should be stressed that in our laboratories we have developed ELISAs which have similar sensitivity, specificity and precision to that of conventional liquid-phase RIAs. This has been achieved by employing the principles laid out in this chapter, the major features of which are summarised below.

A different protein must be used for the immunogen and the plate conjugate and to minimise bridge recognition different linking chemistries should also be employed. The plate sensitisation stage is the most critical and the one which generally causes the most problems. Whilst the conditions described here (pH 7 phosphate buffer, 0.1 M) have worked well in our laboratories, full optimisation of these factors may occasionally be necessary.

A plate conjugate involving a large-molecular-weight carrier, e.g. bovine thyroglobulin or poly-D-lysine (670 000 Dalton) is recommended. To attain maximal sensitivity the conjugation ratio should be low to avoid bivalent binding of antibody. A ratio of less than 20 : 1 is recommended for bovine thyroglobulin. The number and concentration of buffer additives should initially be kept to a minimum. Where a blocking protein is required, the type of protein and its concentration should always be determined. In this respect we have found sodium caseinate to be particularly effective in a number of assays.

References

Arends, J. (1971) *Acta Endocrinol.*, **68**, 425.

Beumer, T., Stoffelen, E., Smits, J. & Carpay, W. (1992) *J. Immunol. Methods*, **154**, 77.

Boraker, D. K., Bugbee, S. J. & Reed, B. A. (1992) *J. Immunol. Methods*, **155**, 91.

Bos, E. S., van der Doelen, A. A., van Rooy, N. & Schuurs, A. H. W. M. (1981) *J. Immunoassay*, **2**, 187.

Briand, J. P., Muller, S. & van Regenmortel, M. H. V. (1985) *J. Immunol. Methods*, **78**, 59.

Bullock, S. L. & Walls, K. W. (1977) *J. Infect. Dis.*, **136**, S279.

Butler, J. E., Ni, L., Nessler, R., Joshi, K. S., Suter, M., Rosenberg, B., Chang, J., Brown, W. R. & Cantarero, L. A. (1992) *J. Immunol. Methods*, **150**, 77.

Cantarero, L. A., Butler, J. E. & Osborne, J. W. (1980) *Anal. Biochem.*, **105**, 375.

Catt, K. & Tregar, G. W. (1967) *Science*, **158**, 1570.

Dise, T. & Brunnell, P. A. (1987) *J. Clin. Microbiol.*, **25**, 987.

Engvall, E. & Perlmann, P. (1971) *Immunochemistry*, **8**, 871.
(1972) *J. Immunol.*, **109**, 129.

Franz, B. & Stegemann, M. (1991) In: Butler, J. E. (ed.) *Immunochemistry of Solid-Phase Immunoassays*. CRC Press, Florida, USA, pp. 277.

Geerligs, H. J. Weijer, W. J., Bloemhoff, W., Welling, G. W. & Welling-Wester, S. (1988) *J. Immunol. Methods*, **106**, 239.

Gissendorf, B. (1990) Australian Patent Application Number: 3901458.

Gosling, J. P. (1990) *Clin. Chem.*, **36**, 1408.

Herrmann, J. E. (1981) *Methods in Enzymology*, **73**, 239.

Karush, F. & Hornick, C. L. (1973) *Int. Arch. Allergy Appl. Immunol.*, **45**, 130.

Kemeny, D. M. (1991) *A Practical Guide to ELISA*. Pergamon Press, New York.

Kemeny, D. M. & Challacombe, S. J. (1988) *ELISA and Other Solid Phase Immunoassays*. Wiley, London.

Lewis, J. G., Manley, L., Whitlow, J. C. & Elder, P. A. (1992) *Steroids*, **57**, 82.

Mushens, R. E. & Scott, M. L. (1990) *J. Immunol. Methods*, **131**, 83.

Pesce, A. J. & Michael, J. G. (1992) *J. Immunol. Methods*, **150**, 111.

Porstmann, T. & Kiessig, S. T. (1992) *J. Immunol. Methods*, **150**, 5.

Shalev, A., Greenberg, A. H. & McAlpine, P. J. (1980) *J. Immunol. Methods*, **38**, 125.

Shirahama, H. & Suzawa, T. (1985) *Colloid. Polym. Sci.*, **263**, 141.

Sondergard-Andersen, J., Lauritzen, E., Lind, K. & Holm, A. (1990) *J. Immunol. Methods*, **131**, 99.

Stenberg, M. & Nygren, H. (1988) *J. Immunol. Methods*, **113**, 3.

Tijssen, P. (1985) *Practice and Theory of Enzyme Immunoassays*. Elsevier, Amsterdam.

Tsang, V. C. W., Wilson, B. C. & Maddison, S.E. (1980) *Clin. Chem.*, **26**, 1255.

Vogt, R. F., Phillips, D. L., Henderson, L. O., Whitfield, W. & Spierto, F. W. (1987) *J. Immunol. Methods*, **101**, 43.

Voller, A., Bidwell, D. E. & Bartlett, A. (1979) *The Enzyme Linked Immunosorbent Assay (ELISA)*. Dynatech, Guernsey, UK.

8

Standardisation of immunoassays

M. J. WARWICK

Zeneca Pharmaceuticals, Macclesfield

Introduction

The purpose of this chapter is to outline some of the commonly used calibration procedures with the emphasis on practical aspects of assay calibration. However, an effort has been made to provide information that may help readers understand the ideas behind the different approaches. For those who wish to delve deeper, references are also given to many of the excellent papers which discuss the theoretical aspects of assay calibration, curve fitting etc. The discussion of standardisation has been approached from a historical point of view since fashion for, and use of particular techniques has changed with increasing knowledge and with increasing computing power.

Immunoassays like all analytical methods give a fixed response to a given amount of analyte. The response units (i.e. cpm, optical density) will depend on the particular detection mechanism employed and this data must be converted into suitable units, usually mass of analyte per unit of matrix, e.g. ng/ml. This conversion is achieved by standardisation or calibration of the assay and normally involves the estimation of a calibration function, or standard curve, from the standard series. The standard series is a collection of samples of known and increasing concentration of the analyte in the matrix of interest. The calibration function is an equation relating assay response to sample concentration, and is estimated from the determined responses of the standards.

The actual response achieved for a given concentration of analyte usually, for a variety of reasons, varies with time (e.g. from day to day). It is therefore necessary to repeat the standardisation process at intervals determined by the known or expected stability of the assay response. Generally, this involves one standard curve for each day's work or batch, but it could be more or less than this. The intention is to ensure that there is no significant effect of assay batch on the concentrations determined.

Immunoassays are characterised by a non-linear relationship between response and concentration of analyte, and this relationship is affected by a large number of variables. This is problematic since standardisation is most reliable when there is a simple, explicit and reproducible model of response to concentration. The most convenient model is linear, since this is easy to understand and easy to fit to data, with very little computing power. The development of standardisation of immunoassays is largely about the search for a universally applicable model, and attempts to linearise the relationship.

Every assay has a real underlying relationship between response and analyte concentration, which is a direct consequence of the mechanism of the antibody–antigen interaction. However, response measurements are subject to error, which means that they show deviation from expectation. The approach to determining a calibration function from a set of standard responses generally falls in one of the following three categories:

First, a relationship can be derived based on an understanding of the underlying mechanism of the antibody–antigen interaction. This relationship would directly relate response to concentration using physically relevant parameters, e.g. antibody concentration and affinity, tracer concentration etc. The result will be a model 'imposed' on the data, i.e. the data will be made to fit the model, any deviation being assumed to be the result of random error. Clearly, it is important that the assumed mechanism is appropriate, or else systematic error may be introduced into the calibration.

Second, the 'shape' of the underlying relationship can be assumed, e.g. linear or sigmoid. Again the calibration function is 'imposed' on the data, though here the parameters will have no physical meaning, but simply describe a mathematical relationship. As with modelling the underlying mechanism, it is important that the assumed shape is appropriate, or else systematic error may be introduced.

The third approach is commonly known as 'joining the dots', though some sophisticated mathematical manipulation may be involved. Here it is assumed that the data, on balance, reflects an unknown underlying mechanism, and the calibration function is derived from the data points alone with no assumptions about its form. In this approach it is important that the errors are small and random, since any systematic error in the calibration data will be reflected in the calibration function.

We will look at each of these approaches in turn, though first some basic understanding of the immunoassay process will be required.

Standard curves from a simple analogy for radioimmunoassay

RIA is often described as a process involving a limited number of binding sites in the presence of excess tracer. It is not difficult to understand the reason for the non-linearity of RIA standard curves when the nature of the process is clear. An analogy for RIA might be that of pouring water into a series of tubes, each one representing a fixed number of antibody binding sites (Figure 8.1). An excess of tritiated water, representing the radiolabelled analyte, is poured into the first tube, resulting in the retention of some (the bound fraction) and the loss of the rest (the free fraction). If the volume of the tube is 0.5 ml and 1 ml of tritiated water (containing 20 000 counts per minute (cpm)) is poured into it, then the tube will retain 10 000 cpm. If for the next tube, we mix the 1 ml of tritiated water with 1 ml of unlabelled water and pour the mixture into the tube, it will still contain 0.5 ml, but only 5000 cpm.

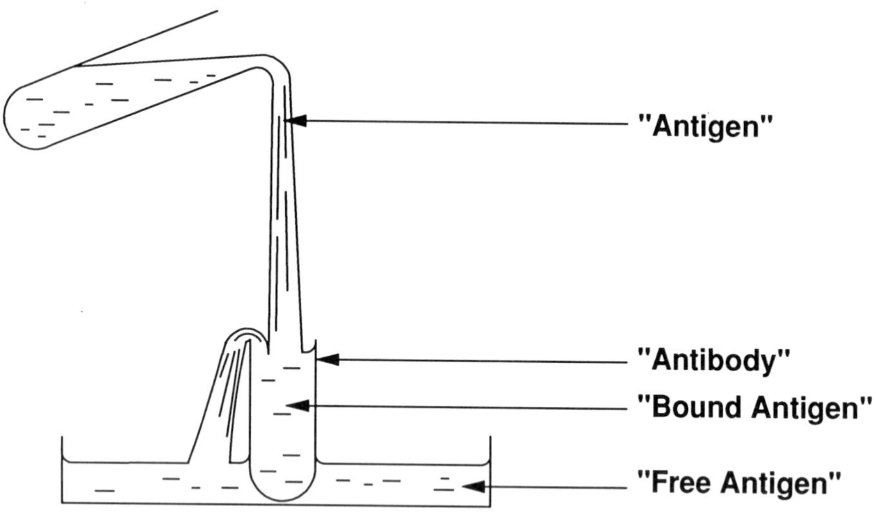

Figure 8.1 A simple analogy for a radioimmunoassay.

Figure 8.2 shows the results of mixing the 1 ml of tritiated water with increasing volumes of unlabelled water before pouring into subsequent tubes. It is clear that the cpm in the tube drops as the amount of added unlabelled water increases, but that the extent of the decrease in cpm gets smaller with each succeeding unit of added unlabelled water. The standard curve (Figure 8.2) of cpm in the tube versus volume of unlabelled water added illustrates the non-linear nature of the response in an immunoassay.

Although it is desirable to use the raw response values, e.g. cpm in the above example, it is possible to transform the response variable in an attempt to obtain a

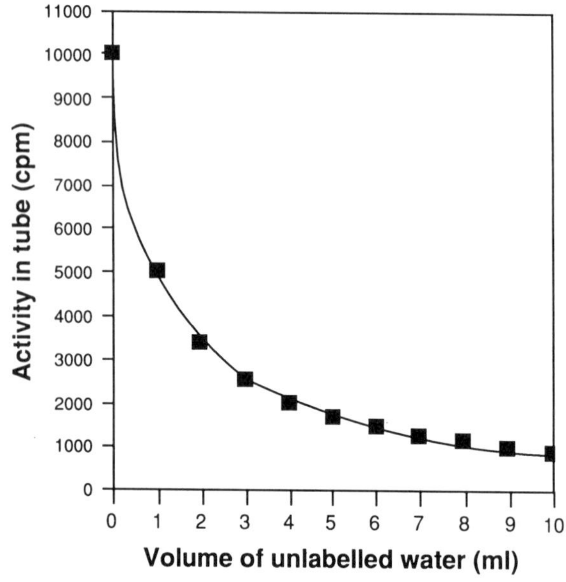

Figure 8.2 Predicted standard curve from a simple analogy of a radioimmunoassay.

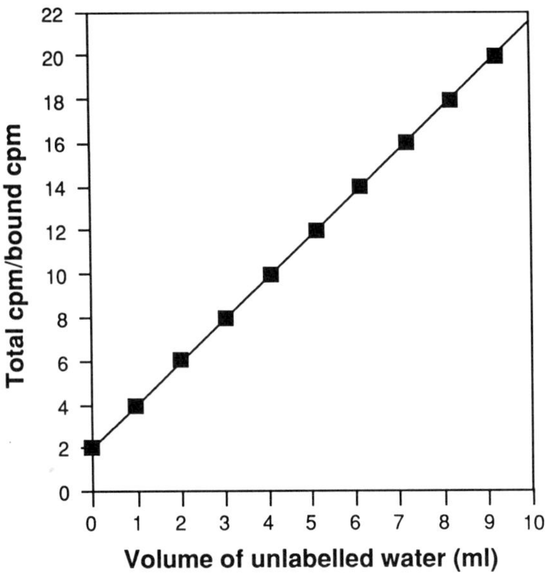

Figure 8.3 Predicted calibration curve from a simple analogy of a radioimmunoassay employing transformation of response to give linearisation.

simpler (linear) calibration plot. Using the model illustrated by Figures 8.1 and 8.2, if the reciprocal of response is taken, and then multiplied by the total counts (T) a new variable is obtained which we can call T/B. A plot of this new response variable against added unlabelled water is shown in Figure 8.3. This is clearly linear with an intercept on the ordinate of 2. This type of transformation was in fact used in the early days of immunoassays (Hales and Randle, 1963) and can be successful today. Do we need anything more complicated? The answer is unfortunately 'yes' and the reason lies in the inadequacy of the analogy we have used (see Ekins *et al.*, 1968 and Yalow and Berson, 1968 for a detailed discussion of the underlying mechanism).

Modelling the mechanism – mass action models for radioimmunoassay

Ideal systems

Antigen–antibody binding is subject to the law of mass action, the reaction reaching an equilibrium between reactants and product, with the ratio of concentration of the reactants and product at equilibrium equal to the equilibrium or affinity constant (K).

$$K = [\mathrm{AbAg}]/[\mathrm{Ab}][\mathrm{Ag}] \tag{1}$$

or,

$$K = B/QP \tag{2}$$

where B = antigen or antibody binding sites bound at equilibrium, P = free antigen at equilibrium and Q = free antibody binding sites at equilibrium.

Now $Q = q - B$, where q equals total antibody binding sites, therefore,

$$K(q - B) = B/P \tag{3}$$

which is the Scatchard equation (Scatchard, 1949). A plot of B/P against B is linear with a negative slope of K and intercept on the ordinate of Kq.

Further manipulation of the mass action equation (Hatch *et al.*, 1976) gives:

$$p_a = (qT/B) - (T/K(T - B)) - p^* \tag{4}$$

where p_a = added unlabelled analyte and p^* = added labelled analyte, T and B are the total added and bound cpm respectively.

Like the relationship derived from the simple analogy, this equation is linear in T/B, but only if the second term $(T/K(T - B))$ is zero, which will occur if K is infinite. However, for all real values of K there is no linear relationship between added analyte and reciprocal bound. This finding reflects a weakness in our original analogy, since a tube of 0.5 ml will always retain (bind) 0.5 ml when excess water is poured into it. This is not true of antigen–antibody interaction where, for all real values of K, even in the presence of excess antigen there will be both free antigen *and* free antibody binding sites at equilibrium.

What then is the relationship between antibody sites filled and changing antigen concentration? If $p = p_a + p^*$ then $P = p - B$, and substituting in equation (3) gives $B = K[(q - B)(p - B)]$. This is a quadratic in B which on expanding gives

$$0 = (KB^2) - B(1 + Kp + Kq) + (Kpq) \tag{5}$$

Parameters p and q in equation (5) are usually of the order of $1/K$ and, on observation, it is clear that plots of bound antigen against antigen concentration will be hyperbolic (Ekins *et al.*, 1968).

An illustration of this is shown in Figure 8.4 using a 2500 cpm of a tritium tracer (equivalent to 20 pg or 40 fmol for a molecule with a molecular mass of 500 Daltons and a specific activity of 30 Ci/mmol). In the presence of 30 fmol of antibody

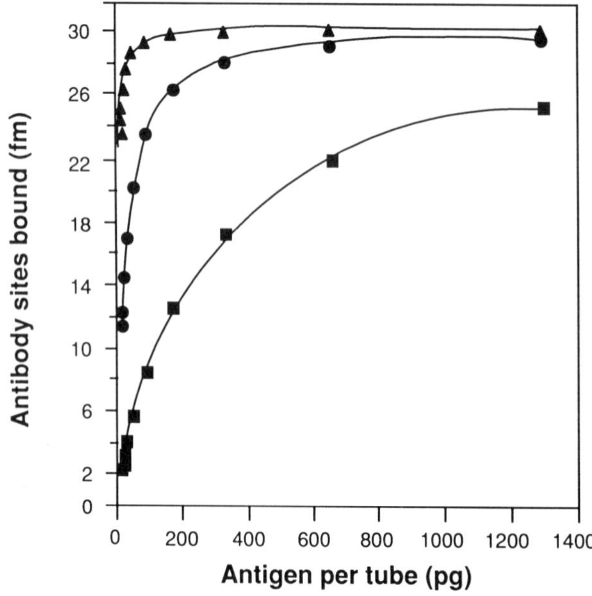

Figure 8.4 Estimation of filled antibody sites, at different concentrations of antigen, for three antibodies with different affinity constant (l/mol). ■ = 1×10^9, ● = 1×10^{10}, ▲ = 1×10^{11}.

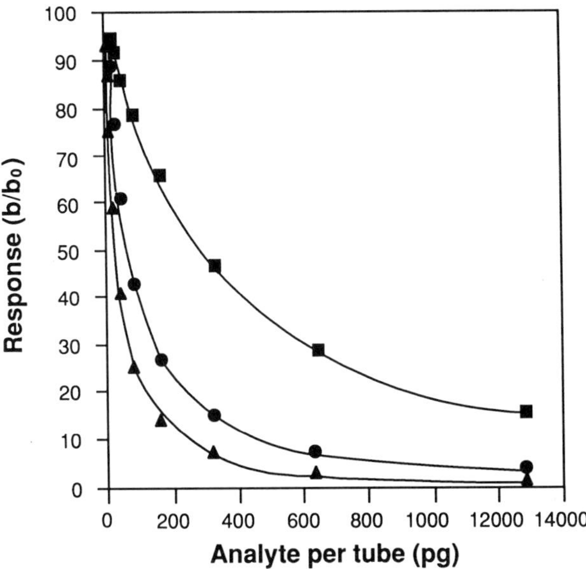

Figure 8.5 Simulated calibration plots generated using antibodies with different affinities. ■ = 1×10^9, ● = 1×10^{10}, ▲ = 1×10^{11}.

binding sites, the concentration of antibody sites filled is shown for increasing concentration of analyte and for antisera with different affinities. For a typical affinity (1×10^9 l/mol) the simulation shows that as expected the number of antibody sites that are occupied in the presence of excess tracer are a small fraction of the total, only increasing to about 85 per cent of the total for a 70-fold increase in antigen. In a typical immunoassay, this implies that as unlabelled antigen is added to the system, both displacement of labelled antigen and increased binding of both labelled and unlabelled antigen occur simultaneously.

The displacement hyperbolas, or calibration curves derived from the same data are shown in Figure 8.5. They are clearly of the same form as predicted by the simple analogy but the shape is dependent on the affinity as well as the tracer and analyte concentrations. The plots also illustrate the potentially greater sensitivity and shorter dynamic range as affinity increases.

The above approach based on simulations is very effective and recommended to anyone involved in immunoassay; it allows a clear graphical illustration of the effects of changing parameters in the model. The necessary programs are relatively easy to write but, if required, immunoassay simulation software can be obtained from the author.

The effect of non-ideal aspects of immunoassay

The discussion so far has highlighted the complexity of the antibody–antigen interaction, even when we are considering an ideal system. The theory suggests there are relationships that are more exact representations of the mass action model than reciprocal bound plots. For example, from a Scatchard plot (equation 3) we can obtain q and K, if we know the concentration of labelled analyte (p^*). Substitution into equation (4) should allow us to work out unlabelled analyte (p_a) for any binding figure. However, the assumptions (Rodbard, 1978) of the ideal immunoassay model are:

- the antibody consists of a single class of homogeneous binding sites
- the tracer is homogeneous and univalent, and identical to the unlabelled analyte in terms of its affinity for the antibody
- the mass of the tracer (p^*) is known perfectly
- the reaction system reaches equilibrium
- the separation of bound and free analyte is perfect and does not affect the pre-existing equilibrium

Most of these conditions are rarely achieved in typical immunoassays, often resulting in non-linearity of Scatchard plots (Rodbard *et al.*, 1971; Rodbard and Catt, 1972). A typical example is shown in Figure 8.6, where the probable cause of non-linearity is the existence of heterogeneity in the antibody population. In spite of these problems Walker and Keane (1977) have used Scatchard plots for assay calibration. They give several examples where the Scatchard plot has exhibited a good fit to the data, and suggest ways to 'compensate' for the presence of other low-affinity binding proteins.

Relationships, other than the ideal model given in equation (5), have been derived by Ekins *et al.* (1968). A model which allows for a single antibody population with different affinities for the tracer and analyte, takes the form of the following third-order polynomial:

$$(K^*/K_a)R^3 + (K_a q + K^*q - K^*p^* - K_a p_a - 1)R^2 + (K^*q - K^*p^* - K^*p_a - K^*/K_a - 1)R - 1/K^*q = 0 \qquad (6)$$

where K^* = affinity constant for tracer, K_a = affinity constant for analyte and $R = P/B$.

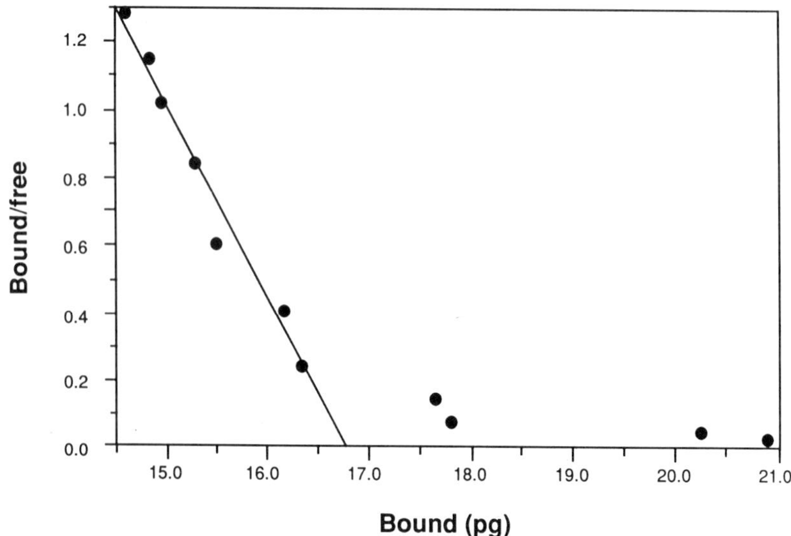

Figure 8.6 Typical Scatchard plot for a polyclonal antiserum raised against a small-molecular-weight antigen.

For the situation of multiple binding sites, Ekins' equation (6) has been rearranged by Finney (1983) to:

$$B/P = N + \sum (K_i q_i T/K_i(p^* + p_a)(T - B) + T) \quad (7)$$

where N = response at infinite dose (non-specific binding, nsb).

For an antiserum containing two antibodies, this also results in a third-order polynomial. These relationships are complex, with multiple parameters, and difficult for routine use except where significant computing power is available. However, Wilkins *et al.* (1977) have shown that the ideal, single binding site model can be a good approximation for non-ideal assays. They have succeeded in using the model to fit calibration curves for several analytes using non-linear regression techniques to fit values to K, q, p^* and N, though these fitted values do not necessarily reflect the true underlying values. It is worth noting that where the mechanism is described by higher order polynomial equations the resulting calibration curves can exhibit much more complicated shapes than simple hyperbolas.

Clearly, attempting to model the underlying mechanism for real assays can be both mathematically and computationally complex. Though these models have been used they are not normally convenient for routine use.

Modelling the shape – logistic models for immunoassay calibration plots

Although consideration of the underlying mechanism provides some simple, linear models for dose interpolation, these are not always exact and not of general utility. The more complex relationships derived from the law of mass action, though providing physically meaningful parameters, are still difficult to fit in the routine laboratory. The second alternative involves fitting an equation to standard responses which describes a shape rather than the mechanism. Logistic fits, commonly used in immunoassay, fall into this category.

Logistic functions and their logit transformations pre-date immunoassay and have been used extensively in fitting bioassay response data (Finney, 1974) where it is common for a plot of response versus log dose or stimulus to be sigmoidal. There is no fundamental equation for a sigmoid and logistic functions belong to a family of functions which can be used to describe sigmoid curves (Finney, 1974). The logit transformation of response is itself related to response by a symmetrical sigmoid, resulting in a linear relationship of logit transform to dose (Rodbard, 1978). RIAs exhibit a sigmoidal relationship of response with log dose and can be fitted by equations similar to those used for other bioassays.

Linear (logit/log) calibration plots

It is possible to derive from the law of mass action (Walker and Keane, 1977) an equation

$$p = [((1 + e^w)q)/e^w B_0] - [(1 + e^w)/K(1 + e^w(1 + B_0))] \quad (8)$$

where B_0 = binding at zero dose of analyte, w = logit transformation of binding = $\log_e[(B/B_0)/(1 - B/B_0)]$.

At infinite affinity (saturated binding sites) the second term becomes zero and the equation reduces to $p = (q/e^{w}B_0) + (q/B_0)$ which on re-arranging and taking logs gives:

$$w = \log_e q - \log_e(pB_0 - q) \tag{9}$$

This equation predicts a linear relationship of transformed response (logit) with the log of analyte concentration.

Finney (1976) states that 'experimental results do not readily discriminate between different sigmoid equations, and reasonable alternatives will commonly lead to essentially the same conclusions'. Consequently, it is not necessary to use the exact equation derived from mass action considerations and the equation typically used is

$$\text{logit}(y/1 - y) = b(\log_e c - \log_e p_a) \tag{10}$$

where $y = B/B_0$, c = the dose halfway between asymptotes, b = slope of the curve at c.

Use of this approach for RIA was first suggested by Rodbard *et al.* (1969) and, because of the use of an empirical equation related to, but *not* derived from an approximation of the mass action law, it is often referred to as a semi-empirical model. Logistic equations used to fit RIA calibration plots make no mechanistic assumptions about the underlying process. The only assumption is that the response versus log dose curve will be a symmetrical sigmoid. Considerations of the mass action law suggests this is often, but not exclusively the case.

Log–logit transformations are theoretically only linear when all antibody sites are occupied (i.e. the antibody has infinite affinity), but as shown by the simulated data in Figure 8.7, these semi-empirical equations do not suffer from the systematic curvature of reciprocal bound plots and provide a good fit to the data. This type of calibration plot was initially used manually with special log–logit paper (Rodbard *et*

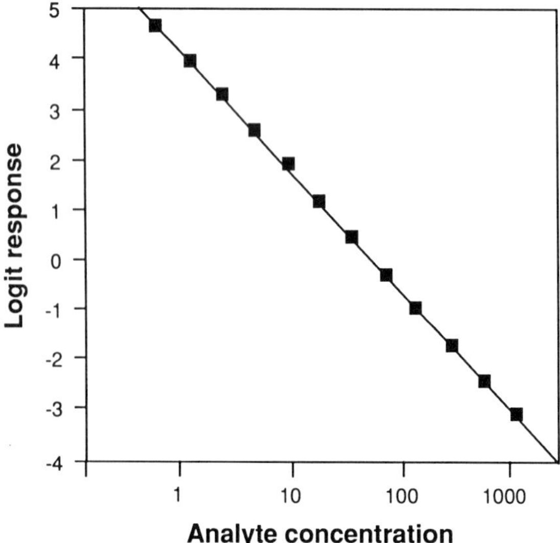

Figure 8.7 Simulated calibration plot fitted using a logit transformation of response. Based on an antibody with an affinity constant of 1 × 10^{10} l/mol.

al., 1969). Later Rodbard and Lewald (1970) described automatic analysis by computer of log–logit calibration plots. Their paper is also a very good overview of the principles and problems associated with this curve fitting procedure.

The log–logit approach became popular and successful for many immunoassays, and was especially favoured with the arrival of cheap desk-top calculators capable of simple linear regression. There are however, problems with this procedure. The first is that the two values of binding, zero dose (B_0) and non-specific binding (N), are used to transform the response, and are therefore assumed to be known exactly. Since they are subject to the same errors as other standards, this is never true, and small errors in these values have been shown to affect linearity (Hatch *et al.*, 1976). A second problem is found when binding sites of different affinity are present in the antisera; this has been shown to lead to curvature in the log–logit plot (Rodbard, 1978).

The second problem can be illustrated with simulations of the type used above, employing the same 40 fmol/tube of a tracer but this time adding 30 fmol of antibody with an affinity of 1×10^{11} l/mol *plus* 300 fmol of an antibody with a relatively low affinity of 1×10^{8} l/mol. The resulting log–logit plot is shown in Figure 8.8 along with the curve produced by the same system without the low affinity antibody for comparison. It can be clearly seen that, for the system with two antibodies, the deviation from linearity at high concentrations is pronounced. This result is expected from our knowledge of the fact that antibody binding sites fill up as antigen concentration goes up (see Figure 8.4). The low affinity antibody acts as a reservoir of binding sites which progressively affect displacement of tracer as the concentration of antigen increases.

Several methods of adjusting the log–logit standardisation were tried in an attempt to cope with the non-linearity occasionally seen. These included manual adjustment of the values of B_0 and nsb (Hatch *et al.*, 1976) and use of quadratic and

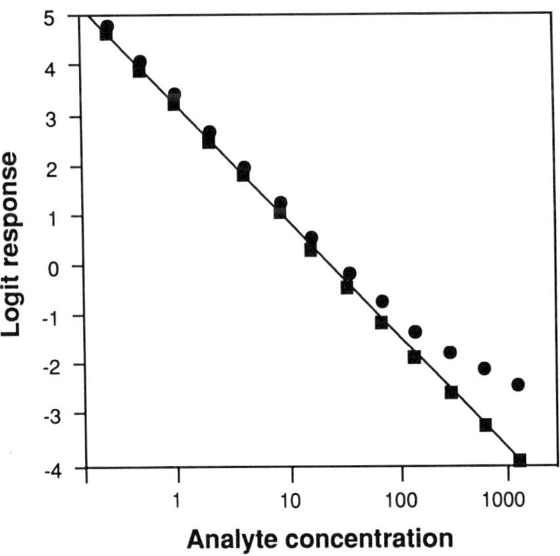

Figure 8.8 Simulated calibration plot fitted using a logit transformation. The data show the response for an antiserum containing a single antibody (■) and an antiserum containing the same antibody but with a second antibody of lower affinity added (●).

cubic functions to fit the curved plots (Murata *et al.*, 1983; Nisbet *et al.*, 1986). However, these mathematical manipulations complicate the original simplicity of the approach and these corrections have never been very popular.

Non-linear logistic calibration plots

A logical extension of the log–logit procedure was to use its logistic equivalent; fitting the sigmoid curve itself rather than attempting to linearise it. This approach was first suggested by Healy (1972) and has the advantage that all four parameters (hence the name four parameter logistic) are fitted rather than just the two (b and c) of the log–logit equation. The form of the 4PL equation most commonly encountered is algebraically equivalent to the logit–log equation (10), i.e.

$$\text{response} = d + [(a - d)/(1 + (p_a/c)^b)] \tag{11}$$

where b and c are as defined for equation (10), a = binding at zero dose (B_0) and d = binding at infinite dose (non-specific binding, nsb).

Other forms of the 4PL equation are also found (Finney, 1976), and these are all functionally if not algebraically equivalent. The 4PL model is a sigmoid with asymptotic values approximating to B_0 and nsb; it is symmetrical about its midpoint. The advantage of the 4PL fit is that it fits a and d as well as fitting c and b, therefore does not rely on experimentally determined values and thus avoids the problems sometimes encountered with the log–logit method. It is important to note that the 4PL fit is not a better model for the immunoassay process, merely that the manipulation of four parameters, rather than the two of the logit–log approach introduces flexibility into thc model.

This flexibility can be illustrated by refitting the simulated data of Figure 8.8 with and without heterogeneity of affinity of binding sites. Figure 8.9 shows a 4PL fit of the data, where both curves pass satisfactorily through all of the data points. Table 8.1 shows the difference between the parameters for the system with and without the second low-affinity antibody; the major change is in the fitted value of the nsb (parameter d).

In general, the 4PL procedure can fit calibration curves whenever the log–logit approach can, and on many occasions when the latter cannot. Consequently, the

Table 8.1 RIA simulation parameters for 4PL fits to data for single and mixed antibody systems

Parameter	One antibody*	Two antibodies**
a	1539	1593
b	1.065	1.022
c	28.3	30.4
d	7	114

* 30 fmol of antibody with $K = 1 \times 10^{11}$ l/mol.
** 30 fmol of antibody with $K = 1 \times 10^{11}$ l/mol plus 300 fmol of antibody with $K = 1 \times 10^{8}$ l/mol.

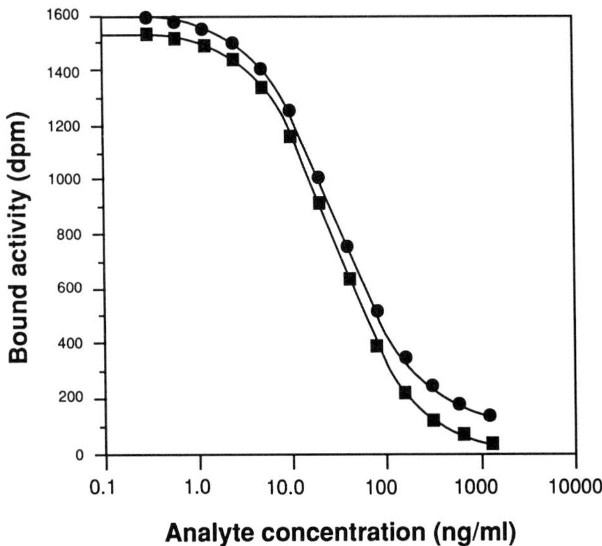

Figure 8.9 Simulated calibration plot from Figure 8.8, using a four parameter logistic (4PL) fit. The data show the response for an antiserum containing a single antibody (■) and an antiserum containing the same antibody but with a second antibody of lower affinity added (●).

4PL procedure has replaced the log–logit wherever the necessary computing facilities are available. In theory the 4PL approach requires the use of non-linear regression, with the necessary extra sophistication in computer facilities, but this has been solved by fitting the equation two parameters at a time. For the first iteration, the experimentally determined values of a and d are used, with b and c being fitted using a log–logit procedure. The determined values of b and c are then used to calculate

$$u = 1/(1 + (p_a/c)^b) \tag{12}$$

for all analyte values. The terms a and d then become parameters in a linear equation relating response to u, and can be estimated using linear regression. The cycle of determining b and c followed by a and d is repeated until a satisfactory fit is obtained. This approach is often used in commercial packages for RIA data reduction (e.g. RiaCalc, Pharmacia). In spite of this simplification the 4PL procedure is computationally more complex than the log–logit approach. Nisbet *et al.* (1986) reported processor times for log–logit of 2 seconds but over 30 seconds for the 4PL. Readers should be aware that the algorithm used to determine the line of best fit of the 4PL model to the data set can influence the quality of the fit. For example, using the asymmetric data described below, a reasonable 4PL fit is obtained using RS1 (BBN, Cambridge, USA) but not with RiaCalc (Pharmacia).

The 4PL logistic method demands that the curve be symmetrical around its midpoint. Occasionally, this requirement is not fulfilled and the 4PL gives a poor fit to the data, particularly around the asymptotes (Figure 8.10). Figure 8.11 shows how a more general form of the logistic equation, called a five parameter logistic (5PL) overcomes the problem (Finney, 1983). The equation for the 5PL is typically represented as

$$\text{response} = d + [(a - d)/(1 + (p_a/c)^b)^e] \tag{13}$$

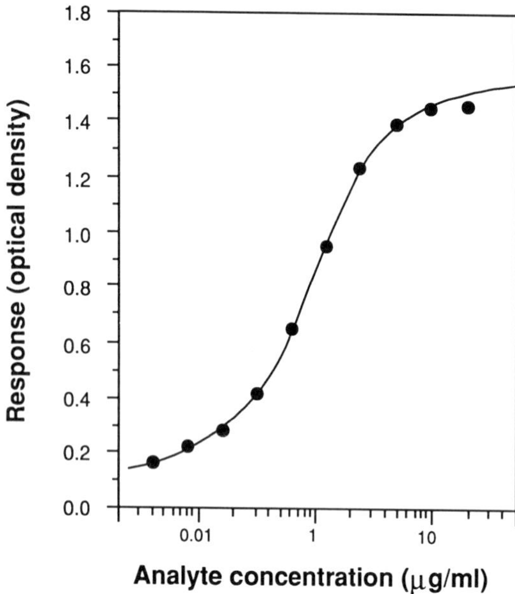

Figure 8.10 A four parameter logistic (4PL) fit of an asymmetric standard curve, using data from a non-competitive ELISA procedure.

and reduces to the 4PL of equation (11) when $e = 1$. Table 8.2 gives the parameters for the 4PL and 5PL fits in Figure 8.11. The differences between the values of c illustrate one of the properties of the logistic equations in that the parameter is actually the turning point of the sigmoid, and only corresponds to the value of the

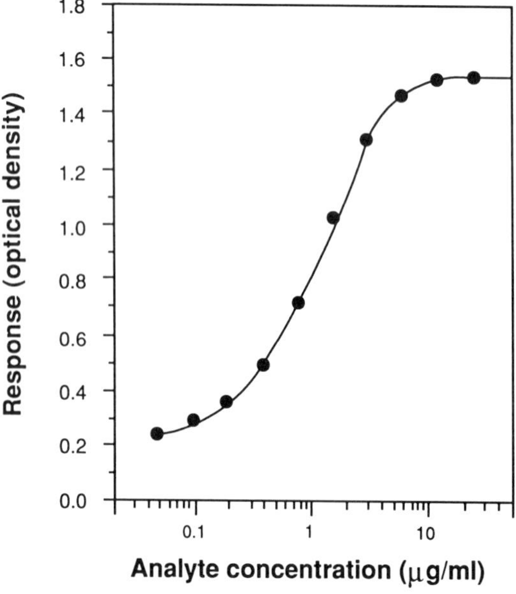

Figure 8.11 A five parameter logistic (5PL) fit of the asymmetric standard curve shown in Figure 8.10.

Table 8.2 Parameters of 4PL and 5PL fits to an asymmetric dose response curve

Parameter	4PL fit	5PL fit
a	1.565	1.542
b	−1.396	−1.813
c	1.190	2.080
d	0.232	0.189
e	—	0.502

ED_{50} when the sigmoid is symmetrical. The 5PL example shown (Table 8.2 and Figure 8.11) was fitted in MultiCalc (Pharmacia). This uses a procedure similar to a 4PL, fitting the parameters *b* and *c* followed by *a* and *d* alternately. Parameter *e* is fitted last using Simplex optimisation. Significant extra computing power is required. On an IBM PS/2 (model 55SX) the 4PL procedure took 24 seconds while the 5PL took 90 seconds.

The data in Figures 8.10 and 8.11 are real data from a non-competitive immunoenzymatic assay, which is equivalent to an immunoradiometric assay. The assay is for a high-molecular-weight protein species using one antibody bound to a solid phase, which captures the analyte, then, after removing the matrix, a second antibody binds to another antigenic site on the analyte. Clearly the amount of second antibody bound is directly proportional to the analyte concentration. Detection is achieved using an enzyme-linked indicator antibody which is specific for the second antibody. The result is a rising response with increasing dose, which is completely opposite to a competitive radioimmunoassay. It should be noted that the logistic equations fit this type of dose response curve equally well, the only difference being in the sign of the exponent (*b*).

In the case of the data in Figures 8.10 and 8.11, the reason for the asymmetry is probably related to practice. During assay development it was found that there was a significant matrix effect (variation in nsb between samples from different individuals) which was minimised by keeping the concentration of indicator antibody as low as possible. For assays of this type, all reagents should be in excess, so that response is determined only by analyte concentration. The response for this assay at the low asymptote concentration is determined largely by the analyte–first antibody–second antibody interactions, whereas at the high asymptote concentration it is progressively more influenced by the second antibody–indicator antibody interaction. This calibration plot provides a good example of how analytical practice can influence the 'shape' of the calibration plot, showing that the commonly found sigmoid cannot be assumed.

Modelling the data – empirical models for immunoassay calibration plots

Thus far we have only considered calibration functions using modelled fits, based on the mass action mechanism or sigmoidal relationships of response to log dose. Dose response curves can also be fitted using totally empirical or interpolated methods (Rodbard, 1978) where no assumption on the shape of the curve is made. The sim-

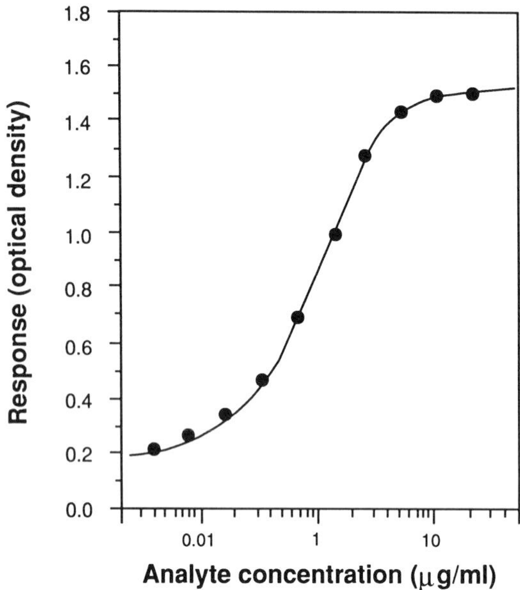

Figure 8.12 The asymmetric standard curve of Figure 8.10, fitted using a spline function.

plest of these is to join up the standard responses with straight line segments, which must obviously lead to significant bias for responses between data points. However, as we have seen, the latter problem can be minimised by using a simple transformation of response to produce a near linear calibration plot (e.g. reciprocal bound versus linear dose). Alternatively, a polynomial may be used to describe the whole curve, though these are not always reliable, being prone to oscillation between data points (Rodbard, 1978). All empirical methods have in common the *absence* of any model for the underlying process and no pre-supposed mechanism, they simply find the function that best describes the data points. The parameters in empirical equations are usually unstable from assay to assay and have no physical significance.

The most versatile, and most commonly used empirical method is a spline function. Spline functions have been described as computerised flexicurves and were first suggested for use in immunoassays by Vikelsoe (1973) and Marschner *et al.* (1974). In effect the whole curve is described by a series of polynomials of low order, which individually relate to a small portion of the curve. Each polynomial is constrained to have the same co-ordinates as its neighbour at 'knots' (usually the standard values) so that they all join up. A further constraint is that neighbouring polynomials should have the same first derivative at the 'knots' making a continuous curve and avoiding 'kinks'.

In theory a spline function can be made to fit any series of points, though this is undesirable since it would even pass through points exhibiting gross error. In practice, spline functions used for immunoassay dose response curves are derived from weighted data, enabling data points exhibiting high error to have reduced contribution towards the fit. They can also be smoothed, to avoid maxima and minima within the curve, and constrained to have a single turning point.

Good accounts of the principles of spline functions are given by Pilo *et al.* (1982) and Rawlins and Yrjonen (1978). The latter describe the algorithm used in RiaCalc

(Pharmacia). Contrary to what one might expect, spline functions are computationally straightforward, and do not require high computing power. Fitting the data for Figures 8.10 and 8.11 using a spline function took less than 2 seconds of processor time (IBM PS/2, model 55SX) and produced an excellent fit to the data (see Figure 8.12).

Errors in fitting immunoassay calibration plots

In the presentation so far, we have only considered sets of data that are without error. In practice of course, observed responses consist of the expected response *plus* an error component. The error will have many contributing factors (Rodbard and Lewald, 1970) and it will almost certainly be related to the expected response, i.e. the error will not be constant at all points on the curve. This non-constancy of error is referred to as heteroscedasticity and has important implications when fitting calibration functions to responses from standard series. In simple regression procedures it is assumed that the error is constant at all points on the curve; if significant heteroscedasticity exists, weighted regression may be required. In the latter procedure the contribution of individual points to the final fitted function is reduced in proportion to the response variance at each point.

It is important to realise that the degree of heteroscedasticity in the response depends not only on the detection procedure and assay errors, but also on any transformation of the response. Figure 8.13 compares the heteroscedasticity of two linear transformations of response (reciprocal bound and logit) with that of the raw data. The severe heteroscedasticity seen at the extremes of the range is typical for linear transforms of immunoassay data.

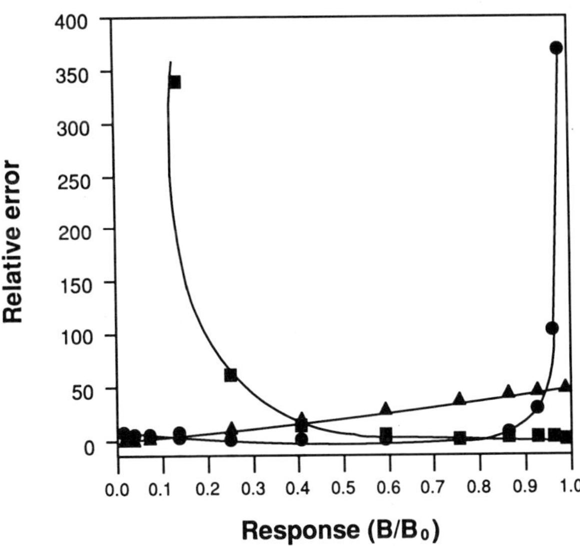

Figure 8.13 Simulated data illustrating the effect of two different response transformations on heteroscedasticity. Relative error is the variance at each response divided by the minimum variance. ▲ = untransformed data, ■ = reciprocal bound transformation and ● = logit transformation.

Weighted regression is the norm, though not an exclusive practice in immunoassay calibration curve fitting. The information for the weights can be obtained from 'binning' the observed errors for standards and unknowns in that batch if replicate analyses are carried out (Finney, 1976; Rodbard, 1981). This involves combining the error estimates for all samples and standards in a narrow concentration range (typically from half way between one pair of standards to half way between the next pair). The combination is a better estimate of the variance (and therefore weighting factor) over that part of the calibration. Alternatively, weights can be established from a known smooth function describing the response error relationship for the particular response measurement in use. Where the function is well established, e.g. for logit transformed responses, it is the recommended approach (Rodbard, 1978).

Error is present in all real data which results in a proportion of the variance of the data being unaccounted for by the calibration function. This is known as the residual variance and can, if replicate analyses of standards have been carried out, be partitioned into true error variance and error because of lack of fit of the calibration function. This is often expressed as a variance ratio in immunoassay data reduction packages and its significance can be tested using standard statistical procedures. The results of such a test should be viewed with caution. Most models are approximations and it is a general rule that the more precise the assay the more likely a significant lack of fit will be observed. It is also not a good way to compare different models. Spline functions for example are designed to fit data with less regard for the 'correctness' of individual data points than mass action models or logistic fits. Consequently, they would be expected to be less prone to lack of fit to the actual data. The best approach is to compare the effect of the fitting procedure on results for quality control samples over several batches (see the chapter on quality control). A very good explanation of all aspects of regression can be found in Massart *et al.* (1988).

Comparison of approaches to fitting immunoassay calibration plots

There are some very good overviews of immunoassay calibration plot fitting procedures (e.g. Rodbard, 1978) and many papers that compare different models for one or several assays. The only clear conclusion that can be made from these reports is that there are no general rules; however, there are some clear indications. Finney (1983) and Raab (1983a) have shown that, for several assays, a 4PL fit is more reliable and more versatile than a single binding site mass action model. Though the latter should be able to cope with some asymmetry, Raab found that when the 4PL fit failed, a 5PL procedure was more likely to work than the mass action model.

When comparing logistic and spline fits there is a tendency to regard the latter as inferior, but without much evidence. Finney (1983) calls spline functions overparametised and, though there is certainly instability of parameters from batch to batch, this need not effect the results. Pilo *et al.* (1982) found that spline functions worked just as well as a 4PL fit though they were less reliable on extrapolating below the lowest standard concentration (not something that should be done in any case). Kraupp *et al.* (1986) in a very good paper, found spline functions to be as good as 4PL fits when the error in the response estimates was small, but inferior at high scatter. They also found them to oscillate at low doses. Rawlins and Yrjonen (1978) suggest splines should be particularly good for asymmetric calibration curves.

A recommended approach to standardising immunoassays

There is very little objective data which clearly indicates a best approach to standardising immunoassays. The following recommendations should therefore be viewed as a guideline only, although they have worked well in the author's laboratory. As a general rule, new immunoassay procedures should be standardised more carefully during initial use. This allows a body of data to be established to which results can be compared when changes of procedure are made. Established assays and purchased kits should have such data available and recommendations given with the assay are best followed.

Number of standard concentrations

As few as four standard points have been successfully used when fitting data using the single binding site mass action model (Wilkins *et al.*, 1977) though a minimum of eight has been recommended (Dudley *et al.*, 1985). The usual number is between eight and twelve. Raab (1983b) suggests the number of concentrations should be at least twice the number of parameters in the model, i.e. 8 for 4PL and 10 for 5PL. Empirical fits such as spline functions benefit from higher numbers of standards to reduce the effect of error in individual points. In my laboratory we generally use 10 standards excluding zero.

Partition of standards

Generally, standards are partitioned with each standard at twice the concentration of the previous one. This is the approach I use, modified only if less than four standards fall on the near-linear part of the sigmoidal log dose response curve.

Replication of standards

The primary reason for replicating standards is to minimise the standard error of the response. However, the resulting information on response errors can also be used to weight the regression, provided error information is also available from unknowns. Replication also allows an estimate of the significance of any lack of fit; if this is an aim, then more than duplication may be required to gain the requisite degrees of freedom. Raab (1983b) recommends that there should be twice as many standard replicates as unknown replicates, although this practice does not seem that common. It is good practice to at least duplicate standards and unknowns for all new immunoassays, to accumulate the information so that objective decisions can be made when the assay 'comes of age'.

Raggatt (1989) discusses how much information is required in order to make a statistically valid judgement between the use of duplicates or singletons. Raggatt's concern lies with the clinical chemistry determinations where a 'blunder' would be undetected with singleton estimates of unknowns. The result of a misdiagnosis could be costly. In other analytical areas, such as the generation of elimination profiles of drugs from plasma or herbicides from plant tissue where multiple samples are taken, the risk associated with the analysis of singletons is much less. In these circumstances 'blunders' would be visible from the mass of related data. Analysts will need to assess the risks and make a judgement, albeit subjective, for their own area of work. Whatever the respective policy for unknown samples, careful investigation should be made on the effect of reducing the number of standard replicates, especially with regard to between batch error.

The necessity for replication of other standards such as B_0 and nsb depends very much on the fitting procedure used. Where they are used to transform the response such as the logit transformation, accurate estimates of their response values are essential, possibly with four or five replicates. With the 4PL fit for example, where the asymptote values are fitted rather than the measured values, replication or even determination of B_0 and nsb is much less important.

Calibration function

If a modern, sophisticated immunoassay data reduction package is available then linear transformations of response can be avoided; as stated earlier linear transforms often lead to an increase in heteroscedasticity. Four parameter logistic fits are a good first choice and will be found to fit data for a large number of immunoassays. If the log dose response curve is asymmetric, use a 5PL or spline function. The 5PL fit is preferred if there is high error in the responses. Comparisons between fits are best made over several batches. Analysis of variance should be used to estimate within and between batch error of quality control samples using each fit in turn. Comparisons of errors generated for each fit should allow the best approach to be identified (see the appendix of Chapter 10 for details of a simple one-way Anova procedure).

Weighting

It is common practice to use weighted regression for immunoassay calibration plots. The source of data for the weights in a particular assay may be taken from error information within that assay. Alternatively it can be obtained from some smooth function relating response variance to response. In the latter case, there must be some mechanism for checking for gross outliers in estimates of response for standard samples. The need for weighting should, however, be investigated in conjunction with different calibration models; if it can be avoided, so much the better.

Response measurement

Although the logistic equations can fit response in several formats, the raw counts should be fitted rather than normalised response (Finney, 1976). It is not possible to improve the quality of the response estimate by transformation, but it can be made worse. Calibration plots can of course be *displayed* using any of the normalised responses (B/T, B/B_0 etc.). Fitting the raw response data improves the chances of avoiding the need to weight the data.

Dose scale

In general, the sigmoid log dose response curves are easier to appreciate, and with which to understand changes. However, if results close to zero are of interest, then a linear dose scale should be used. The latter allows the zero standard (B_0) to be employed in regression analysis, which may improve the definition of the asymptote.

Future options for fitting immunoassay calibration plots

For the future, Rodbard (1978) states that 'although new methods for dose interpolation are likely to appear, these will most probably represent relatively minor technical refinement of existing procedures . . . since virtually all major techniques of mathematical, statistical and numerical analysis have already been applied to RIA'. This seems a very bold statement, but, even if true, further options for routine analysis are likely to become available with increasing computing power. It is now common for detectors to be linked directly to microcomputers, but they may in the future share a more powerful computer. This may bring options such as multi-binding site mass action models and multi-parameter logistic fits; whether they are actually needed remains to be seen.

References

DUDLEY, R. A., EDWARDS, P., EKINS, R. P., FINNEY, D. J., MCKENZIE, I. G. M., RAAB, G. M., RODBARD, D. & ROGERS, R. P. C. (1985) *Clin. Chem.*, **31**, 1264.

EKINS, R. P., NEWMAN, G. B. & O'RIORDAN, J. L. H. (1968) Theoretical aspects of 'saturation' and radioimmunoassay. In: HAYES, R. L., GOSWITZ, F. A. & MURPHY, B. E. P. (eds) *Radioisotopes in Medicine: In vitro Studies.* US Atomic Energy Commission, Oak Ridge, Tennessee, pp. 59–100.

FINNEY, D. J. (1974) *Statistical Methods in Biological Assays.* Griffin, London.

(1976) *Biometrics*, **32**, 721.

(1983) *Clin. Chem.*, **29**, 1762.

HALES, C. N. & RANDLE, P. J. (1963) *Biochem. J.*, **88**, 137.

HATCH, K. F., COLES, E., BUSEY, H. & GOLDMAN, S. C. (1976) *Clin. Chem.*, **22**, 1383.

HEALY, M. J. R. (1972) *Biochem. J.*, **130**, 207.

KRAUPP, M., MARZ, R., LEGENSTEIN, E., KNERER, B. & SZEKERES, T. (1986) *J. Clin. Chem. Clin. Biochem.*, **24**, 1023.

MARSCHNER, I., ERHARDT, F. & SCRIBA, P. C. (1974) Calculation of the radioimmunoassay standard curve by 'Spline function'. In: *Radioimmunoassay and Related Procedures in Medicine.* International Atomic Energy Agency, Vienna, pp. 111–122.

MASSART, D. L., VANDEGINSTE, B. G. M., DEMING, S. N., MICHOTTE, Y. & KAUFMAN, L. (1988) *Chemometrics: A Textbook*, Data Handling in Science and Technology, Volume 2. Elsevier, Amsterdam.

MURATA, A., OGAWA, M., MATSUDA, K., KITAHARA, T., NISHIBE, S., KUROKAWA, E. & KOSAKI, G. (1983) *J. Immunoassay*, **4**, 407.

NISBET, J. A., OWEN, J. A. & WARD, G. (1986) *Ann. Clin. Biochem.*, **23**, 694.

PILO, A., ZUCCHELLI, G. C., MALVANO, R. & MASINI, S. (1982) *J. Nucl. Med. Allied Sci.*, **26**, 235.

RAAB, G. M. (1983a) *Clin. Chem.*, **29**, 1757.

(1983b) Validity tests in the statistical analysis of immunoassay data. In: HUNTER, W. M. (ed.) *Immunoassays for Clinical Chemistry*. Churchill Livingstone, Edinburgh, pp. 614–623.

RAGGATT, P. R. (1989) *Ann. Clin. Biochem.*, **26**, 26.

RAWLINS, T. G. R. & YRJONEN, T. (1978) *Int. Lab.* Nov/Dec, 55.

RODBARD, D. (1978) Data processing for radioimmunoassays: An overview. In: NATELSON, S., PESCE, A. J. & DIETZ, A. A. (eds) *Clinical Immunochemistry: Chemical and Cellular Basis and Applications in Disease*, Current Topics in Clinical Chemistry, Volume 3. American Association of Clinical Chemistry, Washington, pp. 477–494.

(1981) Mathematics and statistics of ligand assays: An illustrated guide. In: LANGAN, J. CLAPP, J. J. (eds) *Ligand Assay: Analysis of International Developments in Isotopic and Non-isotopic Immunoassay*. Masson, New York, pp. 45–101.

RODBARD, D. & CATT, K. J. (1972) *J. Steroid Biochem.*, **3**, 255.

RODBARD, D. & LEWALD, J. E. (1970) Computer analysis of radioligand assay and radioimmunoassay data. In: *Steroid Assay by Protein Binding*. Second Karolinski Symposium on Research Methods in Reproductive Endocrinology, pp. 79–192.

RODBARD, D., BRIDSON, W. & RAYFORD, P. L. (1969) *J. Lab. and Clin. Med.*, **74**, 770.

RODBARD, D., RUDER, H. J., VAITUKAITIS, J. & JACOBS, H. S. (1971) *J. Clin. Endocrinol.*, **33**, 343.

SCATCHARD, G. (1949) *Ann. N.Y. Acad. Sci.*, **51**, 660.

VIKELSOE, J. (1973) *Acta Endocrinologica* (Suppl 177), 100.

WALKER, W. H. C. & KEANE, P. M. (1977) Theoretical aspects of radioimmunoassay. In: ABRAHAM, S. E. (ed.) *Handbook of RIA Clinical and Biochemical Analysis*, Volume 5. Marcel Dekker, New York, pp. 87–130.

WILKINS, T. A., CHADNEY, D. C., BRYANT, J., PALMSTROM, S. H. & WINDER, R. L. (1977) Non-linear least-squares curve-fitting of a simple theoretical model to radioimmunoassay dose-response data using a mini-computer. In: *Radioimmunoassay and Related Procedures in Medicine*. International Atomic Energy Agency, Vienna, pp. 399–423.

YALOW, R. S. & BERSON, S. A. (1968) General principles of radioimmunoassay. In: HAYES, R. L., GOSWITZ, F. A. & MURPHY, B. E. P. (eds) *Radioisotopes in Medicine: In vitro Studies*. US Atomic Energy Commission, Oak Ridge, Tennessee, pp. 7–41.

9

Validation of an immunoassay

R. A. BIDDLECOMBE

GlaxoWellcome Research and Development, Beckenham

B. LAW

Zeneca Pharmaceuticals, Macclesfield

Introduction

Validation is necessary to demonstrate the performance and reliability of a method and to determine the confidence that can be placed in the results it generates. Method validation in most areas of analytical science is governed by regulations such as those from the Federal Drug Administration (FDA) in the case of pharmaceutical analysis and the Environmental Protection Agency (EPA) in the analysis of agrochemicals and pesticide residues. The pharmaceutical industry regulations have tended to be the most stringent and the recently published Washington Conference Report (Shah *et al.*, 1992) is probably the most up to date view of analytical method validation. It is likely that this report will form the basis of future FDA formal guidelines for analytical method validation within the pharmaceutical industry and it has been adopted as the basis for the discussions presented here.

Many of the published guidelines are biased towards chromatographic techniques although many of the principles, procedures and requirements are common to all types of analytical methodologies. It is important to be aware of the fact that guidelines are continuously being updated and made more rigorous. Regulators also tend to assess submissions on the basis of current guidelines, not necessarily the guidelines that were in place when the work was carried out. It is important therefore to keep up to date with the regulations on method validation, anticipate any proposed changes and to work to the highest standards wherever possible.

For those working within a regulatory environment such as Good Laboratory Practice (GLP), method validation will probably involve defining a validation protocol which must be followed. At some stage, data supporting the assay will need to be presented either to a customer, a regulatory authority or even in a publication. It is strongly recommended therefore that all experiments used to make claims or draw conclusions about the validity of the method are written up in the form of a method validation report. This report will contain information supporting the standard operating procedure (SOP) which should also be written for the method. The latter is essential in ensuring that all laboratories and workers perform the assay in the same manner and to the same high standard.

A method report should stand on its own, but comparisons with other methods or laboratories may be necessary, especially when analysis has been conducted at more than one site or different analytical approaches have been adopted. Unless a method is used on a regular basis, such that its continued validity can be demonstrated, it may be necessary to carry out and document limited validation work to demonstrate the validity of the method prior to re-establishing it for routine use.

The parameters that need to be assessed to characterise fully the performance of an analytical method are: accuracy, precision, sensitivity, specificity, suitability of calibration model and robustness. Stability of the analyte, although somewhat method independent, is normally included as part of the validation package. A series of experiments used to validate each parameter of an immunoassay will be presented, however these experiments are not usually carried out in isolation. In the section on experimental plan it will be shown how these experiments can be grouped together to generate the required data with the minimum amount of experimental work.

The validation of an assay involves the application of a number of statistical routines, some of which are a little more specialised than the standard t-test widely used in analytical science. For a good general introduction to statistics and how they are applied to analytical chemistry the reader is referred to the book *Statistics for Analytical Chemistry* (Miller and Miller, 1989).

Response function

The first step in validation of an assay is the verification of the selected calibration model to ensure it adequately describes the relationship between response variable (Y value) and analytical concentration (X value), in each of the matrices studied. For a fuller discussion on the theoretical aspects of curve fitting the reader is directed to the previous chapter. A number of basic assumptions are made about the data when fitting a standard curve.

1 The curve chosen, correctly describes the data
2 The concentration values are known without error, i.e. all of the variability is the result of the measurement process not the preparation of standards etc.
3 The assay errors are independent of one another. This suggests that calibration standards are prepared from separate dilutions of a stock solution, not from serial dilutions of a single stock solution. (The simpler manipulations involved with the latter procedure make this the favoured option in some laboratories)
4 The variance in the Y residuals is relatively constant, i.e. there is homogeneity of variance

The analyst should be aware of these assumptions and as part of the validation, show through data analysis that they have not been grossly violated. Points 1 and 4 can be addressed by examining the residuals (the difference between the observed and fitted Y value) for a minimum of six standard curves. In the authors' laboratories it is normal practice to run duplicate standard curves for the precision and

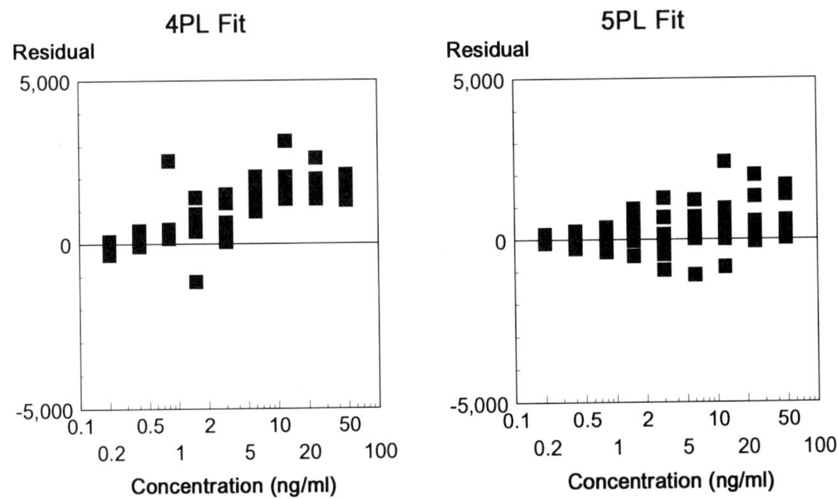

Figure 9.1 Residuals (observed value – fitted value) for assay calibration plots fitted using two different routines, 4PL and 5PL.

accuracy assessment (four assays in all) and pool this data for residual analysis. A plot of raw residual or studentised residual (raw residual divided by the estimated standard error) against concentration (on a log axis) will show how well the model describes the data. This analysis will provide the necessary evidence that the distribution of errors from the fitted value shows homogeneity of variance and that the curve is a reasonable fit to the data. An example of residual plots is shown in Figure 9.1. In this example using raw residuals, the four parameter logistic (4PL) fit shows a clear positive bias at high concentrations. The five parameter logistic (5PL) fit, however, seems to fit the data better; the positive bias is not so noticeable, although the homogeneity of variance is not quite as good.

However, appropriate selection of the calibration model and its verification are a regulatory requirement. This is particularly important for linear fits where variable types of weighting can easily be employed. Most immunoassay data reduction packages offer very poor or at best 'black box' type non-linear curve fitting routines (Gerlach *et al.*, 1993). The analyst often has very little control over the process and has to accept what is offered. In practice, however, a robust 4PL fit is generally capable of fitting most RIA data.

Precision

The precision of the assay is a measure of the random error and is defined as the agreement between replicate measurements of a defined sample (see Chapter 10). Precision is expressed as the percentage coefficient of variation (%CV) or the Relative Standard Deviation (RSD) of the replicate measurements. Most bio-analysts claim to measure and report intra- (within-assay) precision and inter- (between-assay) precision. The first of these is measured by repeatedly assaying a number of samples, typically low, medium and high (with respect to the assay range) in a single assay. The inter-assay variation would be determined by analysing the same samples in several assays. Although giving a measure of assay variability the inter-assay

Table 9.1 Raw concentration data (μg/ml) for determination of assay precision at one concentration

Occasion	Replicate 1	Replicate 2	Replicate 3	Replicate 4
1	0.050	0.049	0.057	0.050
2	0.047	0.038	0.057	0.047
3	0.056	0.052	0.058	0.054
4	0.052	0.051	0.062	0.052

precision as described above is actually a measure of the total assay variation since it has both an intra- and an inter-assay component. To obtain an accurate measure of the assay precision (intra-, inter- and total) the following procedure is recommended.

A minimum of four spiked samples are prepared covering the assay calibration range. These samples are then analysed at least four times in an assay and the assay is repeated on four separate occasions. Increasing the number of samples, replicates or assays, especially the last of these, will result in the generation of more meaningful and reliable data. After the analysis has been carried out a data set similar to that in Table 9.1 can be generated for each concentration studied. These data sets are analysed using one-way analysis of variance (ANOVA) as described in Chapter 10. This form of data analysis can be carried out simply using a spreadsheet program. It will give the total assay variability (%CV) as well as the intra- and inter-assay components of this variability. The ANOVA analysis will also indicate whether the intra- and inter-assay variations are significantly different. The ability to diagnose where the major assay error lies can be a useful tool in directing improvements in the analytical procedure. For example a high inter-assay variation in contrast to a low intra-assay variation could, for example, indicate problems in the preparation of the standards for each assay batch.

The level of acceptable total analytical imprecision will depend on the use to which the assay is put. Several proposed definitions are to be found in the literature. Harris (1979) recommends that the analytical error should be equal to or less than one half of the biological within-subject variation. Stewart and Fraser (1989) make recommendations based on the therapeutic concentration or pharmacokinetics of a pharmaceutical agent. Shah *et al.* (1992) recommend that the total assay CV should not exceed 15 per cent, except at the lower limit of quantification (LLOQ) where it should not exceed 20 per cent. The precision data together with the accuracy data provide an important bench-mark for subsequent assay performance and for any transfer of method.

Accuracy

The accuracy is a measure of the systematic error or bias and is defined as the agreement between the measured value and the true value. Accuracy is usually reported as % bias which is calculated as:

$$\% \text{ bias} = \frac{\text{measured value} - \text{true value}}{\text{true value}} \times 100$$

When working with real samples, the true value is not known making it difficult to determine the extent of assay bias. One of a number of approximate methods therefore has to be used. One approach that is adopted widely is to employ the data for spiked controls generated in the assessment of the assay precision. Comparing the overall mean obtained from the repeat analysis of spiked control samples with the expected or spiked values is the normal method for calculating percentage bias. However, as this method is really comparing one set of spiked samples with another (i.e. standards with spiked controls) the result merely indicates the precision of the spiking and is not really a true indicator of accuracy.

The best measure of accuracy is obtained by comparing with a reference method if available. It is important that this reference method has itself been validated and fully characterised and it should be preferably a physico-chemical method, such as a high-performance liquid chromatographic (HPLC) procedure. Since immunoassay methods are often developed because the alternatives such as HPLC lack the requisite sensitivity, a direct comparison of the techniques is not always possible. However, providing dilutions are accurately carried out, samples can be assayed using the reference method and then diluted for analysis by immunoassay. It is very important to carry out such comparisons using real samples not spikes, since the bias in immunoassays is often caused by non-specific interference or cross-reactivity which may not be apparent with spiked samples.

When comparing two techniques it is recommended that at least 20 samples are assayed using the two methods. To avoid the data being biased by high concentrations and to avoid recourse to the complications of weighting, the concentration range should be relatively narrow, around 20-fold. The most commonly used approach for analysing such data, is to plot one set of results against another and carry out least squares regression on the data. The reference method, which is assumed to be error free, or at least to have less error than the immunoassay method, is plotted on the x-axis and the slope, intercept and the correlation coefficient of the regression line are calculated. If both methods give identical results the regression line will have a zero intercept, and a slope and a correlation coefficient of one. In practice this never occurs: even in the absence of any bias, random errors would ensure that identical results are not obtained. The significance of any deviation is assessed by estimating the 95 per cent confidence limits for the slope and intercept to see whether the calculated values differ significantly from the ideal values of 1 and zero respectively (Miller and Miller, 1989). If the correlation coefficient is low then it is probable that one or both of the methods has poor precision, and it is likely that the analysis will fail to show a difference even if one is present.

Two important assumptions are made in employing this form of analysis. First, the line of regression of y on x is calculated assuming that the errors in the x values are negligible (all errors are assumed to occur in the y direction). This is clearly not the case since every method has a degree of random error. Second, it is also assumed that the errors in the y direction are constant, i.e. they do not vary with concentration, and that all the points thus have equal weighting when the slope and intercept are calculated; again this is not strictly true for an immunoassay method.

Despite the violation of these assumptions, this approach works reasonably well in practice (Miller and Miller, 1989) and it has been used widely in the authors' laboratories.

An alternative approach is to assay a smaller number of samples (approximately six) at least six times by each method. The precision of the measurements is first checked to show that the level of precision is similar for the two methods (F-test on the standard deviation). If this is so, then any difference in the means are compared using a t-test. There can be some difficulty in interpreting this data when some concentrations show a difference and others do not. To overcome this problem compare the mean concentration for the two methods using the paired t-test. To ensure that the data is not biased by high concentrations, the individual data points should be normalised by dividing a pair of concentration values by the average of the pair. If the data analysis shows the difference to be significant then the reference value can be considered to be true and the bias calculated.

Recovery

Recovery is often confused with accuracy although these two concepts are quite separate. Recovery is generally only studied with indirect methods, i.e. where the test analyte is extracted prior to analysis. Under these circumstances it is important, and also a regulatory requirement, to demonstrate consistent analyte recovery across the concentration range. The recovery is estimated by analysing spiked control samples against unextracted standards (Recovery (%) = (Measured value/Theoretical value) × 100). This data is easily generated by comparing extracted standards (i.e. a set of standards put through the extraction process) with a set of unextracted standards. Occasionally this can cause a problem because of the absence of matrix from the unextracted standards. If this is the case, then the unextracted standards should be prepared in an extract of blank matrix.

Limits of quantification

Limits of quantification (LoQ) or the working range of an assay are generally defined as the highest and lowest concentrations which can be determined with an acceptable degree of precision. Thus several workers can use the same assay and justifiably claim different LoQs since they may be using the assay for different purposes and have different requirements in terms of acceptable data quality. The likely LoQs are best determined by using a precision profile as described in Chapters 6 and 10. Although data can be employed from assays containing real samples, to ensure accurate definition of the precision across the calibration range, the precision profile is best generated by repeat analysis of a calibration series (typically 10 times). To obtain clear limits it is necessary to include at least one standard outside the proposed or expected upper and lower LoQ.

Limit of detection or sensitivity

It is common practice to determine and quote the sensitivity or limit of detection (LoD) of an assay, although as more workers become attuned to the concept of working ranges and limits of quantification (LoQ) (as discussed in the preceding section) the usefulness of LoD is diminishing. There are various methods of defining assay sensitivity, such as the concentration when B/B_0 equals 0.5 or 0.8, i.e. the ED_{50} or ED_{80}, or even the slope of the calibration curve. To try to impress with the lowest possible LoD some workers will quote confusingly the mass of analyte in the assay tube rather than sensitivity equivalent to the concentration of analyte in the original sample. Some care is therefore necessary in interpreting LoD data.

The most useful and most commonly understood meaning of sensitivity is the minimal detectable concentration (MDC). The MDC is the lowest concentration of analyte which can be distinguished at a stated level of probability from a sample containing no analyte.

One approach to determining the MDC (Rodbard, 1978) is to measure the response from a number of blank samples, typically 20 to 50, depending on the degree of variability. The mean response (in any units: cpm, B/B_0 etc.) from these samples is calculated along with the standard deviation. The MDC is that concentration which has a response equal to the mean response of the blank samples less 2 standard deviations. This is shown diagrammatically in Figure 9.2, any concentration above this value has a 95 per cent probability of being a true positive result. This simple approach does have one limitation however: if several samples are spiked at the MDC (calculated as above) and analysed, approximately half of these will give a result which falls below the MDC. This is the result of the fact that there is inherent imprecision in this determination, and a concentration at the MDC has its own confidence interval which may or may not be the same as that for a blank sample. This problem can be overcome by analysing the same control samples as above, with and without added compound, spiked at various concentrations around the expected MDC. Technically this approach can be very demanding since it involves the accurate preparation of separate standard solutions using up to 50 or so individual blank samples. The concentration of analyte where the confidence interval does not overlap that for the zero concentration standard is then defined as the MDC (Figure 9.3). This concentration will always be higher than that determined by the simpler approach above. The simpler approach only eliminates false

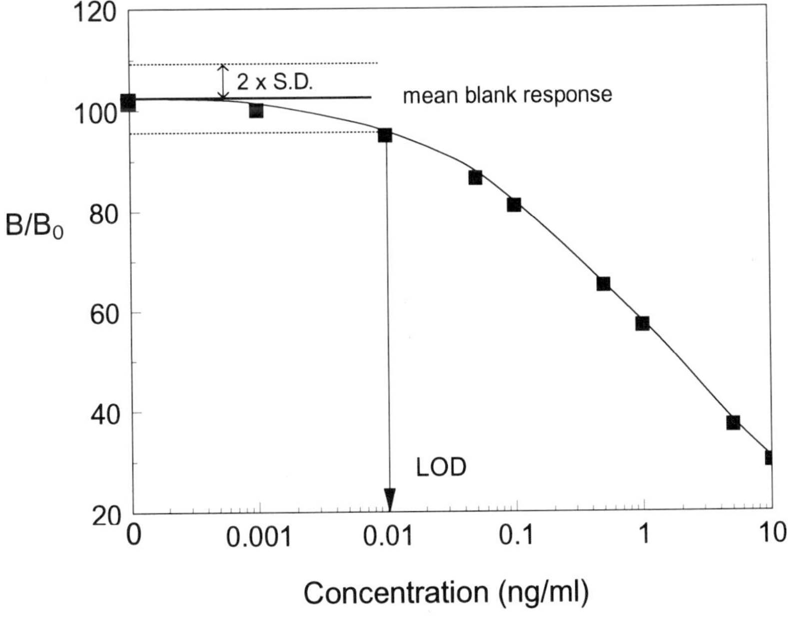

Figure 9.2 Determination of limit of detection (LoD) based on the analysis of blank samples.

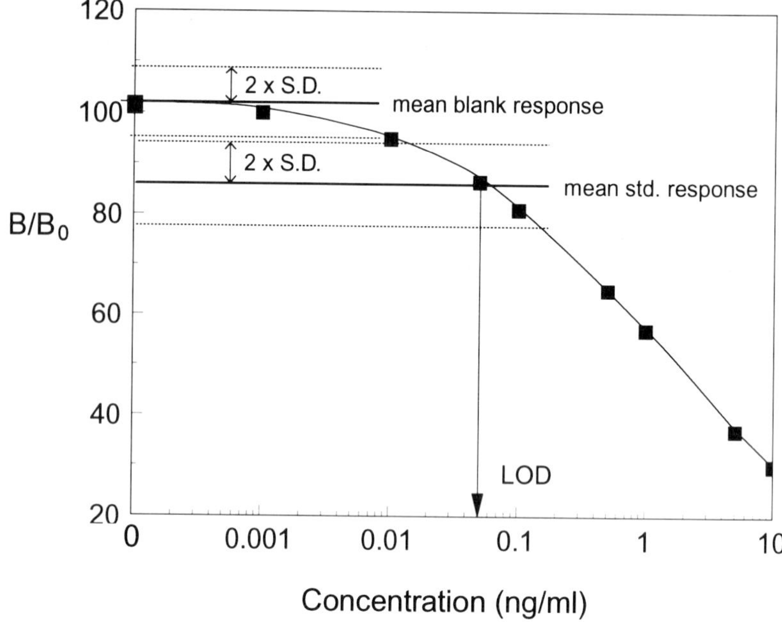

Figure 9.3 Determination of limit of detection (LoD) based on the analysis of blank samples and the precision of the blank and standard estimates.

positive results whilst the more complex procedure eliminates both false positives and false negatives. The former is the more common requirement for most analytical work and this approach has been adopted in our laboratories.

It must be remembered however that although it may be possible to distinguish very low concentrations from zero, the imprecision of such measurements may be so high that they are of little practical value other than to indicate that analyte is present.

In either of the approaches described above no consideration is given to the possible variability in the calibration graph, for example. It is recommended therefore that any conclusions arrived at in the initial experiment are checked out by analysing a subset of blank samples giving low, medium and high responses in at least one further assay.

In the area of pharmaceutical development and clinical chemistry it is often necessary to assay samples from subjects exhibiting various disease states, which may adversely affect the performance of the immunoassay. One example would be renal failure where the levels of plasma proteins and various inorganic ions may be raised significantly to such an extent that they interfere with antibody binding and affect the assay result. If such a scenario is envisaged then it is recommended that control samples from such individuals are analysed to determine the LoQ for that particular subgroup.

Specificity

The specificity of an immunoassay is dependent on the selectivity of the antibodies used and hence it can never be established unequivocally. The quality of the assessment is very much dependent on the compounds tested and the methods used. Practically specificity is best assessed in two ways. First it is important to show that metabolites, analyte degradents and, in the case of pharmaceuticals, other co-administered drugs have low and acceptable levels of cross-reactivity.

Potential cross-reactants, i.e. metabolites, endogenous compounds and co-administered drugs, are usually tested according to the method of Abraham (1969). A calibration series of the test material in question is prepared (at concentrations up to 100-fold higher than the standard series) and assayed under normal assay conditions. The resulting curve is compared with that given by the standard material for which the assay was designed. Cross-reactivity is usually expressed as the relative dose required for 50 per cent displacement of the maximum tracer binding (Figure 9.4), or in mathematical terms:

Cross-reactivity

$$= \frac{\text{concentration of standard required to give 50\% inhibition}}{\text{concentration of competitor required to give 50\% inhibition}} \times 100$$

Thus in the example shown in Figure 9.4 the percentage cross-reactivity for compound A is equal to $X_1/X_2 \times 100$ and for compound B, $X_1/X_3 \times 100$.

It is clearly impossible to examine every substance for cross-reactivity and in practice only related compounds or co-administered drugs in the case of pharmaceuticals are tested. In the authors' experience it has been found useful to evaluate structural analogues of the standard material (where these are available) since these can give information on which substances are likely to cross-react. This is

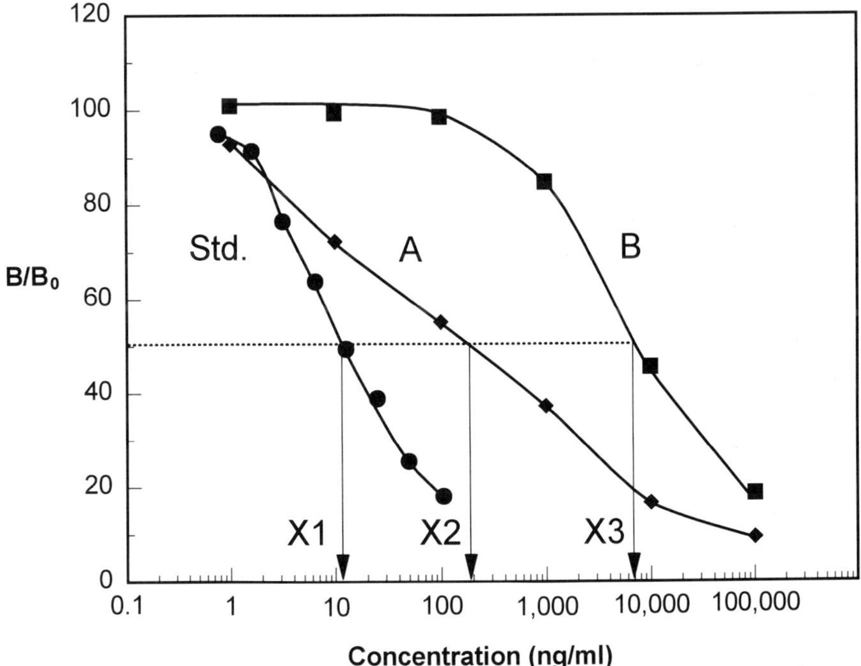

Figure 9.4 Calibration curves for a standard (□), and two cross-reactants A(◆) and B(■) showing different types of curve.

particularly useful when it is difficult to isolate or produce metabolites. When interpreting results it is important to consider cross-reactivity in terms of molar concentration, particularly when the molecular weights of the compounds differ substantially, for example the case with conjugates such as glucuronides.

Not all cross-reactants give displacement curves parallel to the standard curve, i.e. the percentage cross-reactivity is not the same at all concentrations, such as compound A in Figure 9.4. The 50 per cent displacement method would give 6 per cent cross-reactivity, when clearly the level of cross-reactivity at lower concentrations is much higher. Indeed, although the 50 per cent displacement method is the method most often used, it has the disadvantage that it takes little account of the region of highest cross-reaction at low antigen concentration and it underestimates the degree of cross-reactivity. The limitations of the 50 per cent displacement method and two alternative methods, the $CR_{1\,ng}$ method and the 10 per cent error method, are discussed by Pratt (1978). The $CR_{1\,ng}$ method expresses cross-reaction as a ratio of displacements caused by 1 ng of both antigens. Under certain circumstances this can give a more reliable estimate of cross-reactivity, the arbitrary 1 ng level means the method is not universally applicable. The 10 per cent error method expresses cross-reactivity as the ratio of the initial gradients of the two curves, giving a more reliable estimate of cross-reactivity when the curves are non-parallel. All three methods were used to analyse the data for compounds A and B in Figure 9.4, and the resultant cross-reactivity estimates are presented in Table 9.2. Providing calibration curves are parallel the 50 per cent displacement method is acceptable; if certain compounds give non-parallel curves then the results should be qualified or other methods used.

The second approach to demonstrating specificity involves showing that analyte in real samples will give a curve parallel to the standard curve. Once again this approach is particularly useful when there are no metabolites available for analysis. A range of samples containing a high concentration of analyte (approximately equal to the top standard) are selected. Ideally these should be from different individuals and at different times after dosing in the case of pharmaceuticals, or from independent samples in the case of other analyte types. These samples should be serially diluted (typically $\times 2$) so that the expected concentrations cover the assay calibration range. They are then assayed against a standard calibration series. Assuming the original high concentration value (undiluted sample) is correct, the responses for the diluted samples are plotted against the expected concentration alongside the calibration graph. Certain types of non-specific interferences (Perlstein *et al.*, 1980) or the presence of some metabolites (e.g. compound A in Figure 9.4) may give curves that are non-parallel when compared with the standard curve. An alternative and more exact method of analysing the data is to plot the expected against the observed concentration. The degree of parallelism and the significance of

Table 9.2 Cross-reactivity estimates (%) derived from the data presented in Figure 9.4, using three different methods

Compound	50% inhibition method	10% error method	$CR_{1\,ng}$ method
A	6.0	100	100
B	0.3	0.2	0.3

any deviation can then be checked by performing linear regression analysis. The slope and intercept are calculated and the values compared with the ideal of 1 and 0 using the appropriate statistics (Miller and Miller, 1989).

Stability

Stability data are required to show that the concentration of analyte in the sample at the time of analysis corresponds to the concentration of analyte at the time of sampling, e.g. sample collection, storage or processing do not affect concentration. This view is endorsed by the Washington guidelines (Shah *et al.*, 1992) which emphasise that environmental conditions, matrix material or procedural variables should be studied for their effect on analyte concentrations. Generation of the stability data, although an important part of the validation, is method independent and the majority of this work may be carried out separately, particularly the long-term studies. As a minimum, sufficient work should be carried out as part of the validation to provide one month's stability data for the analyte in the sample matrix under normal storage conditions. This would allow routine analysis to begin, with further data being generated on an ongoing basis.

It is a common occurrence in the analytical literature to find statements to the effect that 'the analyte was stable for x weeks when stored at room temperature'. No definition of stability is given nor is the experimental design or the statistical method used for the assessment reported. The procedure recommended here for stability assessment is that of Timm *et al.* (1985). This approach has the advantage that it takes into account the precision of the assay, there is a clearly defined confidence interval and the analyst sets a level of instability that is relevant to the use to which the data is to be put. Timm and co-workers (Timm *et al.*, 1985) recommend the study of two or three concentrations covering the range of interest. These samples are prepared in bulk and stored as sub-aliquots at the required storage temperature with each aliquot capable of giving at least six analyses. At the required stability time point an aliquot is removed from storage and analysed (six times) alongside six aliquots of freshly prepared samples at the same concentration. It is important that the same matrix sample is used for both the stored and fresh samples. The geometric means of the fresh and stored samples are calculated along with the percentage difference and the 95 per cent confidence limits for the stored aliquots. If the confidence limits bracket the expected concentration there is no significant degradation. If the upper or lower confidence limits do not bracket the expected concentration and the limits are equal to or greater than 90 per cent of the expected concentration, there is significant but not relevant degradation. Degradation of greater than 10 per cent is generally considered relevant.

With biological samples there are two other areas where it is necessary to show evidence of stability. The first is heat inactivation which is carried out on all high-risk samples (e.g. HIV positive). Spiked samples at three concentrations would be assayed before and after heat inactivation and the data treated as described above.

The second area of study is the effect of repeated freeze–thawing. For the freeze–thaw experiment two approaches can be taken based on the perceived stability of the analyte under the freeze–thaw conditions. If it is believed that the analyte concentration will not change, then a sample can be prepared, subjected to four freeze–

Table 9.3 Experimental plan for the generation of the minimum validation data for a pharmaceutical agent

Occasion	Format	Number of samples	Day
	Prepare 2 analytical stock solutions Prepare calibration standards in matrix Prepare control samples (C1, C2, C3, C4) in matrix		−1
1	Standards × 2 (beginning and end) Spiked controls (C1, C2, C3, C4) × 4	16	0
2	Standards × 2 (beginning and end) Spiked controls (C1, C2, C3, C4) × 4	16	1
3	Standards × 2 (beginning and end) Spiked controls (C1, C2, C3, C4) × 4	16	2
4	Standards × 2 (beginning and end) Spiked controls (C1, C2, C3, C4) × 4	16	3
5	Standards × 1 20 blanks 6 clinical samples Metabolites	 20 6 ?	
6	Standards × 1 Co-administered drugs Other possible cross-reactants	 ? ?	
	Prepare fresh analytical stock solutions Prepare fresh controls (C1, C2, C3, C4)		30
7	Standards × 1 Old spiked controls (C1, C2, C3, C4) × 6 New spiked controls (C1, C2, C3, C4) × 6 Freeze–thaw (3 cycles) (C1, C2, C3, C4)	 24 24 4	30

thaw cycles and assayed against freshly prepared samples. If it is thought that some decrease in the analyte concentration may occur or the experiment previously outlined has shown a significant change, then the freeze–thaw samples can be assayed after each freeze–thaw cycle. Using either approach six separate determinations should be carried out on the processed and fresh samples. Once again the data would be analysed using the method of Timm *et al.* (1985).

Stability experiments are normally carried out using spiked samples as opposed to real ones. There is one area however where the alternative approach may be more appropriate. This is where the analyte of interest is obtained from a living system, as in clinical chemistry or pharmaceutical bioanalysis. As part of the elimination process in living systems, many exogenous and endogenous compounds undergo conjugation with sugars, such as glucuronic acid, and also sulphate. Some of these conjugates, particularly the *O*-ester glucuronides of carboxylic acids can be relatively unstable, especially in a basic environment such as stored urine. Decomposition of such conjugates in a sample could result in a gradual increase in concentration of the analyte with time. If it is believed that such labile metabolites are likely to be formed then suitable samples should be generated at the earliest opportunity and the stability studied.

Experimental plan

The minimum experimental work required to validate an immunoassay is presented batch by batch, in Table 9.3. In this particular example the analyte of interest is assumed to be a drug compound. It is assumed in setting up these experiments that the analyte has good stability under the normal storage conditions, i.e. at least 30 days. The experiments as outlined will generate sufficient data, including one month's stability, to give the necessary confidence to allow sample analysis to be started. This is very much the start of the validation process since this type of approach does place a heavy emphasis on the ongoing monitoring of assay performance once routine analysis has begun.

Initially two independent stock solutions of analyte are prepared. Using two separate plasma pools, one stock solution is used to generate standards and the other control samples for determination of precision and accuracy. The concentrations of two of the control samples should be set at the expected or desired limits of quantification of the assay, and the other two positioned over the calibration range. The control samples should be sub-aliquoted to allow analysis as per Table 9.3 and stored under normal storage conditions. Analysis of the results from these samples using one-way ANOVA will give a good indication of the overall assay precision and allow limits of quantification to be set. By comparing the found concentration with the expected some indication of the assay accuracy can be assessed. Finally new stock solutions are prepared and fresh controls generated using the same batch of matrix to allow stability to be confirmed. The same samples are also subjected to repeated freeze–thawing (three cycles) and compared with the untreated samples.

Conclusion

Method validation is often considered to consist of two phases. Phase one described here is the initial validation carried out prior to sample analysis. From this work statements can be made regarding accuracy, precision, sensitivity, specificity etc. This is the bench-mark for the assay. Phase two is the application to real samples which is the start of an ongoing validation of the assay where confidence is built up and the assay is shown to be robust.

References

ABRAHAM, G. E. (1969) *J. Clin. Endocrinol.*, **29**, 866.

GERLACH, R. W., WHITE, R. J., DEMING, S. N., PALASOTA, J. A. & VAN EMON, J. M. (1993) *Anal. Biochem.*, **212**, 185.

HARRIS, E. K. (1979) *Am. J. Clin. Pathol.*, **72**, 374.

MILLER, J. C. & MILLER, J. N. (1989) *Statistics for Analytical Chemistry*, 2nd Edition. Ellis Horwood Ltd, Chichester.

PERLSTEIN, M. T., CHAN, D. W. & BILL, M. J. (1980) *Ligand Quarterly*, **3**, 34.

PRATT, J. J. (1978) *Clin. Chem.*, **24**, 1869.
RODBARD, D. (1978) *Anal. Biochem.*, **90**, 1.
SHAH, V. P., MIDHA, K. K., DIGHE, S., MCGILVERAY, I. J., SKELLY, J. P., YACOBI, A., LAYLOFF, T., VISWANATHAN, C. T., COOK, C. E., MCDOWALL, R. D., PITTMAN, K. A. & SPECTOR, S. (1992) *Pharm. Res.*, **9**, 588.
STEWART, M. J. & FRASER, C. G. (1989) *Ann. Clin. Biochem.*, **26**, 220.
TIMM, U., WALL, M. & DELL, D. (1985) *J. Pharm. Sci.*, **74**, 972.

10

Quality of immunoassays and quality control procedures

M. J. WARWICK

Zeneca Pharmaceuticals, Macclesfield

Introduction

All analytical methods used for quantitative analysis should be subject to validation procedures which have been described in detail in Chapter 9. Initial validation experiments are carried out before first use of the assay, thereby helping to establish boundary conditions and the quality to be expected in the data. However, it should not be assumed that these experiments justify all subsequent use of the assay; for this, ongoing validation in the form of a quality control (QC) policy is essential. A QC policy tests the results, usually from a number of replicates of QC samples (where the concentration of the analyte is already known) against established QC rules. If the QC data conforms to the rules, the assay is considered to be in specification and the data generated acceptable for the use for which it is intended.

Analysing samples for which the concentration is already known is a complete waste of time, unless the action adds to the value of your product. QC samples only have value if their satisfactory analysis demonstratively provides the required level of confidence for the whole assay batch, or their unsatisfactory analysis reflects a true error in the method. There is no statistical process that can be applied to these QC data to provide an unequivocal answer; interpretation is *always* necessary. This implies there is a learning curve to getting the maximum value from quality control samples, a process which cannot be circumvented. The investment of time however is well worth it.

Unlike the chapter on standardisation, there will be no recommended set of QC rules, those that are discussed are merely examples. What will be demonstrated is that there is no ideal QC policy for all assays, it depends what the data is to be used for, and on the quality and stability of the assay itself.

The aims of a QC policy

The aim of quantitative analysis is to produce a result which is an accurate reflection of the true concentration of the analyte in the matrix. However, all analytical methods produce results which consist of an analyte-related response plus an error component. The use of an assay implies that the inherent level of error is acceptable. A quality control policy must therefore indicate when the level of error has become unacceptable. It should have a high level of error detectability, but it must be insensitive to the acceptable level of error, i.e. it should have a low false rejection rate. It is the decrease in 'quality' that must be detected, not the level of 'quality'. The QC process must be as cost effective as possible, and reasonably simple and easy to operate. With the modern computer support available on detection instruments, the data reduction aspects should wherever possible be automatic. A well designed QC procedure is an ongoing validation process, confirming earlier results or indicating where modifications are required. Ideally, it should indicate the nature of any error that occurs (see Montgomery, 1991 for a fuller discussion)

The aims described so far are commonly known as internal quality control. External quality control procedures, which are commonly used in clinical chemistry, are designed to ensure the quality of data is independent of the laboratory which generates it. This chapter will consider only internal quality control. Finally, it should be emphasised that quality control is not an option, it is part of good laboratory practice in every sense. Regulatory authorities are demanding higher standards, and all customers have a right to expect analysts to be able to justify their results.

Precision, bias and accuracy

If the principal aim of a QC policy is to indicate when an assay method has decreased in 'quality', it is clearly important to know the initial (presumably acceptable) 'quality'. One of the most important attributes of an assay is accuracy; in order to monitor this parameter we need to describe its components, precision and bias. Figure 10.1 illustrates these in a manner that may be familiar. The four series of concentric circles represent targets, and the black dots are shots at the target, each shot representing a replicate analysis of a sample. When these shots, or analytical results, are grouped close together (i.e. the two targets on the left), then the process is precise; when the spread of the shots around the centre shows a tendency to one side or another (top left and bottom right), the process is biased.

Imprecision is the result of random perturbations in response in every direction so that, overall, there is no general tendency in any direction; these perturbations are often referred to as random error. Bias is a result of systematic error, or the tendency for a result to deviate from the true value in a particular direction. Inaccuracy arises as a result of both random and systematic error (bias) and can be expressed mathematically (Schwarz, 1982) as:

$$\text{inaccuracy} = \sqrt{[(\text{standard error})^2 + (\text{bias})^2]} \qquad (1)$$

Standard error represents random error of the mean estimate and is the standard deviation divided by the square root of the number replicates.

The formula is not necessarily exact but it illustrates how each error component may affect inaccuracy (see Ekins, 1983 for a fuller discussion). If the assay is imprecise and samples are analysed only once (i.e. as singletons), the random error component may be the dominant cause of inaccuracy; however, the contribution to inaccuracy from this source of error can be reduced by increasing the number of

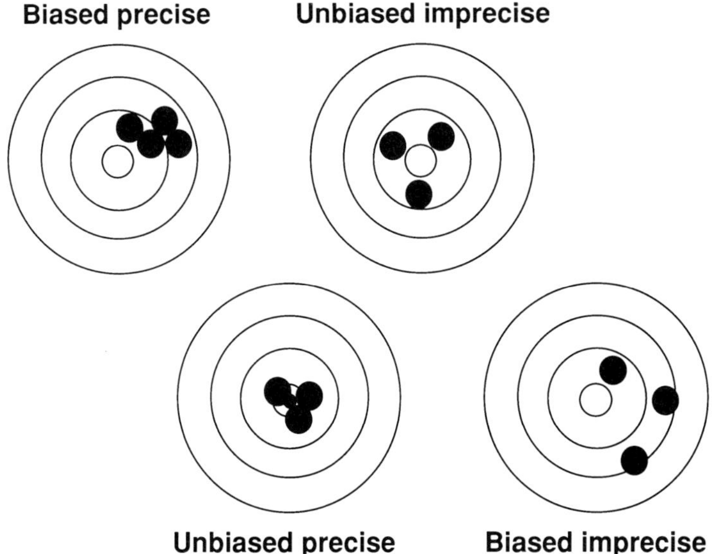

Figure 10.1 Analogy for precision and bias in analytical methods.

replicates. If the assay has a large bias, then any number of replicates will not reduce the resultant inaccuracy. If sufficient replicate analyses are carried out so that the standard error is only a small fraction of the bias, then inaccuracy is approximately equal to bias, which is sometimes how it is defined.

It is clear from the above description that a good QC programme should be sensitive to changes in both random and systematic error.

Response error relationships and the precision profile

All types of analytical methods exhibit random error in the response and for most methods the extent of this error is proportional to the response. This relationship between error and response can be described by a function known as the response error relationship (RER). There are many contributing sources to the response error in immunoassay (Schwarz, 1982), but the relationship can be simply illustrated by considering the counting errors alone. The measurement errors in radioactive decay processes have a Poisson distribution, one of the properties of which is that the variance of any response is equal to that response. Other terms used to describe this error are standard deviation (SD) or coefficient of variation (CV) of response (standard deviation as a percentage of the response). For an error process with a Poisson distribution:

$$\text{SD of response} = \sqrt{\text{response}} \tag{2}$$

$$\text{CV of response (\%)} = \text{SD of response} \times 100/\text{mean response} \tag{3}$$

Figures 10.2 and 10.3 show the response error relationships, plotted in terms of variance and CV respectively, for the simulated standard curve shown in Figure 10.4. The results are typical of immunoassays; variance or absolute error generally increases with response but, when error is expressed as a proportion of response (i.e.

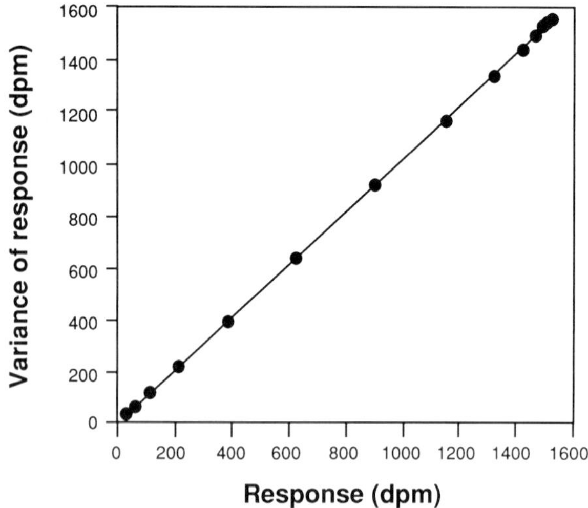

Figure 10.2 Response error relationship, using variance of the responses from the simulated standard curve of Figure 10.4. dpm = decays per minute.

as CV), proportional error is often higher at low responses. Although the simple RER of Figure 10.2 is linear, the presence of other sources of error may result in more complex relationships (Raab, 1981).

Since the calibration function is non-linear (Figure 10.4), the error in the concentration estimates is not a linear function of the error in response. Examination of Figure 10.4 shows that the slope of the calibration function varies continuously along its length; clearly, the lower the slope the bigger will be the error in concentration for a given error in response. A simple way of expressing the relationship is (Ekins, 1983):

$$\text{concentration error} = \text{response error/slope of calibration function} \qquad (4)$$

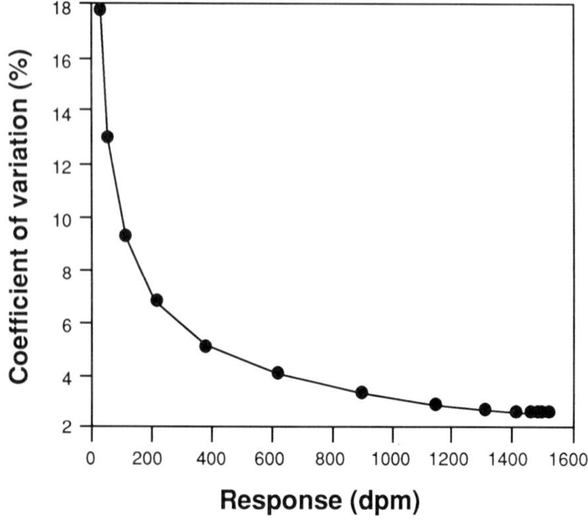

Figure 10.3 Response error relationship, using coefficient of variation of the responses from the simulated standard curve of Figure 10.4.

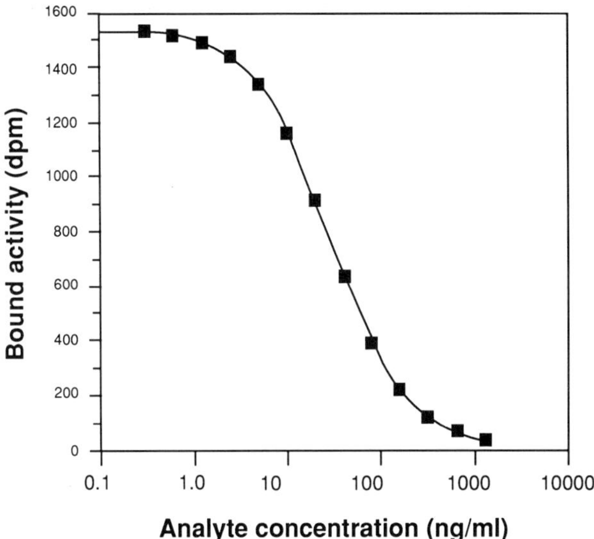

Figure 10.4 Simulated standard curve based on 30 fmol of an antibody with an affinity of 1×10^{11} mol/l and 40 fmol of tracer.

The response error at any response is expressed in the RER. The slope of the calibration function at any concentration is given by the differential of that function. Error in concentration is therefore the response error relationship divided by the differential of the calibration function. When concentration error, expressed as coefficient of variation (CV), is plotted against the log of concentration, the well known precision profile is obtained (Ekins, 1983). Figure 10.5 shows the precision profile obtained for the standard curve of Figure 10.4, using the response error relationship

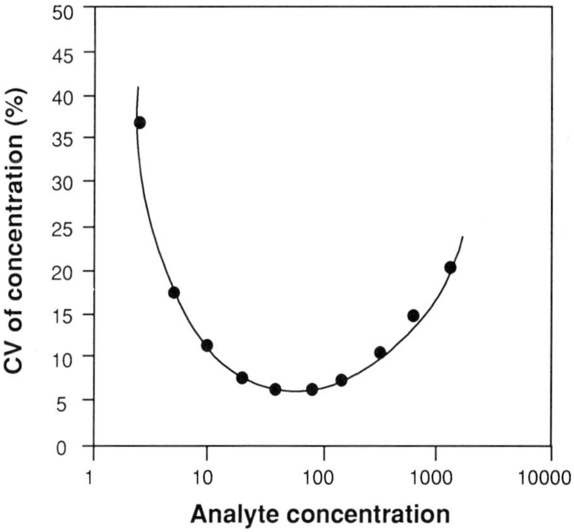

Figure 10.5 Precision profile derived from the response error relationship of Figure 10.2 and the standard curve of Figure 10.4.

of Figure 10.2. The decrease in precision (when expressed as CV) at the extremes of the calibration range is typical of immunoassay methods.

One of the advantages of the precision profile as a descriptor of assay quality is that it can be derived from information contained within a normal assay batch, provided that all standards and samples are replicated; the latter is a common although not an exclusive practice for immunoassays. To obtain a reliable estimate of error at any response level requires a large number of degrees of freedom, implying large numbers of replicates. However, it is possible to pool the information contained in the duplicate results of several different samples. The only requirement is that the variances be homogeneous, which simply means that only error data from samples of very similar concentrations should be pooled. This is usually achieved by setting up concentration 'bins', ranging from halfway between one pair of standards to halfway between the next pair; error data from unknowns are added to the appropriate 'bin'. The median error value for each 'bin' is determined and used in the estimate of the RER.

Limits of quantification

It is clear from the discussion so far, that in order to be confident about the quality of quantitative data produced from our assay we will need to restrict the assay to a reasonable range. Ekins (1983) defines the working range as 'that range within which estimates display acceptable precision'; examination of Figure 10.5 would suggest that this range is somewhere in the middle of the precision profile where the CV of the assay and its rate of change are low. Immunoassays therefore have both lower and upper limits of quantification (LoQ), which are the limits of the working range. It is worth noting that the lower LoQ does not necessarily coincide with the limit of detection (LoD) for the assay. The latter is usually defined as the point where the response is significantly different from that for a true blank. The precision at the LoD however may be very poor.

There are several ways of defining the assay range, most of them subjective. The area between a B/B_0 of 20% and 80% is often advocated, alternatively, that part of the range where the predicted CV on concentration is less than 10% is often used (Ekins, 1983). Though useful guides, there is no sound reason for either of these approaches.

An approach we have used recently employs a form of the precision profile having relative response (B/B_0) as the independent variable rather than concentration. This simple transformation linearises and normalises the scale so that it is the same for all assays. The limits of quantification are defined as the points where the slopes of the tangent to this curve reach 45 degrees. Between these two positions the CV of concentration estimates are reasonably constant, while outside this range imprecision increases rapidly. One advantage of this approach is that it requires no fixed values of precision or response to be assumed. The limits of quantification in concentration units can be obtained from the calibration data. In my laboratory, these limits of quantification are determined during assay validation and, in subsequent routine analysis, QC samples are included at concentrations equal to each of them.

Figure 10.6 shows the precision profile of Figure 10.5 re-scaled as described above. Marked on the figure are ranges based on a CV of 10% and on 20/80%

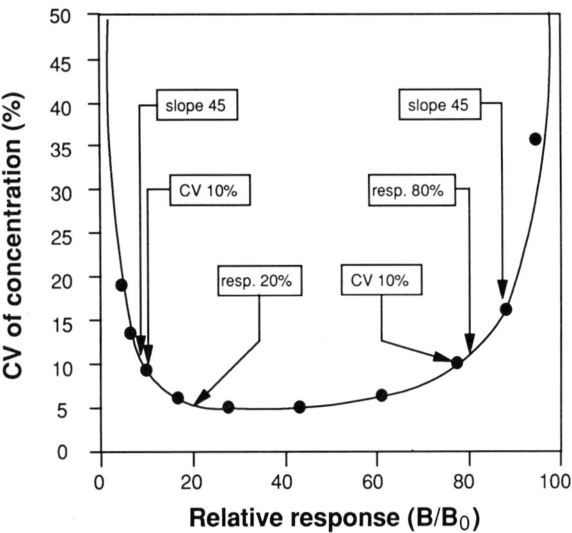

Figure 10.6 Precision profile based on the data in Figure 10.5, re-scaled using relative response as the independent variable. The profile illustrates three different ways of defining the limits of quantification, based on slope of the profile, a CV of 10%, and 20% and 80% of the maximum response.

B/B_0. Also marked are the positions where the slope of the profile reaches 45 degrees. Clearly the assay working range is very dependent on the definition used for the limits of quantification. It is important that the QC policy continually validates this range.

Within and between batch error

The analyses above have established the reliable range of the assay, along with a measure of the error in the concentration estimate throughout this range. Other quality parameters need to be established before there is sufficient information to design a quality control policy for the assay. The absence of inherent bias is difficult to establish unless a reliable reference method is available (seldom the case for new chemical entities) but the validation exercise would be expected to show any gross effects. Sometimes overlooked is the partition of total error into within batch and between batch components. Between batch error is the decrease in precision resulting from re-analysis of samples on different occasions, and it is additional to within batch error. It is not compensated for by calibration in each batch and indeed, it can actually be a consequence of the calibration process.

Rodbard (1974) states that 'the ratio of between batch to within batch variance provides an index of the temporal stability of the system', and Davis *et al.* (1980) suggest that an assay with a between to within batch error ratio of greater than three is unstable. Since instability is what a QC policy is intended to detect, the presence of significant between batch error will affect the design of such a policy. Between batch error is normally viewed as a random component in the overall error of an assay, but for any one batch it represents a systematic error which adds to the within batch error. Because between batch error can never be totally eliminated it is necessary to design rules that avoid false rejection that could follow as a consequence of this error component.

The partition of assay error into within and between batch components is a relatively straightforward process using one-way analysis of variance (ANOVA) on the results of a sample of known concentration analysed repeatedly in each of several batches (any simple statistics textbook will explain this process). During assay validation we routinely use four batches with four replicates per batch, but increased numbers of batches will improve the sensitivity to between batch error. Appendix 1 gives details of the necessary manual calculations. Between batch error may well be different at different concentrations, the experiment should therefore be carried out at a minimum of three concentrations spanning the assay working range. Improved estimates of both within and between batch error can be obtained by incorporating the results of QC samples analysed during routine use of the assay.

The causes of between batch error are such long-term effects as reagent instability, procedural variations (e.g. incubation time), detector ageing and analyst fatigue. However, a commonly overlooked cause is standard preparation and calibration error. The latter can arise when the error in response estimates is such that the line of best fit varies from day to day, even though the mean response for any standard concentration is the same. The one-way analysis of variance approach offers a convenient way of comparing the effects of different calibration curve fitting procedures (4PL, 5PL, spline etc.), weighting schemes and standard preparation and replication protocols. Most of these can be compared using the one set of data, and the effects of the variables on the overall mean concentration, total error, and within and between batch error should be investigated.

QC rules and their 'power functions'

A QC rule is a 'parameter' with acceptability limits which is applied to the results of the QC samples. As long as the parameter is within the acceptability limits, the assay is considered stable. The parameter can be the raw concentration values, their mean, their range or precision. Westgard *et al.* (1977a) and Montgomery (1991) give several examples of such rules. Since the assay and the attendant results will be rejected when the parameter falls outside its limits, the first important characteristic of the rule is that it should not cause assay rejection when no extra error is present, i.e. it should have a low probability of false rejection. Clearly, in the presence of increased error, to be effective the rule must signal assay rejection, i.e. it must have a high probability of error detection. Other desirable characteristics of QC rules are that they should be sensitive to both random and systematic error, need only a small number of replicate analyses and minimal data manipulation. The decision criteria should be clear, unequivocal and simple, also, recording of results should be easy. Needless to say very few rules have all of these attributes.

A 'power function' for a QC rule (or combination of rules) was defined by Westgard and Groth (1979). It is a plot of the probability of error detection against the level of added error. It provides a graphical estimation of both the probability of false rejection and the probability of true error detection at several levels of error. Power functions make possible the simple comparison of QC rules as will be shown below.

Calibration curve parameters

Parameters derived from standard curves are not effective as primary QC measures. Parameters such as percentage bound, ED_{20}, ED_{50}, ED_{80}, slope and residual error are characteristics of the standard curve rather than the assay as a whole. Since the objective of standardising the assay in every batch is to calibrate a varying response, variation in standard curve parameters do not necessarily imply variation in assay error. The trends in curve parameters are, however, worth recording; they may prove to be valuable diagnostic tools when an assay is declared out of control.

Quality control samples

Quality control procedures are normally based on the analysis of QC samples which are treated as unknowns, with the results being interpreted according to one or more rules. The simplest examples of such rules are those based on direct use of the QC results, without data manipulation, as these lend themselves very well to manual quality control procedures. Figure 10.7 shows data from a real example in operation. Here three replicates of a QC sample, nominally at 120 ng/ml, were analysed in each batch; the assay exhibiting a CV of 5%. Over the course of 18 batches, three separately prepared QC pools were used, their actual concentrations being shown as the target value. Limits have been drawn at plus or minus three times the standard deviation and at plus or minus one standard deviation. The two rules (Westgard *et al.*, 1977a) in operation are that:

1 for any one batch no replicate should fall outside plus or minus three times the standard deviation (the so-called 1s3 rule)

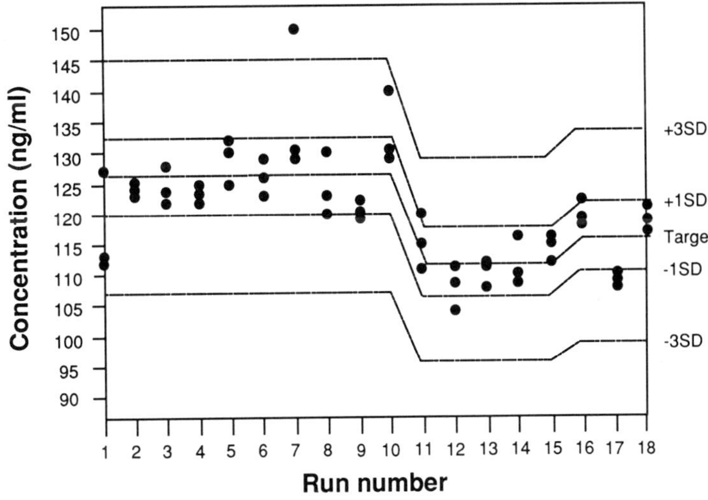

Figure 10.7 A control chart showing the application of quality control rules to the results from three pools of a quality control sample assayed in several assay batches (runs). Three replicate analyses were performed in each batch with the 3s1 and 1s3 rules being applied (see text). Pool 1 had a target value of 126 ng/ml and ran from runs 1 to 10, pool 2 had a target of 112 ng/ml and ran from 11 to 15 and pool 3 had a target of 116 ng/ml and ran from 16 to 18.

2 for any one batch all three replicates should not fall outside either plus or minus one standard deviation (the so-called 3s1 rule)

Referring to Figure 10.7, at run 7 one replicate fails the first rule and at run 17 the three replicates fail the second rule. These assays and all associated data would be rejected.

Although these rules are obviously simple and easy to operate, we need an indication of how good they are at detecting different types of error, or avoiding false rejection. The approach used by Westgard and Groth (1979) was to simulate (using a random number generator) batches of analytical results. Each result belonged to a normal distribution, with a standard deviation equal to the assay error. Further data was also simulated with added extra systematic or random error, then different QC rules were applied to see how often an assay rejection was indicated.

When the probability of error detection was plotted against the amount of error, a 'power function' for the rule was obtained. The probability of error detection indicates the proportion of batches, with that error, which will be rejected. Figures 10.8 and 10.9 show 'power functions' for the 1s3 and 3s1 rules, and their combination, in the presence of different amounts of random and systematic error. Where the extra error is zero the probability of rejection is the probability of false rejection. The added error is scaled as a multiple of the inherent assay error, such that at zero only the assay error is present.

Both rules exhibit a low probability of false rejection as shown by the near zero intercept on the *y*-axis. Figure 10.8 shows that the 1s3 rule is very effective at detecting random error while the 3s1 rule is poor. Both rules detect systematic error (Figure 10.9), although the 3s1 rule is better. Taken together they are even more effective at detecting systematic error. Combinations of rules, e.g. 3s1 and 1s3, where the elements are aimed at different types of error, often give better overall performance. The simulation approach allows the testing of combination rules for their

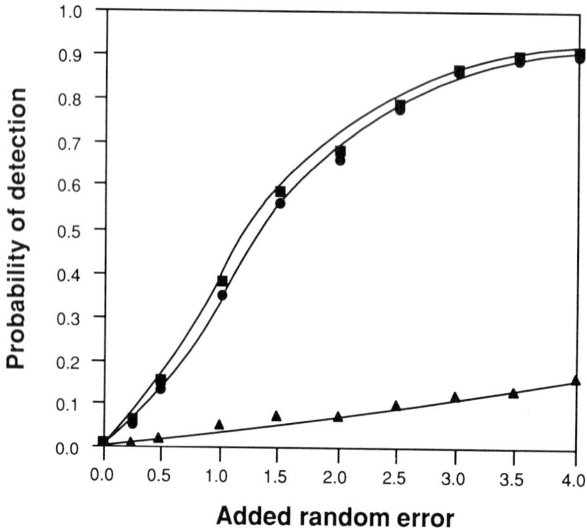

Figure 10.8 Power function for the 1s3 and 3s1 rules and their combination with increasing levels of random error. ● = 1s3 rule, ▲ = 3s1 rule and ■ = combination of the two.

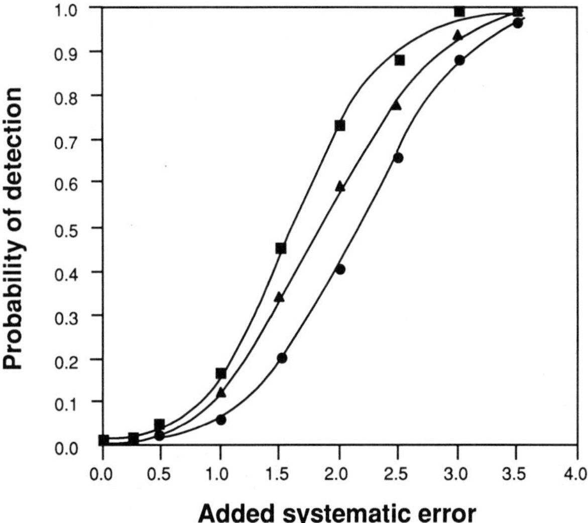

Figure 10.9 Power function for the 1s3 and 3s1 rules and their combination with increasing levels of systematic error. ● = 1s3 rule, ▲ = 3s1 rule and ■ = combination of the two.

effectiveness (Westgard and Groth, 1981) and quite complex combinations can be studied. However, the more complex the rules the more difficult becomes manual application, and automatic computer-based assessment eventually becomes a necessity.

The 'power functions' shown assume that three replicates of the QC sample are analysed per batch: changing the number of replicates in a batch changes the 'power functions'. Figure 10.10 illustrates the effect of increasing the numbers of replicates on the 3s1 rule. As would be expected, increased numbers of replicates give

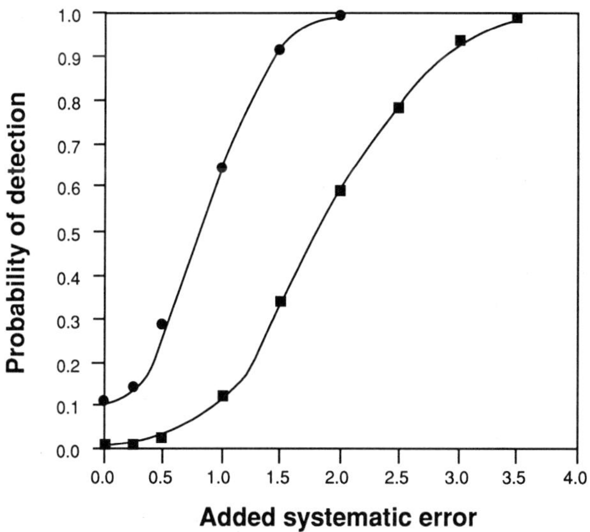

Figure 10.10 The effect of the number of QC replicates per batch on the power function for the detection of systematic error by the 3s1 rule. ■ = 3 replicates and ● = 6 replicates.

increased probability of error detection, but, for this type of rule there is a cost in the increased likelihood of false rejection, shown by the positive intercept on the *y*-axis. Some QC rules do not give increased false rejection with increased replicates (Westgard *et al.*, 1977a) and others are affected to different degrees. However, it is generally the case that increasing the probability of error detection causes an increase in the probability of false rejection.

Relationship of QC rules to assay quality and assay stability

As outlined above, the performance of QC rules will be affected by the presence of between batch error. This error is observed as systematic error within a batch, the extent and direction of which varies from batch to batch. Figure 10.11 shows the effect on the 3s1 rule of the presence of different proportions of between batch error. The simulated data is of the same type as in Figure 10.9, only in this case inherent assay error contains various combinations of between batch and within batch error. For all three sets of data the error components combine to give an overall assay error equivalent to a CV of 10%. In the first data set all the error is within batch, whereas the other data sets have an increasingly higher component of between batch error. Extra systematic error is then added, at various levels, as a multiple of the overall inherent assay error.

There is clearly an increase in the probability for false rejection which tends to increase further as the between batch error component increases. This is accompanied by a decrease in the probability of true error detection, as shown by the shallow curve. Overall this results in an all-round decrease in performance of the rule (Westgard *et al.*, 1979). The decreased performance in the presence of between

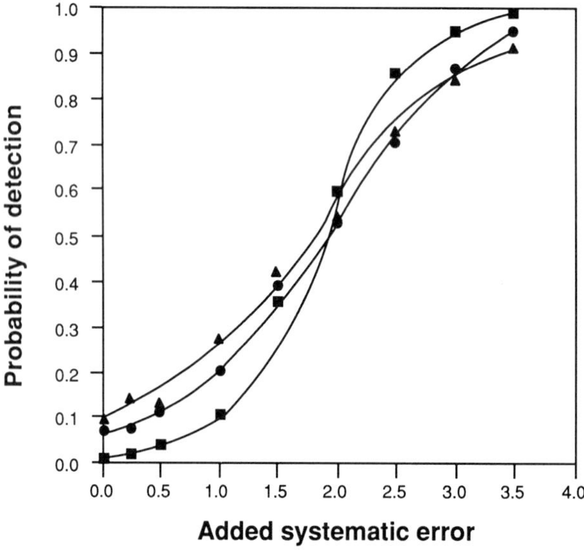

Figure 10.11 The effect of the ratio of between to within batch error on the power function for the detection of systematic error by the 3s1 rule. ■ = ratio of 0 : 1, ● = ratio of 1 : 1 and ▲ = ratio of 2 : 1.

batch error is common to most QC rules but differs in extent. The implication is that a single set of rules will not give the same performance for different assays, and that if a consistent probability of error detection is required, then each assay should have its QC rules optimised.

The following simulated data serves as an example of how QC rules can behave very differently depending on the nature of inherent assay error, and of the extra error the rules are intended to detect. The simulated data in Table 10.1 is for a QC sample of 10 ng/ml, analysed in triplicate in each of 30 batches. The assay has an overall precision (CV) of 10% made up of a 4% within batch error and a relatively high between batch error of 9%. From batch 25 onwards, a 20% positive systematic error was introduced.

The data has been analysed first with the 3s1 rule previously described, using the overall assay CV to set the limits, i.e. the assay batch is failed if all three results

Table 10.1 Simulated analytical data with QC testing by 3s1 and cusum rules

	Analytical results			QC test results			
Batch number	Repl. 1	Repl. 2	Repl. 3	3s1	Cusum		
1	9.9	8.9	8.5		—	9.9	9.4
2	9.5	10.8	9.2		9.9	—	—
3	8.6	10.6	10.6		9.6	—	—
4	9.8	10.5	10.9		—	—	—
5	8.7	7.7	7.1	*	9.7	8.4	6.5*
6	9.9	9.5	8.5		7.4	7.9	7.4
7	10.6	10.8	10.2		9.0	—	—
8	10.8	12.8	11.5		—	11.8	12.3
9	8.9	8.9	8.3	*	10.2	—	9.3
10	12.4	11.9	10.0		—	10.9	—
11	11.1	12.0	13.2	*	10.1	11.1	13.3*
12	9.0	9.4	12.1		11.3	—	11.1
13	9.7	10.7	9.2		—	—	—
14	7.6	8.6	8.1	*	8.6	8.2	7.3
15	10.8	9.5	10.3		9.1	9.6	—
16	9.9	9.8	8.5		—	—	9.5
17	7.7	7.3	9.9		8.2	6.5*	7.4
18	11.9	11.1	11.1	*	—	10.1	10.2
19	9.5	10.4	11.1		—	—	10.1
20	7.5	6.7	8.9	*	—	7.7	7.6
21	11.7	11.6	10.2		—	10.6	—
22	8.8	8.3	8.1	*	9.8	9.1	8.2
23	10.4	10.5	12.4		9.6	—	11.4
24	9.2	10.5	9.9		—	—	—
25	11.9	12.4	11.4	*	10.9	12.3	12.7
26	11.3	11.1	10.5		13.0*	13.1*	12.6
27	11.4	11.0	10.9		13.0*	13.0*	12.9*
28	11.9	13.0	13.5	*	13.8*	15.8*	18.3*
29	13.5	12.9	12.7	*	20.8*	22.7*	24.4*
30	10.1	11.0	10.9		23.5*	23.5*	23.4*

* The nominal QC value is 10 ng/ml and the sample is assayed three times in each batch.

exceed 11 ng/ml or all three are less than 9 ng/ml. Second, a cumulative sum (cusum) rule, described by Westgard *et al.* (1977b), has been used. Using the cusum approach each replicate is treated independently and the rule applied sequentially to each value, ignoring changes of batch. The cusum rule has two sets of control levels. First, the points where it is activated, which we will set at plus and minus one standard deviation (i.e. 9 and 11 ng/ml), and second, two rejection levels, when the assay is deemed out of control, at plus and minus 2.7 times the standard deviation (i.e. 7.3 and 12.7 ng/ml). See Westgard *et al.* (1977b) for a discussion on the choice of activation and rejection levels for this rule.

A cusum level is activated when a QC replicate falls outside one of the control levels (i.e. 9 and 11 ng/ml). At this point the activated control level is subtracted from the replicate value and the difference added to the true QC concentration to form the cumulative sum or 'cusum'. For each subsequent replicate, the difference between its concentration and the activated control level is determined and added to the cumulative sum. If the cumulative sum moves to the other side of the target concentration value, the process is ended. It is re-activated when another QC replicate falls outside a control limit, but the cumulative sum begins again at the true QC concentration. When the cumulative sum crosses a rejection level, the assay is deemed out of control. The more familiar way of setting limits for cusum rules, using a V-mask, is described by Kemp *et al.* (1978).

Returning to Table 10.1, all detected failures by either rule are marked with an asterix. Careful examination of the data allows the expected between batch error to be seen clearly. This is indicated by the general closeness of the replicates within a batch, but the often large differences between batches; for example compare batches 9 and 10. Given the high between batch error component, this is expected and must be accepted. This between batch error explains the regular and repeated false rejection by the 3s1 rule in batches 1 to 24. The rule is designed to detect systematic error and it sees the between batch error as such. Worse still, is the fact that when the systematic error is added, in batches 25 to 30, the rejection rate of the 3s1 rule does not increase significantly. For this data set the 3s1 rule has proved ineffectual, it has given false rejections and false acceptances and would have long since been ignored by the analyst.

The cusum rule is also appropriate for detecting systematic error. For the same set of data it is again affected by the between batch error, showing three failures in the first 20 batches. However, these failures occur at single replicates and are clearly not part of any trend. After batch 25 every replicate gives an out of control signal with a steadily increasing cumulative sum. The added extra systematic error is clearly and unequivocally indicated.

These limited results are not intended to demonstrate a general superiority of the cusum over the 3s1 rule, only that in this data set, with these particular errors, the one rule is successful and the other not. The example is intended to show that the general utility of a QC rule cannot be assumed, its usefulness clearly being affected by the nature of the assay error.

Westgard and Groth (1983) have used a predictive value theory for quality control. This seeks to relate the frequency of errors as detected by the QC policy to the predictive value of reject and accept indicators. Their analysis indicates that at high error frequency (greater than 10%) the most important factor of the QC policy is the probability for error detection, this should be given prominence even at the expense of a raised probability of false rejection. Where the frequency of errors is low, in order to avoid a high proportion of these being false, the probability of false rejection should be low, even at the expense of a lowered probability of error detection.

It is a common experience that newly developed assays have a high error rate since the short-term nature of the validation process cannot have tested all variables. As experience of the method grows, the error rate falls as more of the variables are brought under control and the analyst becomes familiar with the method. The results of the predictive value theory suggest that, in order to maintain the same confidence, the QC policy for an assay may need to be adapted during its lifetime.

Recommendations

Simulation of data such as that in Table 10.1 is a very useful way of examining the properties and performance of QC rules, with different sorts and extents of inherent assay error. A full and rigorous analysis requires expert input and an understanding of the techniques involved. However, a relatively simple analysis can be carried out and is thoroughly recommended for analysts to understand the advantages and limitations of different quality control approaches. Appendix 2 gives details of how to generate normally distributed random numbers containing different sorts of errors. The necessary software can be written on a spreadsheet or in a package such as RS/1 (BBN Software Products Corporation, Cambridge, USA) but can be supplied via the author if required.

A recommended approach to quality control of immunoassay is not easy to make. A good paper (Westgard *et al.*, 1984) has outlined an approach to developing quality control procedures for clinical chemistry assays, though some aspects are not necessarily relevant to other environments. However, the following general comments can be made.

Assay 'quality'

The inherent error of the assay procedure must be known. This includes precision, bias, limits of quantification and within and between batch errors. Some between batch error is inevitable (from preparation and aliquoting of standards for example, however, every effort should be made to reduce this to a minimum. Significant between batch error will adversely affect the performance of any QC policy and the reliability of the assay. An often overlooked cause of between batch error is inappropriate calibration procedures, including the effect of the calibration function as well as weighting, standard partition and replicate numbers.

Critical error

If possible, determine the critical error or the level of acceptable error as defined by the users of the assay results. This may be easier in a clinical chemistry environment where the critical error is that above which the diagnostic value of the data is lost. For more research-based analysis, where new information is being generated, this information is not normally available; the best approach in these circumstances is to adopt some general laboratory standard. An example would be that there must be

90% confidence that error has not risen above a certain factor times the inherent assay error.

Although a 90% probability of error detection sounds convincing, it implies a 10% probability of falsely accepting an assay batch which is in fact in error. This must be judged against the use to which the data is to be put. In the area of forensic drug testing for example a falsely accepted positive result could potentially lead to an unsound conviction! In the pharmacokinetic environment, however, where a single result may be just one time point on a plasma profile of a drug, a 'bad' result would be obvious against the mass of good data and could be disregarded. Clearly the consequences of false acceptance are very different in the two cases.

The cost of false rejection of an assay batch is a problem for all laboratories, but, unlike the examples above there are no risks involved. However the re-analysis of a falsely rejected batch is a waste of time and resources, which in the current cost conscious climate must be minimised or eliminated.

QC rules

Given the inherent assay error, and the user-defined critical error, it is possible to determine which QC rules are appropriate and the number of replicate QC samples which are required (Westgard *et al.*, 1984). Multiple QC rules can be used and these may be connected in parallel (by 'or' statements) or serially (by 'and' statements) (Westgard *et al.*, 1981). Unless adequate computer facilities are available the least number of the simplest rules (i.e. with clear and straightforward limits) should be chosen. In all cases, unnecessary complication should be avoided. It is worth reiterating the point that with well designed QC rules the effort required to reach a given standard of performance is determined by the nature of the inherent assay error.

In spite of the common inclusion of precision profile estimations in modern computer packages for immunoassays, these are not necessarily a first choice for routine quality control. Some packages produce these profiles without confidence limits, which means that it is difficult to decide when the assay is out of control. Although confidence limits can be calculated (Sadler *et al.*, 1988; Chiecchio *et al.*, 1992) it is not a trivial process, requiring understanding of the limitations of the approach taken (Sadler and Smith, 1990).

The use of the response error relationship as a quality control parameter has been reported (Schioler, 1984; Malvano *et al.*, 1989). The latter paper produced 'power' functions of a rule, based on defining the slope of the RER, and its confidence limit, assuming the relationship was adequately described by a straight line. A subsequent paper by the same group (Chiecchio *et al.*, 1992) showed the latter assumption may not always be justified.

In general, more work is required before either the precision profile or the response error relationship become the primary assay acceptance criteria. What circumstances compromise their predictability as QC parameters is a question that particularly needs answering. At the present time, quality control is best performed with QC samples subjected to well defined rules. The precision profile and response error relationship are, however, useful tools for diagnostic purposes when an assay goes out of control.

Some laboratories adopt a fixed QC policy for all assays. This approach is rooted in the need for clear and simple rules, often with manually maintained data records.

It is important to realise that fixed QC rules mean that the probability of error detection and of false rejection will both vary from assay to assay. Although this may not be a problem, it is important that those developing assays should know how various sources of error will affect the operation of the chosen rules.

Interpretation

The most important property of a QC policy is that it should be believable. Limits should be clear and unequivocal, and when breached should result in immediate action. A QC policy where the analyst judges whether to believe the QC results or not is of little use; if the results are not credible then either the assay or the QC policy needs attention.

The future

The immediate future will bring increasing demand from customers and regulatory authorities for QC procedures which give clear assurance on the quality of analytical data. The validation exercise is not acceptable as a guarantee of quality throughout the life of the assay; it provides only an initial assessment of the analytical performance. An effective QC policy not only provides customers with confidence in the data, but also provides information to allow the analyst to improve his or her own performance. To achieve an effective policy the analyst must be able to assess the cost, in terms of the probability of false rejection, and the utility, in the form of the probability of error detection. Whatever the demands, quality control in analytical chemistry is a growth industry.

Appendix 1: The use of one-way analysis of variance to determine within and between batch error

If the analysis of a sample is carried out in quadruplicate in four batches on separate occasions, then an array of sixteen results is obtained. In general, if there are n replicates in each of r different batches, then the following calculations should be performed:

Batch	Replicates	Row sum	Square of row sum	Row sum of sqares
1	$x_{11} \cdots x_{1n}$	R_1*	R_1^2	s_1**
2	$x_{21} \cdots x_{2n}$	R_2	R_2^2	s_2
⋮				
r	$x_{r1} \cdots x_{rn}$	R_r	R_r^2	s_r
	Total	$\boldsymbol{T}$	$\boldsymbol{R^2}$	$\boldsymbol{s}$

* $R_1 = (x_{11} + x_{12} \cdots + x_{1n})$

** $s_1 = (x_{11}^2 + x_{12}^2 \cdots + x_{1n}^2)$

After calculating the basic statistics, the table below is used to determine the analysis of variance:

Source of errror	Sum of squares (A)	Degrees of freedom (B)	Mean square
Between batch	$\sum (R^2/n) - (T^2/rn)$	$(r - 1)$	A/B
Within batch	$s - \sum (R^2/n)$	$(rn - r)$	A/B
Total	$s - (T^2/rn)$	$(rn - 1)$	A/B

The hypothesis, that there is no significant batch-to-batch contribution to assay variance, is then tested by dividing the between batch mean square by the within batch mean square. If the resulting ratio is greater than the 5% point of the F distribution, where numerator degrees of freedom $= (r - 1)$ and denominator degrees of freedom $= (rn - r)$, then the hypothesis is rejected and a significant between batch component to assay variance has been shown to exist.

Total coefficient of variation (CV) = [$\sqrt{}$(Total mean square)/mean] $\times$ 100

If there is a significant between batch contribution to assay variance then:

Within batch CV = [$\sqrt{}$(Within batch mean square)/mean] $\times$ 100

Between batch CV = ($\sqrt{}$[(Between batch mean square

− Within batch mean square)/n]/mean) $\times$ 100

Appendix 2: The generation of simulated assay results belonging to a normally distributed population of given mean and standard deviation

In order to test the performance of QC rules, data must be generated which simulates the inherent assay errors and various added errors. The simpler approach is to assume that errors are normally distributed and increasing error adds to the spread of the distribution or alters its mean value.

Most software packages, including spreadsheets, provide a random number generator which provides numbers from a square distribution between the values of 0 and 1. If 12 such numbers are generated and summed (to give the value a) then the following equation produces a single number from a normal distribution:

$$[(a - 6) \times b] + c$$

where b is the standard deviation and c the mean of the distribution.

Several such numbers can be generated, corresponding to the number of QC replicates in an assay batch. Extra random error can be added by increasing the value of b, and systematic error by increasing the value of c.

To simulate independent within and between batch error, a number c^* is generated by

$$[(a - 6) \times b^*] + c$$

where b^* is the between batch standard deviation and c is the true QC concentration. c^* is then used to generate the QC replicates of a single batch by

$$[(a - 6) \times b] + c^*$$

where b is the within batch standard deviation, a new c^* being generated for each batch.

References

CHIECCHIO, A., GIGLIOLI, F., MALVANO, R., RINGHINI, R., MANZONE, P. & BO, A. (1992) *J. Immunol. Methods*, **147**, 211.

DAVIS, S. E., MUNSON, P. J., JAFFE, M. L. & RODBARD, D. (1980) *J. Immunoassay*, **1**, 15.

EKINS, R. P. (1983) The precision profile: Its use in assay design, assessment and quality control. In: HUNTER, W. M. (ed.) *Immunoassays for Clinical Chemistry*. Churchill Livingston, Edinburgh, pp. 76–105.

KEMP, K. W., NIX, A. B. J., WILSON, D. W. & GRIFFITHS, K. (1978) *J. Endocrinol.*, **76**, 203.

MALVANO, R., CHIECCHIO, A., BO, A., MANZONE, P. & RINGHINI, R. (1989) *J. Nucl. Med. and Allied Sci.*, **33**, 7.

MONTGOMERY, D. C. (1991) *Introduction to Statistical Quality Control*, 2nd edition. John Wiley, New York.

RAAB, G. (1981) *Appl. Statist.*, **30**, 32.

RODBARD, D. (1974) *Clin. Chem.*, **20**, 1255.

SADLER, W. A., SMITH, M. H. & LEGGE, H. M. (1988) *Clin. Chem.*, **34**, 1058.
(1990) *Clin. Chem.*, **36**, 1346.

SCHIOLER, V. (1984) *Scand. J. Clin. Lab. Invest.* (Suppl 172), **44**, 87.

SCHWARZ, S. (1982) Strategy and organization of intralaboratory radioimmunoassay quality control. In: *Radioimmunoassay and Related Procedures in Medicine*, International Atomic Energy Agency, Vienna, pp. 447–524.

WESTGARD, J. O. & GROTH, T. (1979) *Clin. Chem.*, **25**, 863.
(1981) *Clin. Chem.*, **27**, 1536.
(1983) *Amer. J. Clin. Pathol.*, **80**, 49.

WESTGARD, J. O., GROTH, T., ARONSSON, T., FALK, H. & DE VERDIER, C.-H. (1977a) *Clin. Chem.*, **23**, 1857.

WESTGARD, J. O., GROTH, T., ARONSSON, T. & DE VERDIER, C.-H. (1977b) *Clin. Chem.*, **23**, 1881.

WESTGARD, J. O., FALK, H. & GROTH, T. (1979) *Clin. Chem.*, **25**, 394.

WESTGARD, J. O., BARRY, P. L., HUNT, M. R. & GROTH, T. (1981) *Clin. Chem.*, **27**, 493.

WESTGARD, J. O., GROTH, T. & DE VERDIER, C.-H. (1984) *Scand. J. Clin. Lab. Invest.* (Suppl 172), **44**, 19.

11

Assay problems and troubleshooting

B. LAW

Zeneca Pharmaceuticals, Macclesfield

Introduction

Even following the guidelines laid out in the previous chapters, anyone developing or running an assay will inevitably encounter problems, it would be dishonest to say anything different.

The 'breakdown' of any assay suggests that some variable has gone out of control. If it is not obvious what this variable is, and as a consequence it is difficult to get the assay working effectively again, then the assay contains some uncontrolled variable(s). In an ideal world these factors would have been identified and/or eliminated by following the procedures laid out in the chapters on assay development and validation. Time spent at the development stage using well planned experiments to investigate the major assay variables such as incubation temperature, incubation time, batch of protein additive etc., is time well spent, as this should ultimately reduce assay down time. However, to investigate every conceivable assay variable could take many months if not years of experimental work. Such investigation needs to be balanced against the likelihood of the assay failing, the consequences of this and the time taken to re-establish the assay.

The examination of the between batch error (see Chapters 6 and 10) and the influence of assay variables on this, can help focus on those factors which are unstable or worthy of more attention and are likely to cause problems in the future.

One must accept that problems will occur even in the most well developed and robust of assays if only because they are operated by humans. The aim of this chapter therefore is to help solve those problems through their timely identification, solution and prevention, with the emphasis very much on prevention. Do not expect to find solutions to all your problems or even descriptions of all the possible problems. Such a task would be impossible given the diversity of both immunoassays and the way they are performed. Furthermore most analysts prefer to forget the problems and concentrate on their successes, so that well documented problems of failed assays, where the problem has been worked through and solved, are few and far between.

What you will find in this brief chapter are examples of some of the common and more interesting problems, and ways in which these can be identified and eliminated, but most importantly prevented.

Loss of binding

One of the commonest problems in immunoassay work is the sudden and inexplicable loss of binding. This can happen for a number of reasons, such as decomposition of tracer, decomposition of the antisera, or separating agents going 'off'. Another possible reason is that one or other of the reagents has become contaminated with analyte, effectively suppressing all binding. The usual answer to such a problem is to systematically replace all the reagents one at a time until the malfunctioning reagent is identified and can be replaced.

Choosing where to start is often dictated by experience or some knowledge of the assay characteristics. If the assay procedure is lengthy (i.e. it takes several days to produce results) then it may be necessary to set up several assays in parallel each involving a different reagent variable. Typically B_0, nsb and a mid-point standard would be set up for each reagent change.

A scientist new to immunoassays would expect such a scientific approach to lead to a rapid diagnosis of the problem; unfortunately in the world of immunoassay this is not always the case. Many days, if not weeks have been wasted as analysts check through assorted batches of reagents, setting up various controls in an attempt to diagnose an assay malfunction. Then, suddenly, one day the assay starts to work again for no apparent reason. This is most frustrating and it is one of the factors that gives immunoassay the image of a 'black art'. In scientific terms it must be put down to the assay containing an uncontrolled and non-obvious variable.

To avoid any delay and get the assay up and running as quickly as possible, analysts frequently adopt the pragmatic approach and simply discard all the reagents, prepare a fresh set and start again. Although this is dissatisfying for the true scientist, who is keen, through experiment and application of the scientific method, to solve the problem in a logical manner, it is necessary to admit that this is often the best approach.

Shifted calibration curves

Problems with standards

A commonly encountered assay problem is shown in Figure 11.1. It is seen that the calibration curve is shifted either to the right or to the left of its usual position. This would usually be signified by a change in the assay parameters, such as the ED_{50}, ED_{80} etc., and/or a change in the values of the QC samples. One such incident displaying the above symptoms occurred in the author's laboratory and in its diagnosis and solution were a number of useful lessons.

A well controlled assay suddenly started to give ED_{50} values which were significantly lower than normal, i.e. the curve was shifted to the left. The deviation was not consistent but it was always between 60 to 80% of the accepted value. A similar deviation was shown in the ED_{20} and ED_{80} values. There was no change in the B_0

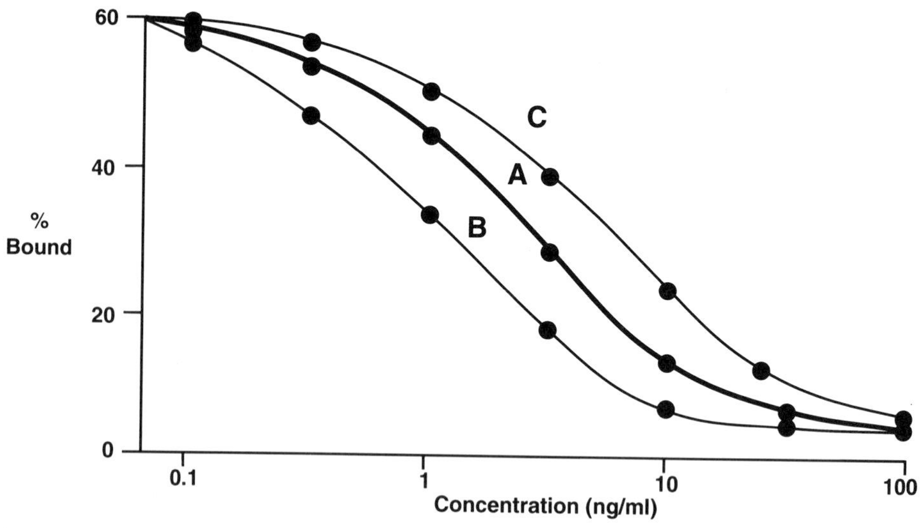

Figure 11.1 A typical calibration curve (A) is shown along with curves, which because of one of a number of problems appear more potent (B) or less potent (C).

value and the batch of control plasma used to prepare the standards had not changed; so a matrix effect could be ruled out. All the evidence pointed to the standards being too potent, although there had been no change in their method of preparation.

As the analyte was relatively unstable, as well as being in short supply, the standards were prepared fresh for each assay. Typically a stock solution was prepared by weighing out around 5 mg of analyte and then dissolving this in the appropriate amount of buffer to give a 1 mg/ml solution. This stock solution was then further diluted in buffer to give a 0.1 mg/ml spiking solution which was used to generate the plasma standards.

After some investigation the problem was eventually tied down to the automatic pipette that was used to dispense buffer for preparation of the stock solution. Although the pipette was being correctly set to give the desired amount of buffer (approximately 5 ml, depending on the exact mass of analyte), it was actually jamming such that it always delivered 3.7 ml. Thus the standards were always too concentrated. As different amounts of compound were weighed out each time, but always dissolved in 3.7 ml of buffer, the actual concentration of the stock solution varied from assay to assay. After repairing the pipette and getting the assay back on the rails a number of changes in procedure were put in place.

Most laboratories calibrate their pipettes on a regular basis (approximately once every six months or so). The above problem however suggests that as well as this formal checking, it is probably worth carrying out a quick check of any critical pipetting apparatus on a more regular basis.

A check on the spiking solution prior to the preparation of the standards was also instituted. This was carried out by recording the UV spectrum of the compound and determining the absorbance at a preset wavelength. Although this is common practice in the author's laboratory it had been omitted in the present assay for two reasons. First, the assay procedure was reasonably short with an incubation period of only 30 min, hence any problems would rapidly become apparent. Second, because the UV properties of the compound were relatively poor – there was no clear lambda max and the molar extinction coefficient was very low – it was believed that the use of the UV check would be of limited value. In the example described above an error of 20 to 40% would have been readily apparent and several wasted assays and a number of wasted days trying to track down the problem could have been avoided.

Contamination problems

A problem which was superficially similar to the above, but which had a very different cause is shown by the calibration graphs in Figure 11.2. In this instance as well as the calibration series appearing too potent, the binding at zero dose was also reduced. This problem had all the hallmarks of contamination by analyte of either the standards (including the zero standard) or the assay buffer. The fact that the QCs were giving roughly the correct concentrations, despite the distorted calibration graph, suggested that it was not the standards alone which were contaminated.

In this particular instance the assay procedure was relatively complex because of the presence in the samples of significant amounts of cross-reacting metabolites. To eliminate this cross-reactivity problem the samples were 'cleaned-up' using a fully automated multistage procedure. The samples and standards were passed through a solid-phase extraction cartridge and the eluent collected and blown to dryness. After redisolution the extracts were injected on to an HPLC system where they were chromatographed and the eluent fraction corresponding to the analyte of interest collected and taken for off-line RIA analysis.

After a period of investigation the problem was shown to be the result of the HPLC eluent being recycled during the previous analytical run, rather than being

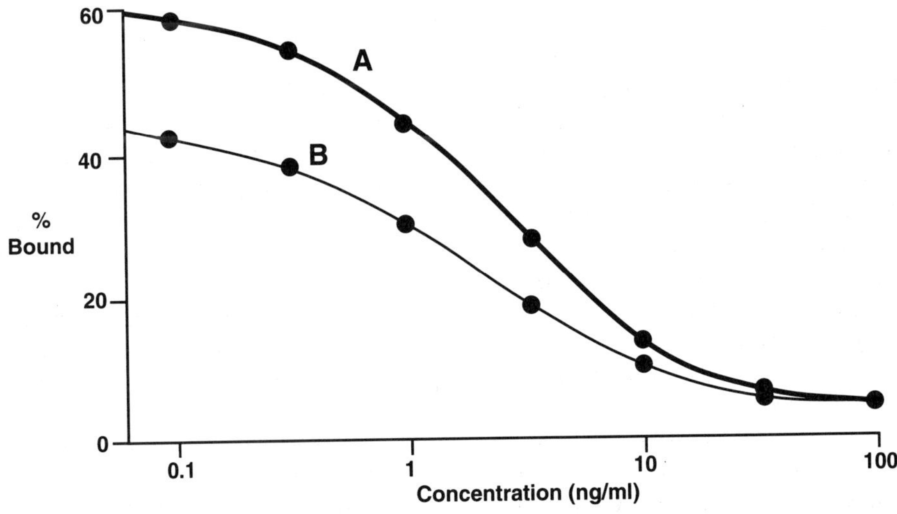

Figure 11.2 A typical calibration curve (A) is shown along with a problematical curve (B) which has been shifted to the left and the binding at zero analyte concentration reduced.

run to waste as was normal practice. Consequently a considerable concentration of the waste cross-reacting metabolites had built up in the eluent and this contamination effectively suppressed the tracer binding in all subsequent assay tubes.

The diagnosis of this particular problem was only achieved by considering the assay procedure as a whole and effectively working through the method and eliminating all those stages where contamination could not have occurred.

Poor precision

To anyone involved in immunoassay work it is generally accepted that no two operators work in the same way. An assay which works well for one or a number of analysts can in another's hands fail completely. This is particularly frustrating to those who developed the assay, but more so to the poor individual who cannot get the assay to work. Once all the obvious things such as using the wrong reagent or conditions have been eliminated, the only foolproof method of diagnosing the problem is for a highly experienced and astute individual to sit down with the analyst in question and watch them perform an assay from start to finish. For the person doing the watching this is a mundane and tedious task but it is essential that the individual does not let his or her concentration lapse or a crucial manipulation, such as the over-vigorous shaking of an antibody reagent leading to foaming and imprecise pipetting, could be missed. It is also essential that the assay is performed very much as it would be in normal practice and that no operations are simplified or missed out for the sake of expedience.

What points to look for? This is a most difficult question to answer as it depends very much on the particular problem under scrutiny. An obvious and simple thing to look at is pipetting technique and how this could affect precision. Is the pipette being held so that all the reagents are fully dispensed into the bottom of the assay tubes? Depending on the technique adopted it is sometimes possible to leave small droplets of sample or reagent near the mouth of the assay tube, which, as a result of limited ferocity of mixing do not get incorporated into the bulk of the incubation mixture. Alternatively with some of the modern automated pipettes, the force with which the reagent is dispensed can often make the liquid fly out of the tube after hitting the bottom. This phenomenon could also result in reagent being left high and dry on the inside top of the assay tube.

Few analysts operate in the same way, we all sit differently, hold pipettes differently etc. Unless someone is actually doing something wrong, it is pointless making them change. What is essential, is that providing the technique is acceptable it should be used consistently throughout the work.

Pipettes and the way they are used are not the only source of assay imprecision as is indicated in the following example. Figure 11.3 shows the raw counts for the duplicate analyses of a series of standards (pairs 1 to 10) and a series of samples (pairs 11 to 32). The assay had been working well in the hands of an experienced operator but after a four month lay off the same operator could not seem to get good reproducibility. The data in Figure 11.3 indicate a high degree of what appears to be random error resulting in poor agreement (difference greater than 5% of mean) between the following sets of duplicates: 2, 3, 5, 7, 13, 15, 20, 21, 23, 29 and 32. Superficial examination of this data, and that from related assays supported the

29993 29973	1890 1895	● 4408 4171	3298 3500
● 1234 1468	5897 5789	3330 3359	● 2395 2459
● 9956 11798	● 4568 4272	● 4367 4673	
10313 10257	3467 3498	3497 3588	
● 8430 8001	● 2612 2792	2912 2793	
6349 6543	8903 8809	6349 6243	
● 4288 4596	2523 2775	4408 4593	
3330 3340	2156 2099	3450 3590	
2613 2595	1800 1796	● 2309 2169	
2191 2134	● 6345 6543	7856 7900	

Figure 11.3 Raw data from a gamma counter showing pairs of duplicate tubes. Pairs 1 to 10 are the calibration series and pairs 11 to 32 samples. The pairs showing poor duplication (>5%) are highlighted (●).

view that the assay or operator had developed a high random error component, with no obvious cause.

Most analysts work in a fairly systematic manner which is often dictated by the instrumentation and racks used for the assay. For example, assay tubes are frequently set up in blocks of 10 or 20 as these are convenient numbers to work with. Furthermore, when carrying out large assays, the assay batch may be broken down into small sub-batches to fit in with centrifuge or centrifuge rack capacity.

Systematic examination of the data in Figure 11.3 in the light of the above comments allowed the problem to be diagnosed rapidly, and in this instance it was shown to be the result of a gamma counter malfunction. In this particular assay a multi-well gamma counter was used in the end point detection. When the data in Figure 11.3 are re-presented, but in this instance in blocks of 16 tubes corresponding to the batches counted together in the 16-well counter, a different picture emerges. Examination of the data presented in this way (Figure 11.4) shows that apart from some truly random error (pairs 2, 3 and 20), one of which (2) was associated with the nsb where the counts were low, the poor duplication is always confined to tubes 9 + 10 and 13 + 14 as counted by the 16-well counter. On closer inspection it can be seen that the counts in tubes 10 and 13 are always lower than those in their

29993	2613	2523	2912
29973	2595	2775	2793
1234	2191	2156	6349
1468	2134	2099	6243
9956	1890	1800	4408
11798	1895	1796	4593
10313	5897	6345	3450
10257	5789	6543	3590
8430	4568	4408	2309
▶ 8001	▶ 4272	▶ 4171	▶ 2169
6349	3467	3330	7856
6543	3498	3359	7900
▶ 4288	▶ 2612	▶ 4367	▶ 3298
4596	2792	4673	3500
3330	8903	3497	2395
3340	8809	3588	2459

Figure 11.4 The data from Figure 11.3 presented as blocks of eight duplicate pairs (16 assay tubes) corresponding to the batches of tubes counted together in the 16-well gamma counter. The individual tubes of each batch (numbers 10 and 13) which show systematic error are highlighted (▶).

respective duplicates 9 and 14. A quick check of the counter using an ^{125}I source clearly showed that wells 10 and 13 were out of calibration and reading low by around six per cent. Thus the cause of the problem in this instance was clearly instrumental.

There are two clear messages to be learnt from this example. The first, which reiterates the point made earlier, is always carry out routine calibration checks on all equipment, especially when it has not been used for several months. The 30 minutes or so spent checking the efficiency of the 16 wells could have saved several days of generating worthless numbers.

The second message is equally important but somewhat more difficult to enforce since it relates to the way of looking at the analytical data. The analyst was initially puzzled by the data because as well as the systematic bias of wells 10 and 13, there was also a random error component. This random error, which is present in every assay, gave rise to the high spread for tube pairs 2, 3 and 20. The data was only being considered in terms of a set of standards and a set of samples which disguised the repetition of the errors. It was only through an understanding of assay errors and how an assay is set up and assay tubes manipulated that the true cause of the problem became apparent.

Difficulties in transferring an assay to another laboratory

In this modern age more and more companies are developing an international role and the need to ship assays around the world is becoming increasingly necessary.

An analyst who has successfully run an assay in his own laboratory for a number of years might assume that transferring and establishing an assay half way across the world is a relatively simple matter; anyone who has tried to do this will tell you different.

Although the second laboratory may be able to obtain calibration curves, they may well be different to those from the original laboratory. There will probably be differences in the level of binding, ED_{50}, limits of detection etc. Whilst some of these differences may be minor, many are significant and they can often be traced to the use of different batches of reagents, particularly the buffer additives such as proteins or the prevailing temperature etc. A number of these problems can be minimised by shipping a full set of reagents which are known to work in the originating laboratory, however, other factors can influence the outcome of such an exercise.

Very precise stipulation of all operating parameters is essential. If the assay has been developed and carried out at ambient temperature which was actually 22 ± 1°C then the precise temperature should be stated, not 'room temperature'. A poorly heated laboratory in the UK where the ambient temperature may be 18°C may generate a very different calibration curve to a poorly ventilated laboratory in an equatorial country where the temperature may reach 25 or 28°C.

The assay buffer is a relatively simple factor to change in an assay, either deliberately or accidentally. For example, a buffer may be replaced with another because it is handy and readily available, or as sometimes happens a change is made by the analyst to make the assay effectively his or her 'own'. Accidental changes can occur when the buffer recipe requires adjustment of the final pH with either acid or base. For instance certain pH electrodes do not respond accurately to Tris buffers and consequently the wrong final pH may be obtained. To avoid such problems it is recommended that buffers are prepared from measured ingredients in proportions

Table 11.1 The effect of varying buffer and sodium chloride molarity on binding (B_0) in an assay for epanolol

Buffer* molarity	NaCl molarity	$B_0 \pm$ SD (%)#
0.01	—	15.0 ± 0.3
0.01	0.14	33.0 ± 1.1
0.02	—	16.1 ± 0.1
0.02	0.13	32.8 ± 1.2
0.05	—	19.6 ± 0.4
0.05	0.1	31.5 ± 0.7
0.10	—	27.1 ± 1.5
0.10	0.05	30.8 ± 0.9
0.15	—	30.0 ± 0.6

* Buffer is Tris pH 7.4.

\# $n = 5$.

designed to give the required pH. Although such buffers do not require pH adjustment it is still useful to check the final pH.

Changes to buffer type as discussed previously (Chapter 6), as well as the buffer pH can have a marked effect on assay parameters, a fact which does not appear to be appreciated widely. Of relevance and interest also is the data in Table 11.1 which show how the buffer molarity as well as the addition of sodium chloride can have a very significant effect on binding in an assay for the β-blocker epanolol. In this instance increasing the molarity of the buffer from 0.01 to 0.15 resulted in a marked increase in binding. However a higher level of binding was obtained if the buffer contained a high concentration of sodium chloride relative to the concentration of the buffer salts.

Tight stipulation of operating conditions may initially cause problems for a laboratory attempting to set up a predeveloped assay, especially if the right materials are not readily available. However when finally established it should perform exactly as it did in the originating laboratory.

The avoidance of these types of problems ultimately comes down to training and making all analysts aware of the consequences of small and simple changes. It is also essential that the conditions for the optimal use of an assay are clearly and tightly specified, and wherever possible give the analysts no option but to use the conditions defined.

Conclusions

It needs to be borne in mind that many immunoassay problems seem to be intractable simply because they occur through two things going wrong simultaneously. A typical example could be a change in a reagent accompanied by the introduction of a new operator. Such instances can give confounding results which makes elucidation of the problem all the more difficult.

The only way to tackle such problems is by systematically working through all the assay variables and eliminating those which are of no consequence; to quote Sherlock Holmes 'when the impossible has been eliminated whatever remains however improbable must be the answer'. Such investigation will be aided enormously if the development work and validation have been carried out to a high standard and all the significant factors determined and documented. Investigation of the problem will also be facilitated if good records have been kept of all changes in batches of reagent, buffer salts and even batches of distilled water. It is worth remembering that many problems develop gradually and the symptom can often be correlated with the age of a particular reagent.

It is worth emphasising that immunoassays do not always play by the rules and in many instances the only answer is to throw all the reagents away, make up fresh and start again. Although this is very dissatisfying to the true scientist, in immunoassay pragmatism often wins. Ask any experienced immunoassayist on how many occasions they have spent days if not weeks trying to diagnose an immunoassay problem only to have the assay come right spontaneously!

Glossary of common terms used in immunoassay

Accuracy: This is the degree by which a measured value agrees with the true value. It is frequently used interchangeably with bias.

Adjuvant: A material added to an immunogen to enhance the immune response (q.v. Freund's).

Affinity: The strength of the interaction between the antibody and the antigen.

Affinity constant (*K*): The equilibrium constant for the reaction between an antibody and an antigen. It is equal to the ratio of the rate constants of the antibody–antigen association and dissociation, and it has the units l/mol.

Antibody: Glycoproteins of the immunoglobulin class. There are five distinct classes of antibody IgG, IgM, IgA, IgE and IgD, based on the number of basic units.

Antibody binding site: This is the variable region of the Fab fragment which interacts with the antigen. Its size can vary up to that corresponding to four amino acid units or around 600 $Å^2$ in the case of a large antigen.

Antibody titre: The dilution of antiserum, either working dilution or final dilution, in the assay tube that binds a given mass of labelled compound, typically 50%.

Antigen: A molecule that will interact and bind specifically to an antibody.

Antigenic determinant: That part of the antigen which is recognised and bound by the antibodies.

Antiserum/a: In its strict sense it is the serum obtained from the blood of an immunised animal which contains antibodies.

Avidity: Frequently confused with affinity on which it is dependent. It is actually a measure of the stability of an immune complex brought about by multiple binding. It has little importance in the immunoassays of small molecules.

Blocking buffer: A buffer added to an ELISA assay (q.v.) usually containing a protein to prevent non-specific binding to the plastic surface.

Boosters: The inoculations following the primary immunisation.

Bridge: The chemical linking group between the hapten and carrier protein in a conjugate, or the hapten and labelled molecule in a tracer.

Carrier/carrier protein: The large-molecular-weight material, typically a protein such as bovine serum albumin or keyhole limpet haemocyanin, to which a hapten must be chemically linked in order for it to elicit an immune response.

Conjugation labelling: A means of labelling a molecule through reaction with a molecule which is already labelled, e.g. Bolton–Hunter reagent.

Cross-reactivity: The degree to which molecules related to the analyte will bind to the antibody.

ED_{20}, ED_{50}, ED_{80}: ED stands for Effective Dose and the terms are used to define the dose or concentration required to give 20%, 50% or 80% of the maximum calibration response.

ELISA: A generic term used to describe an immunoassay where the tracer is an enzyme and one or other of the reagents is linked to a solid phase.

Epitope: That part of an antigen which binds to the antibody.

Fab: One of two identical parts of an antibody molecule which carries the antigen binding site. It is so named because it is the fragment bearing the antigen binding site.

Fac: The non-variable region of an antibody molecule. The name is derived from the fact that it is the fragment that can be crystallised.

Freund's: A commonly used adjuvant prepared from Arlacel A, a neutral detergent and paraffin oil. It is available in two forms, complete and incomplete, the former containing added mycobacteria.

Immunisation: The process whereby an immunogen (q.v.) is introduced into an animal to elicit an immune response.

Immunogen: A molecule which when injected into an animal will elicit an immune response, i.e. it will produce antibodies. For a molecule to be immunogenic it must have a molecular mass of at least 2000 Daltons and possess a complex and stable tertiary structure.

Gamma-globulin (IgG): See IgG.

Hapten: A low-molecular-weight antigen (typically less than 2000 Daltons) which must be linked to a larger molecule in order to make it immunogenic. It can also be used to describe the derivative of the analyte which is used to prepare the immunogen or tracer.

IgG: The simplest of the antibody molecules which contains only one structural unit, and the most important in relation to immunoassays. It is a glycoprotein of molecular mass 160 000 Daltons, which can be thought of as being Y shaped with the binding sites on the ends of the arms of the Y.

Iodo-tag: A molecule labelled with ^{125}I which can be used to label a drug or any other species for which an assay is desired.

Label: A colloquial expression describing either the labelled molecule, i.e. the tracer, or alternatively the entity that produces the signal, i.e. the enzyme or the radioactive atom.

Limit of detection (LoD): That concentration of analyte that can be distinguished from zero with defined confidence.

Limit of quantification (LoQ): That concentration of analyte that can be determined with a given degree of confidence, typically with a CV or relative standard deviation of 15%. The LoQ is usually around three times the LoD.

Logit: A method of transforming immunoassay calibration data to generate a straight line.

Monoclonal antibody: Antibody produced from a single clone using hybridoma and cell culture techniques. Once the clone has been established it can be used to produce a single population of antibodies with defined characteristics, indefinitely.

Non-specific binding (nsb): Binding of labelled analyte to anything other than the specific binding protein or antibody.

Plate conjugate: A conjugate of the analyte (or an analogue) and a large-molecular-weight protein used in an ELISA-type assay to coat the plate with analyte.

Polyclonal antiserum/antibody: The term used to describe antisera or antibodies obtained following standard immunisation procedures. As these sera contain a mixed population of antibodies produced by many clones, no two polyclonal sera will be the same. The antibodies will vary in their specificity and affinity.

Precision: Not to be confused with accuracy, it is the reproducibility of a measurement observed following multiple determinations.

Radioiodination: The process of labelling an analyte with iodine-125 or iodine-131.

Radiotracer: The radiolabelled form of the analyte used in a radioimmunoassay.

Second antibody: An antibody raised against the primary antibody in an immunoassay and used as a separation reagent.

Sensitivity: This is a somewhat ambiguous term which has been given different meanings by different workers. It can be equated to the limit of detection (q.v.) of the assay, or the ability of an assay to discriminate between two similar concentrations. In this respect it would be related to the slope of the calibration graph.

Specificity: This is a term used to describe how susceptible an assay is to interference from substances related or unrelated to the analyte. It is frequently quantified in terms of cross-reactivity (q.v.).

Specific activity: The measure of the amount of radioactivity incorporated into a molecule. It has the units radioactivity/mass, e.g. Ci/mg, Ci/mmol or in S.I. units Bq/mmol.

Spline: An empirical mathematical procedure used for fitting a curve to an immunoassay calibration function.

Totals, total counts: A colloquial term used to describe the total amount of radioactivity that is added to a radioimmunoassay.

Tracer: The labelled analyte in an immunoassay.

Tritiation: The chemical reaction whereby an analyte is labelled with one or more atoms of tritium (q.v.).

Tritium (^{3}H): A radioactive isotope of hydrogen.

Index